Pain Management - Practices, Novel Therapies and Bioactives

Edited by Viduranga Yashasvi Waisundara, Ines Banjari and Jelena Balkić

Published in London, United Kingdom

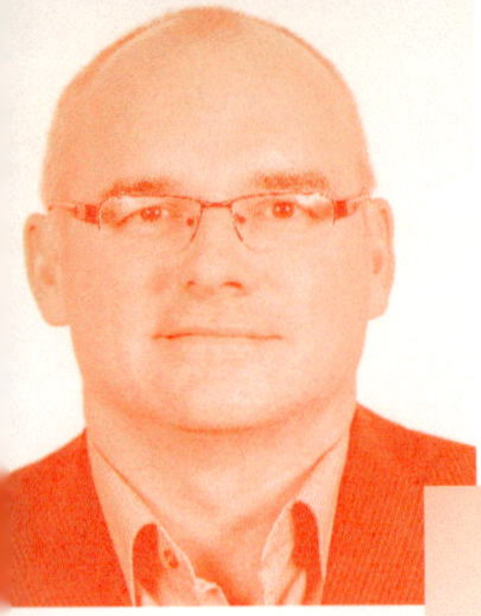
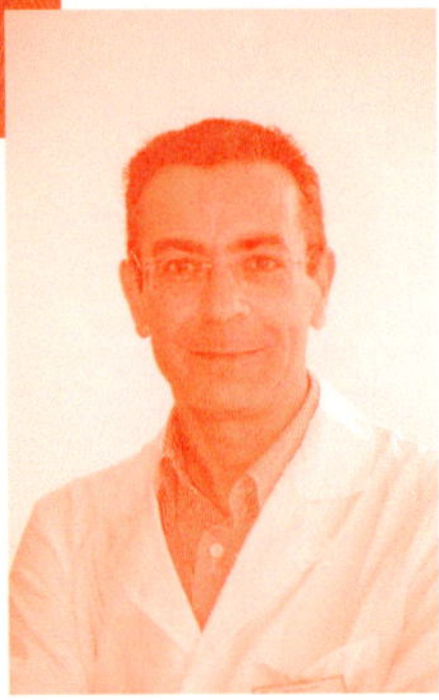
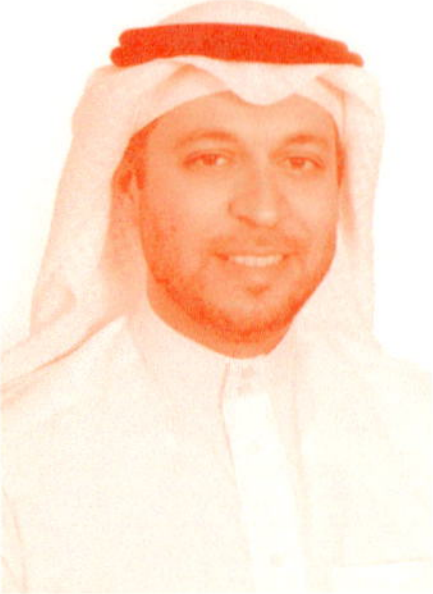
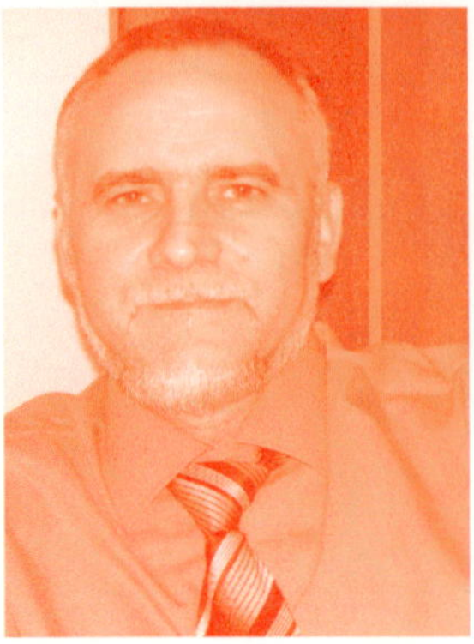
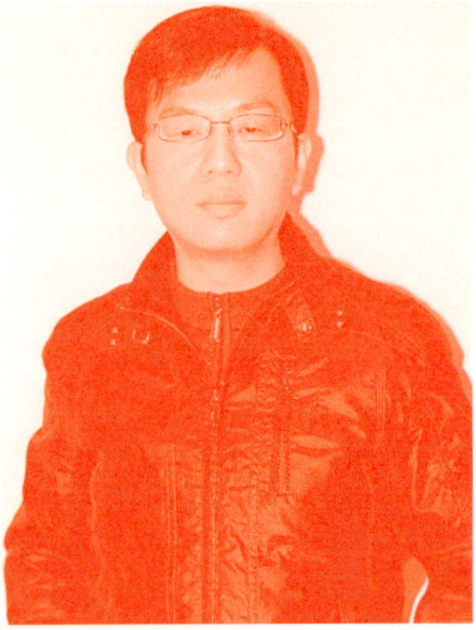
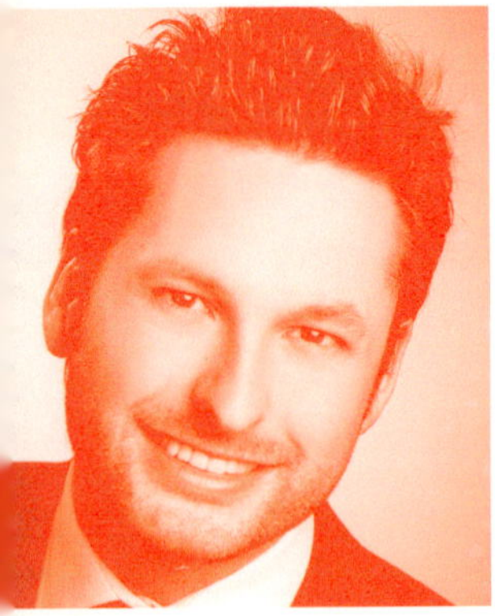
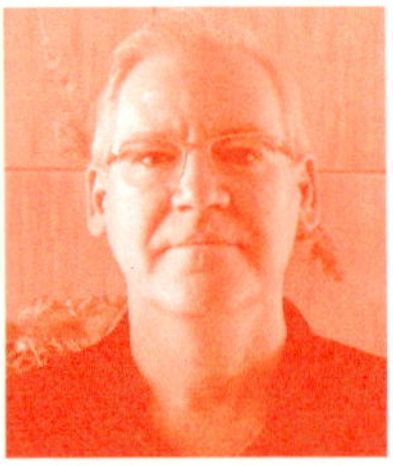

IntechOpen

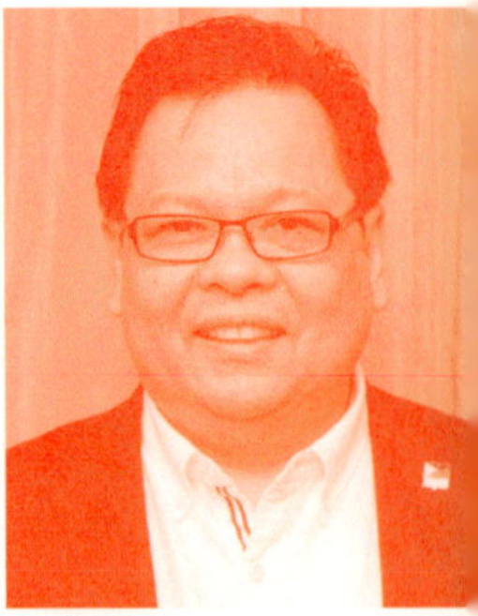
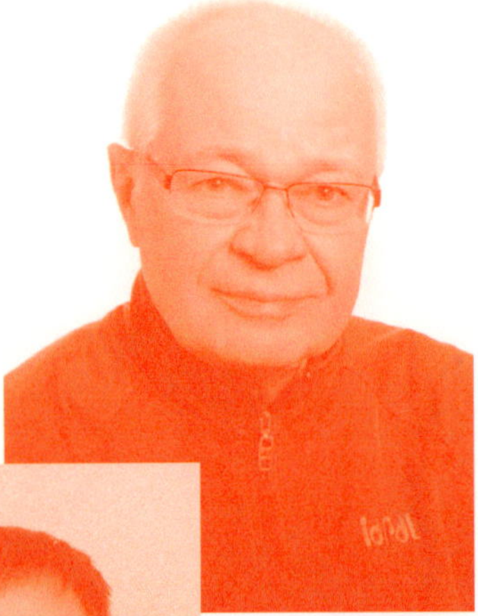
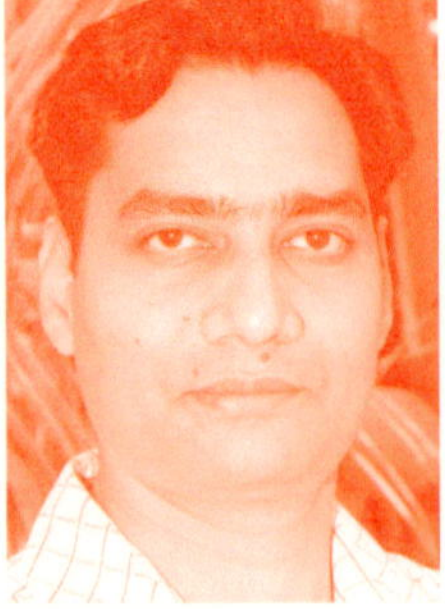
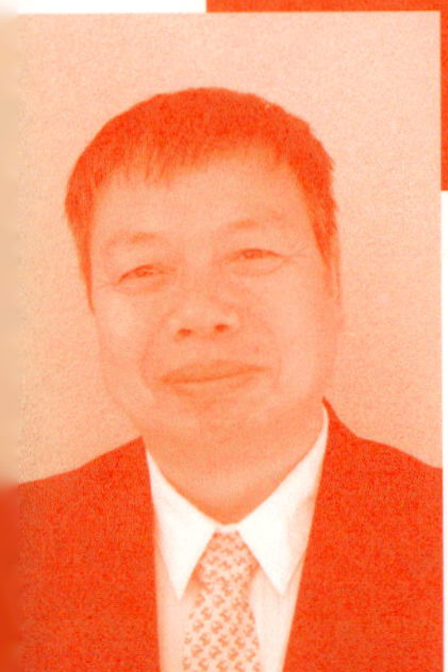
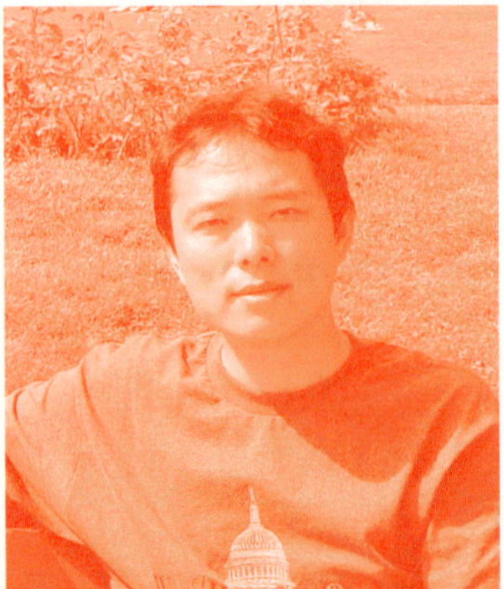
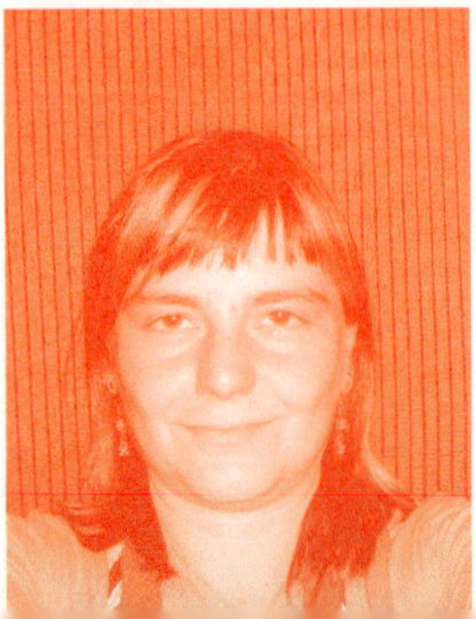

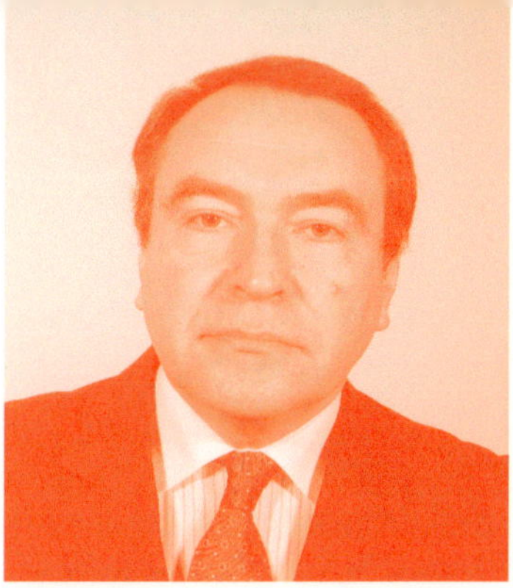
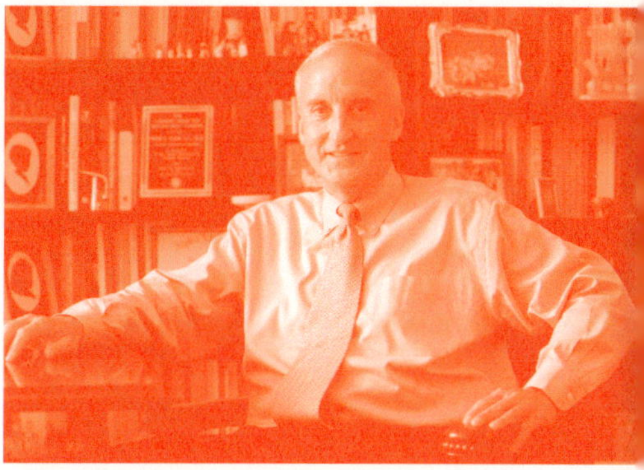
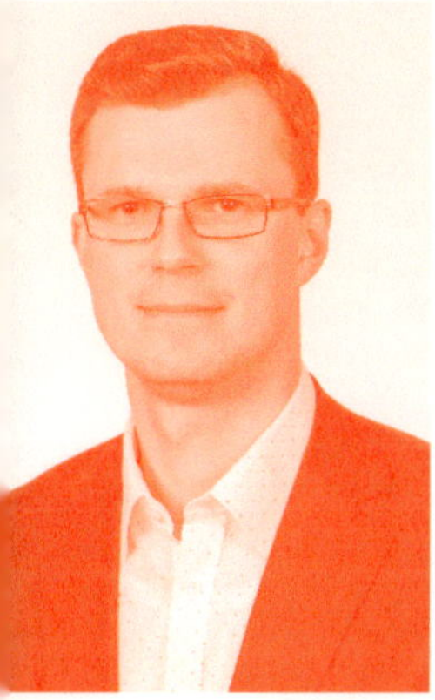
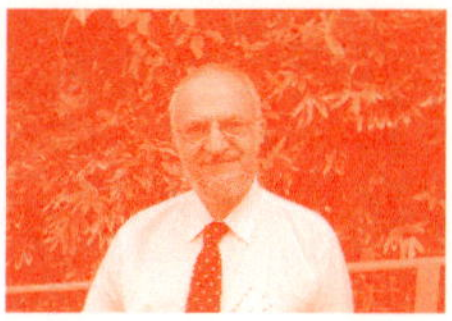
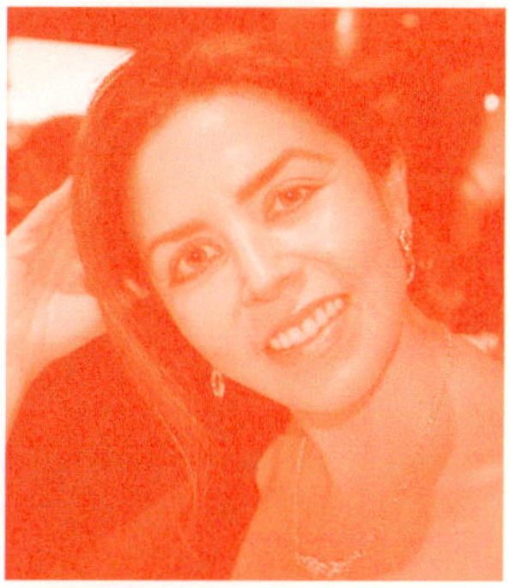

Supporting open minds since 2005

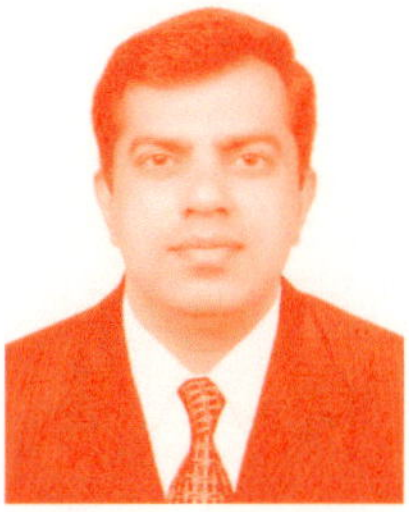
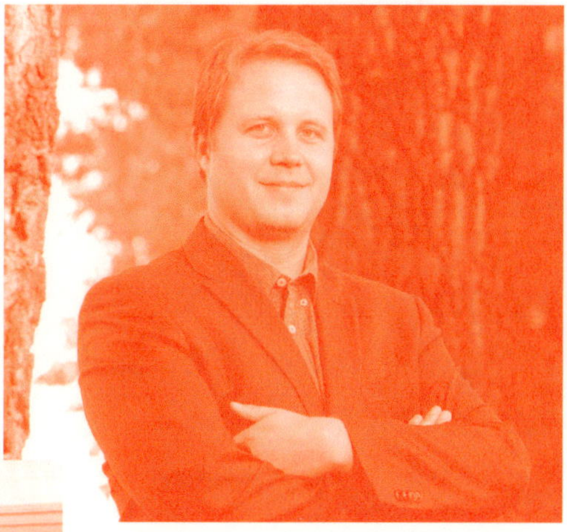
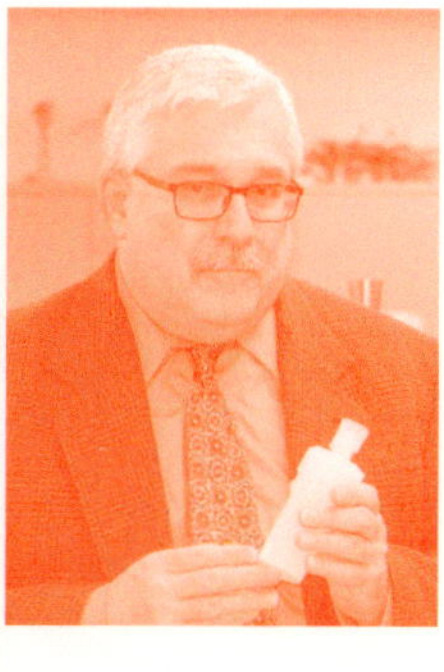
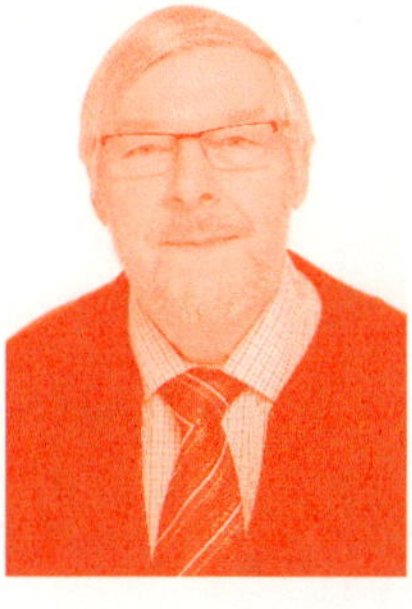
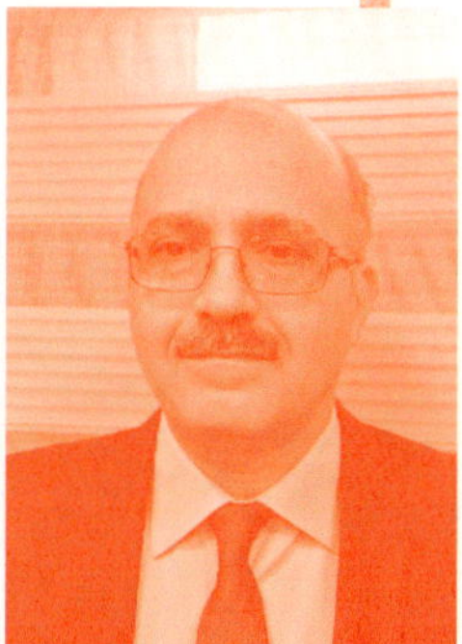
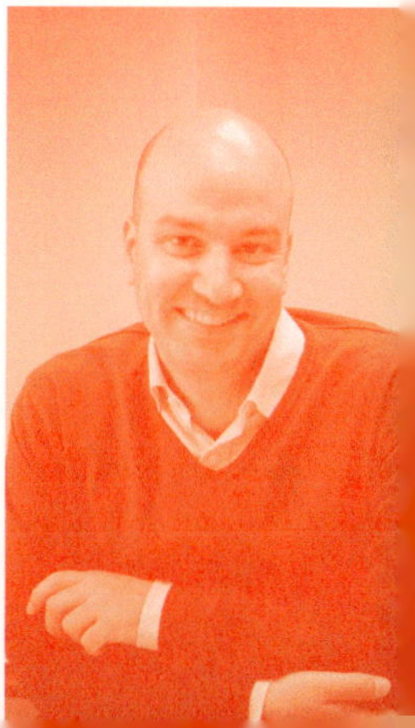
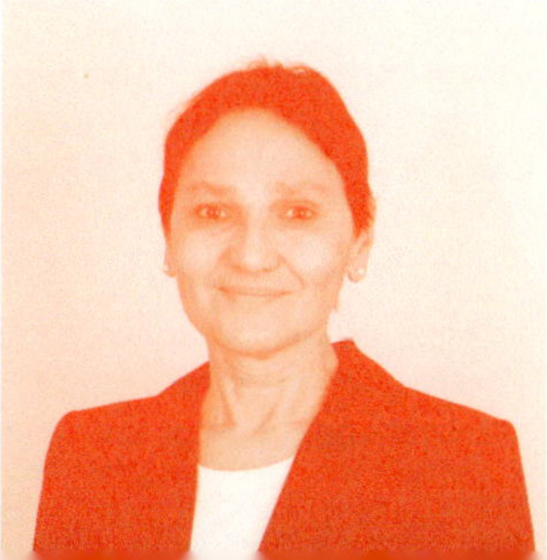

Pain Management - Practices, Novel Therapies and Bioactives
http://dx.doi.org/10.5772/intechopen.87267
Edited by Viduranga Yashasvi Waisundara, Ines Banjari and Jelena Balkić

Contributors
Viduranga Yashasvi Waisundara, Ines Banjari, Jelena Balkić, Teketel Ermias Ermias Geltore, Abiy Tadesse Angelo, Abdulaziz Al-Mahrezi, Asma Al-Shidhani, Srini Chary, Ensa Johnson, Marek Rózycki, Robert Tobias, Coti Phillips, Jessica Oswald, Edwin Contreras, Giustino Varrassi, Antonella Paladini, Shane M. M Heffernan, Gillian E. Conway, Nicholas West, Gillian Lauder, Armen Haroutunian, Tennison Malcolm, Thomas Zouki, Mihai Botea, Melinda S. Seering, Sangini Punia, Ann Ukachi Madukwe, Nnenna Ugwu, Ece Ozdemir Oktem, Seyda Cankaya

First published in London, United Kingdom, 2021 by IntechOpen
IntechOpen is the global imprint of INTECHOPEN LIMITED, registered in England and Wales, registration number: 11086078, 5 Princes Gate Court, London, SW7 2QJ, United Kingdom
Printed in Croatia

British Library Cataloguing-in-Publication Data
A catalogue record for this book is available from the British Library

Additional hard and PDF copies can be obtained from orders@intechopen.com

Pain Management - Practices, Novel Therapies and Bioactives
Edited by Viduranga Yashasvi Waisundara, Ines Banjari and Jelena Balkić
p. cm.
Print ISBN 978-1-83880-026-0
Online ISBN 978-1-83880-897-6
eBook (PDF) ISBN 978-1-83880-898-3

For EU product safety concerns:
IN TECH d.o.o., Prolaz Marije Krucifikse Kozulić 3, 51000 Rijeka, Croatia, info@intechopen.com or visit our website at intechopen.com.

Meet the editors

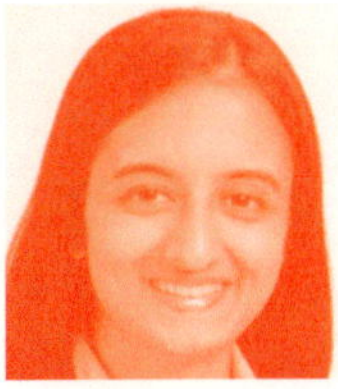

Dr. Viduranga Waisundara obtained her Ph.D. in Food Science and Technology from the Department of Chemistry, the National University of Singapore in 2010. From July 2009 to March 2013, she was a lecturer at Temasek Polytechnic, Singapore, after which she relocated to her motherland of Sri Lanka. There she spearheaded the Functional Food Product Development Project at the National Institute of Fundamental Studies from April 2013 to October 2016. Dr. Waisundara was a senior lecturer on a temporary basis at the Department of Food Technology, Faculty of Technology, Rajarata University of Sri Lanka. She is currently the Deputy Principal of the Australian College of Business and Technology–Kandy Campus, in Kandy, Sri Lanka. She is also the present Global Harmonization Initiative (GHI) Ambassador to Sri Lanka.

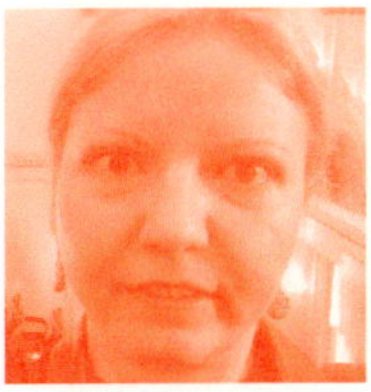

Ines Banjari, Ph.D., is an Associate Professor at the Faculty of Food Technology, University of Osijek, Croatia, where she lectures a number of Human Nutrition courses at undergraduate, graduate, and postgraduate levels (both doctoral and specialist). She received her Ph.D. in Nutrition (Clinical Nutrition specialist) in November 2012 from the Faculty of Food Biotechnology, University of Zagreb, Croatia, and finished her postdoctoral fellowship at the University of Toronto, Faculty of Medicine, Canada. Since October 2019, she has been a guest professor at the Faculty of Agriculture and Food Technology, University of Mostar, Bosnia and Herzegovina. She has also been a guest researcher at the Jagiellonian University Medical College, Krakow, Poland (2019); the University of Oslo, Faculty of Medicine, Norway (2017); the University of Split, School of Medicine, Croatia (2016); and the University of Belgrade, School of Medicine, Serbia (2016). She is currently an expert in Public Health Nutrition for the Association of Schools of Public Health in the European Region (ASPHER) and has been working closely with the European Commission's Joint Research Centre. She is PI of a scientific project with Slovenia (2020–2021) and was PI of a scientific project with Montenegro (2015–2016) and one NATO-funded project (2016–2017). She is also a collaborator on several national and international scientific projects. In 2014, she received the Danubius Young Scientist Award from the Austrian Federal Ministry of Science and Research and the Institute for the Danube Region and Central Europe. In 2016, she received the Young Scientist Award "Vera Johanides" from the Croatian Academy of Engineering. In 2019, she was awarded the International Visitor Leadership Program (IVLP) fellowship from the US Department of State. Dr. Banjari actively volunteers in civic organizations gathering Parkinson's disease patients (Awakening) and oncology patients (OncoPut).

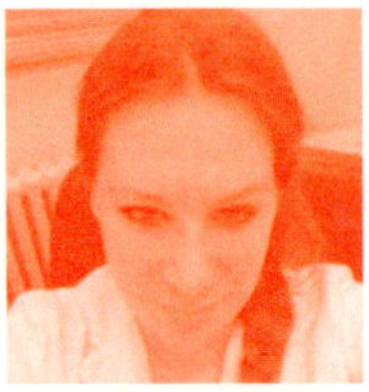

Jelena Balkić, Ph.D., was born in 1982 in Osijek, Croatia. She graduated from the Faculty of Food Technology, University of Osijek, Croatia, in 2008. She received her Ph.D. in Nutrition in 2017 with her thesis on chronic pain management with nutrition intervention. Since 2011, she has been employed at the University Hospital Osijek, Department of Dietetics and Nutrition, where she organizes, coordinates, and supervises the work of the department. She is actively involved in improving dietetics at the hospital by close collaboration with the IT sector on developing nutritional software for the hospital. Patient nutritional counseling is another important aspect of her work. Dr. Balkić has participated in several international and national conferences and is co-author of several scientific publications. She won the best poster award at Štampar Days in December 2019. She is also a collaborator on a scientific project in Slovenia (led by Dr. Banjari).

Contents

Preface

Pain is a distressing feeling often caused by intense or damaging stimuli. The International Association for the Study of Pain defines pain as "an unpleasant sensory and emotional experience associated with, or resembling that associated with, actual or potential tissue damage." In medical diagnosis, pain is regarded as a symptom of an underlying condition. Pain is the most common reason for any individual to reach out for medical support. It is a major symptom in several medical conditions and can interfere with a person's quality of life and general functioning. As such, prevention and management of pain are of paramount importance in remedying any disease.

Pain is part of our lives; it makes us alert, and it is a "signal for danger." However, when pain extends far beyond the healing period, it becomes an independent medical entity known as chronic pain. This book brings new perspectives on pain, particularly the management of pain. It examines the pain from biochemical, pharmaceutical, and clinical angles.

We would like to take this opportunity to thank the authors who have contributed so many wonderful chapters to this book. In addition, our heartfelt appreciation goes to IntechOpen and Author Service Manager Ms. Sandra Maljavac, who supported us throughout the creation and publication of this volume.

This book will be of value to academics conducting pain research in all its complexity, as it contains updated and current content. We have no doubt that readers will find these fresh points of view insightful and astute in moving forward the existing knowledge on pain.

Dr. Viduranga Waisundara
Australian College of Business and Technology – Kandy Campus,
Sri Lanka

Dr. Ines Banjari
Associate Professor,
Faculty of Food Technology,
University of Osijek,
Croatia

Dr. Jelena Balkic
University Hospital Osijek,
Croatia

Section 1

Pain Management - Updates

Chapter 1

What Do We Need to Consider for Pain Management?

Srini Chary

Abstract

Chronic pain in palliative care is viewed as an illness but remains as a subjective symptom. Hence, we must consider genetics, pain experience, coping skills, epigenetic effects, mental health, social determinants of health, interventions, and molecular biology. Acute pain transitions to chronic pain in some individuals following an injury, and there is poor evidence to stop such change. Acute, Chronic, and mixed pain can occur in patients with trauma, cancer, organ failure due to primary illness and other co-morbidities. The response to interventions may include biopsychosocial, non-pharmacological, surgery, radiation, chemotherapy, interventional radiology, pharmacological and depending upon survivorship, consider what is appropriate with peer reviewed medical evidence. Neurobiology is important in relation to physical and psychological issues; it affects an expression of pain. Manageable pain and relief are considered as being Human Right. Lack of adequate knowledge and treatment resources are common for care providers and patients. Cancer and noncancer pain ought to consider collaborating with interdisciplinary palliative approach, palliative care, and end of life care along with acute, chronic, and mixed pain management. Cancer patients with survivorship is increasing and risk management with chemicals, noncancer individuals appear similar. Barriers include health professional education, lack of treatment resources, medical, economic, ethical, and legal reasons. Pain management as an illness, care providers considers patient and family centered approach, useful to the community.

Keywords: pain taxonomy, genetics, epigenetic effects, biopsychosocial, molecular biology, interventions

1. Introduction

As a care provider, we must consider up to date pain management skills beneficial to individual patient. Valuing, dignity and hope along with better therapeutic relationship with the patient, allows us to return home happier at the end of the day. Relief of pain is not effective; health care professionals feel uncomfortable and complain around the world.

In 1967, the world's first purpose-built, St Christopher's Hospice in south London, England by Dame Cicely Saunders, who was a nurse, social worker and became a physician for "end of life care and clinical research" in the United Kingdom. Dr. Robert Twycross and from Canada Dr. Balfour Mount had worked with Dame Cicely Saunders and Dr. Mount came up with a term "Palliative Care" in 1973 which within a short time, the entire world accepted.

World Health Organization (WHO) present definition comprises: "Palliative care is an approach that improves the quality of life of patients and their families facing the problem associated with life-threatening illness, through the prevention and relief of suffering by means of early identification and impeccable assessment and treatment of pain and other problems, physical, psychosocial and spiritual."

More recently "Palliative Approach, Palliative Care and End of Life Care" has been accepted internationally as well as also "Early, Integrated, Collaborative and Inter-professional Care". Advanced care planning, goals of care, and good communication with relevant language and words reduce distress of patient and family (**Figure 1**).

Now palliative care has patients with palliative approach, palliative care, end of life care and survivorship with cancer or organ failure. Dr. Pippa Hawley explained the value of a visual "Bow Tie Model" as a disease management and palliative care triangles can be adopted for cancer and non-cancer interventions [1].

At the end of last century, pain management and scientific research had improved but chronic pain and palliative care specialists with present knowledge were limited in Canada and other parts of the world.

The Gold Standards Framework from the UK has prognostic indicators; general, cancer, and organ failure trajectories, which are important and useful to consider, before treatment plan [2].

In 2007, Boulanger et al., did a study whether chronic non-cancer pain has improved, though more patients were receiving medical analgesics, the changes were minor and could be better in Canada [3].

Genetics play a major role with physical, psychological health or illness and our knowledge and management is improving [4, 5]. Nutrition has a role in pain management and requires learning care providers, patients, and families [6].

Optimal pain management requires history, physical examination, investigations, and appropriate interventions. In the past four to five years "opioid crisis" increased deaths due to the use of illicit fentanyl [7]. "Pain crisis" is an experience of a patient relating to pain and requires immediate interventions, whereas "opioid crisis" relates to substance use disorder or an error with medication or illicit drug use.

IASP, pain and palliative care societies across the world are encouraging physicians and interprofessional team members to consider interventions for pain management, clinical research and in the past three decades, several peer reviewed manuscripts have been published for pain management with such evidence and knowledge, can reduce pain in an individual and community can prosper.

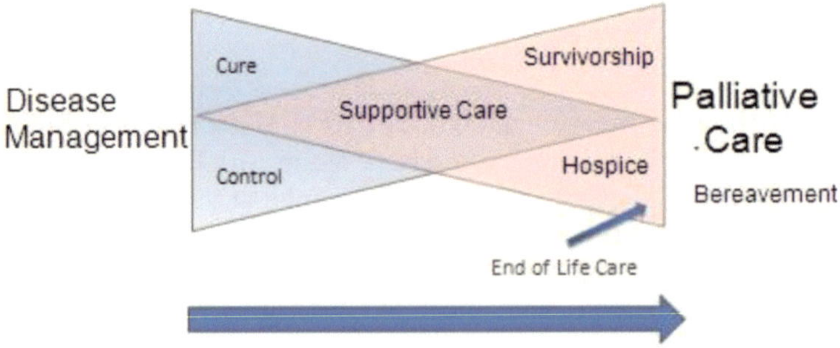

Figure 1.
Bow Tie Model: Bow Tie Model: Palliative care is an interdisciplinary coordination at the time of diagnosis and the timelines can vary in an individual head towards survivorship with cure or illness is controlled and requires supportive care or some individuals can be at the end of life.

2. Optimal pain management

International Association for the study of pain (IASP) has revised, 1979 definition of pain in 2020 considering concepts, challenges and compromises and stated "An unpleasant sensory and emotional experience associated with, or resembling that associated with, actual or potential tissue damage" and is relevant for pain management [8].

Pain perception and expression is associated with molecular biology which includes transmission of signals from an injury, transmitting through spinothalamic tract to thalamus in the brain, in nanoseconds, the signals move to limbic system. Alteration in the limbic system, changes in neurotransmitters, tissue receptors lead to high expression of pain, anxiety, frustration, and major depression.

2.1 Acute pain

Acute pain like "stubbed toe or a needlestick" disappears in a few minutes secondary to the antinociceptive nervous system triggered and the pain stimuli release endorphins within the brain, and enkephalins in the brain stem, which block the transmission of pain signals at different levels and the ion channels are functioning.

However, the acute pain secondary to cell injury caused by pressure, heat, chemicals, or physical stimulus; damaged cells release lysosomes which causes inflammation within hours and magnifies the pain signals through the release of signaling chemicals such as prostaglandins, arachidonic acid and leukotrienes in the nervous system and involves glutamate at low levels. Ion channels may not function appropriately thus endorphins may not be active [9].

Acute nerve injury associated with acute neuropathic pain, e.g., broken bone, amputation.

2.2 Chronic pain

Acute, nociceptive, and inflammatory pain can transition to chronic pain, if the pain persists more than 3 months in an individual. In this period of transition, the ion channel function may not be normal, and endorphins may not be active.

Following an acute injury; infection, crush or nerve injury, degeneration of tissues, micro, macro vascular insufficiency, and cancer the recovery is low, and healing is slower, leading to chronic pain associated with poor quality of life.

Palliative and end of life care, some patients who are dependent, frail and require extensive nursing care may have pain crisis along with delirium. Identifying the difference between the symptoms, pain and delirium, using appropriate pharmacological interventions are useful. Refractory symptoms like delirium, respiratory distress, seizures may need palliative sedation. Patients with pain and agitation may require analgesic and intermittent or palliative sedation [10].

2.3 Cancer and pain

Advanced cancer trajectory leads to end of life, pain crisis or delirium and other co-morbidities need to be considered. However, if patient responds to intervention, almost 50% of them are in survivorship and not end of life, requiring long-term pain and symptom management. Cancer pain is often a "mixed pain" as inflammation around primary or metastasis is common [11].

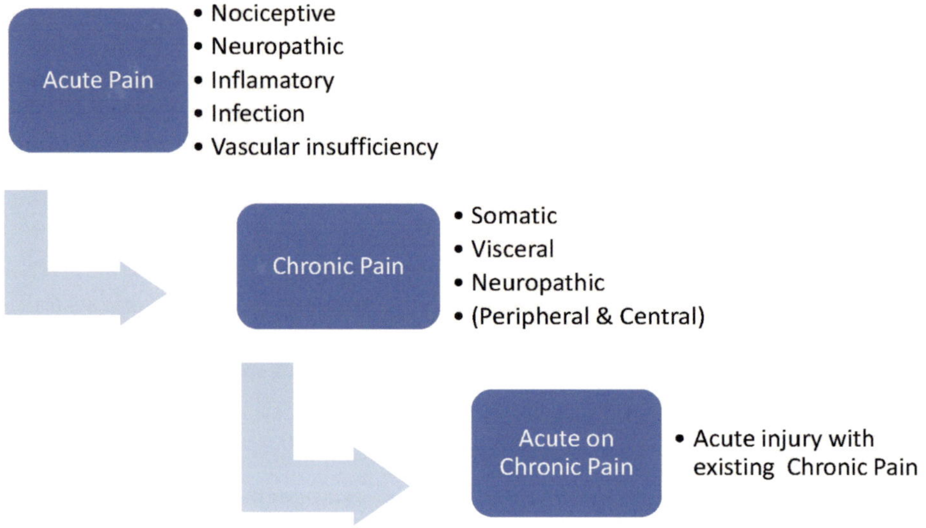

Figure 2.
Pain classification: acute, chronic, and acute on chronic pain.

2.4 Tissue injury, organ failure, comorbidities, and pain

Soft tissue or bone in the elderly have more issues like arthritis, tissue injury and healing can be poor giving rise to the pain. Acute or Chronic kidney disease (AKI or CKD) with comorbidities require pain management and most opioids are excreted through kidney and opioid toxicity is common. Diabetes is associated with neuropathy, likely microvascular insufficiency [12] (**Figure 2**).

2.5 Taxonomy

Nociceptive pain, neuropathic pain and nociplastic pain have been approved by IASP in 2019 and International Classification of Diseases (ICD-11), which the

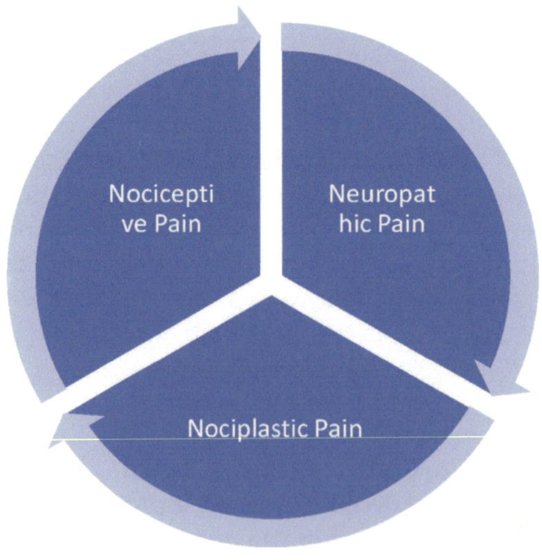

Figure 3.
Taxonomy change in 2019, IASP added "Nociplastic Pain" relating to neuroplasticity and future application of research.

World Health Organization adopted in the same year. These combined efforts have potential benefits for both research and patient care [13] (**Figure 3**).

Neuroplasticity is the change in neuronal pathways and synapses that occurs due to certain factors: behavior, environment, and neural process. Chronic pain has been related to central excitation, wind-up theory and IASP approved Neuroplastic pain; as the brain learning or neuroplasticity and alteration in the function of anatomy for future research an appropriate term [14, 15].

Epigenetic effects, including major depression in an individual related to negative experience associated with poor coping and neuroplasticity secondary to changes in gene–environment, psychosocial environment leading to lower levels of neurotrophic factors altering structural and functional aspects of brain. Such epigenetic effects can be generational [16–17].

3. Principles of pain management

Pain management should include biopsychosocial assessment, pain severity, pain descriptors and planning physical, psychological, spiritual rehabilitation, invasive therapies, and pharmacological interventions for patients with acute, chronic, neuropathic and nociplastic pain. Patients in pain crisis and agitated often require pharmacotherapy initially to manage pain and following that nonpharmacological interventions have a value and can reduce or stop medications.

Acute pain may require anti-inflammatory medications, steroids and opioids, depending upon the extent of injury for a short period, which could be hours to days, which needs to be explained to the patient and family.

Chronic pain is associated with goal setting. If patient's opioid use disorder risk is high by using "opioid Risk Tool" questionnaire, before opioids are being used requires boundary setting, along with written patient agreement document, for opioid therapy [18].

Patients with life expectancy few hours, days or weeks may need more pharmacological interventions, as other interventions non-pharmacological to improve symptoms, may need longer time to respond (**Figure 4**).

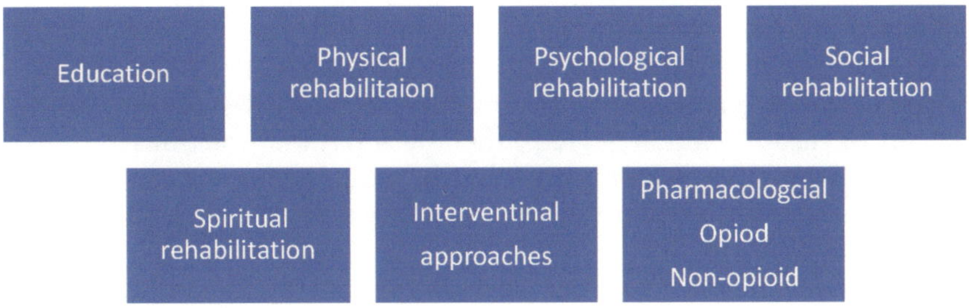

Figure 4.
Pain management includes variety of approaches, which require to improve patient's suffering.

3.1 Education

Individuals with chronic pain, and suffering may benefit with explanation of their pain, which is a subjective symptom along with interventional plan which should include in such education. Such education either individual, or group education, depending upon the choice of the patient. Education can be verbal, written or online [19].

3.2 Physical medicine approach

Somatic, myofascial nociceptive pain can respond to exercise, passive physical modalities (TENS, laser, ultrasound, and massage) along with stretching has value in chronic back, neck and shoulder pain. Elderly, chronic pain, neuropathic, psychosocial and cancer pain patients/individuals may require interprofessional management [20, 21].

3.3 Psychosocial approach

Chronic pain in some patients is associated with alteration in the function and anatomy of limbic system in the brain and prefrontal system is not comfortable.

Cognitive-behavioral therapy (CBT) for chronic pain management has been used widely. Dennis Turk first described in 1983 education, skill acquisition, cognitive and behavioral rehearsal, generalization, and maintenance, and in review 2008 CBT, self-management skills and other suggestions [22].

Vulnerable populations with pain require social and financial rehabilitation along with multidisciplinary engagement.

3.4 Spiritual approach

Spiritual awakening as non-medical approach: meditation seems to benefit self-management skills, emotional improvement, and empowerment. Physical pain and discomfort in an individual may improve, whether neurotransmitters alter to benefit emotions.

3.5 Interventional approaches

3.5.1 Surgery

For patients with a reversible pain diagnosis due to fracture, obstruction, perforation and other causes, surgical intervention is possible and beneficial. Chronic pain improves with deep brain or spinal stimulation, which requires surgery [23].

3.5.2 Radiation therapy

Primary cancer and metastasis either curative or palliative- the intention is to reduce acute or chronic pain. It is a local therapy and initial fractions may increase pain due to inflammation. Systemic injection of radionuclide was used few decades ago for bone metastasis, but at present it is used for thyroid cancer as a primary therapy only [24].

3.5.3 Chemo and immune therapy

Patients with cancer pain receiving chemotherapy, initially the pain may increase due to necrotic tumor and inflammation. After two or three cycles of chemotherapy the tumor may reduce in size and pain may improve along with other symptoms.

3.5.4 Interventional radiology (IR)

Lately nerve mapping is better and anatomically using local anesthetic, steroids or other medications can reduce or stop pain for a few weeks. IR can be used for palliative bone/musculoskeletal and neuropathic pain in the form of cryoablation, microwave thermal ablation, plasma medicated radiofrequency ablation. Vertebroplasty and kyphoplasty along with stent therapy is possible [25].

Sympathetic blockade, stellate ganglion, coeliac and splanchnic plexus, and lumbar plexus block is possible to reduce sympathetically medicated pain and symptoms.

3.5.5 Neuraxial therapy

Palliative and end of life care when the pain is not manageable epidural and spinal analgesia using local anesthetic, opioid, alpha-2 agonist, and other pharmaceuticals to control pain is available [26].

3.5.6 Pharmacological

Non-opioid analgesics such as anti-inflammatory; acetaminophen, NSAIDs and Cox-2 inhibitors are used for acute pain but less effective with chronic pain including neuropathic or nociplastic pain. Such medications are associated with adverse effects and a therapeutic trial is useful in an individual and testing appropriate dose is useful and not harmful.

3.6 Adjuvants, co-analgesics: systemic and topical

Antidepressants and anticonvulsants have been used as systemic adjuvants for chronic pain and neuropathic pain. Number needed to treat (NNT) and number needed to harm (NNH) was adapted from Finnerup et al. in 2005 and 2007. Topical adjuvants include lidocaine patch and capsaicin and ointment and topical formulation with certain local anesthetic, amitriptyline, ketamine, gabapentin, and clonidine have been reported as beneficial for localized pain which is neuropathic in nature [27, 28].

3.6.1 Opioid analgesics

Chronic pain management requires opioids, we need to consider pain diagnosis, risk/benefit of use of opioid in an individual, mental health and behavior. Opioid risk tool has been useful to note the risk and if it is high, consider goals and boundaries, verbal or written signed documents to encourage patient's better behavior [18] (**Table 1**).

Goal setting—Chronic pain—opioids
Restful sleep at night
Brain activity sharp in the daytime
Affect, being better than neutral
Pain reduction by >30%
Improved activity and function
Physical, psychological rehabilitation
Plan for reduction of opioids—if pain improved

Table 1.
Opioid use requires goal setting and needs to be shared with the patient, the first time and reminded on follow-up.

Boundary setting—high risk—opioids
Strict boundary setting is essential
Treatment agreements—(verbal/signed)
Urine drug testing (UDT)
Interval/contingency dispensing

Table 2.
High risk in a patient with opioids or substance and opioid use disorder likely, consider boundary setting and improving behaviour.

What activates glia and immune cells?
Pro-inflammatory cytokines
Chemokines
ATP
Neuropeptides
Prostaglandins
Glutamate
Nitric oxide
Endogenous danger signals

Table 3.
Long-term opioid use can activate glia and immune cells causing tolerance, allodynia, and hyperalgesia and considering how to approach pain management.

Opioids use has been common, and morphine was considered as a "gold standard" for pain management few decades ago along with "no ceiling". Initially, morphine was used for acute pain when the pain was excessive and Twycross, once he was able to establish physiological half-life of morphine, suggested every 4 h, and on the clock. In the early 1980s and before, opioids were short-acting oral pills, liquid, and injectable. Long acting opioids through formulation became available in the late 1980s and 1990s. Now tramadol, oxycodone, codeine, hydromorphone, morphine long acting oral medications along with transdermal fentanyl and buprenorphine are available [29] (**Table 2**).

Several animal and clinical studies have shown codeine, oxycodone, morphine, and fentanyl may have benefit relieving pain for short term but when used long term lead to glial and immune cells activation, leading to tolerance, allodynia, and hyperalgesia [30, 31]. Hydromorphone long-term use has similar effect, opioid neurotoxicity with twitching, myoclonus, unrestful night sleep, and minor agitation. Activation of glial cell is associated with N-methyl-D-Aspartate (NMDA) receptor and release of amino acid, glutamate which is neuroexcitatory [30, 31]. None of the above opioids have NMDA antagonism. Methadone and levorphanol have two racemic mixtures opioid with half-life 7–8 h and non-opioid, NMDA antagonist, norepinephrine, and serotonin re-uptake inhibition. Ketamine has NMDA antagonism but adverse effects in relation to tolerance and mental health issues are high [32] (**Table 3**).

3.6.2 Opioid use

For the use of opioids as analgesics we need to consider pharmacokinetics, active metabolites, half-life, and excretion. "Start low and go slow" has been the principle and in pain crisis either opioid toxicity or pain is not responding requires higher doses. Opioid switch in such states and 20–30% reduction of equianalgesic opioid need to be considered. Breakthrough pain, if it occurs 10% of 24-h dose of the opioid is used as a dose and around half-life such dose is given [33].

The short-term use of opioids may be useful for acute pain, but the long-term use is associated with activation of glial and immune cells with neuroexcitatory chemicals along with tolerance and hyperalgesia [30, 31] (**Figure 5**).

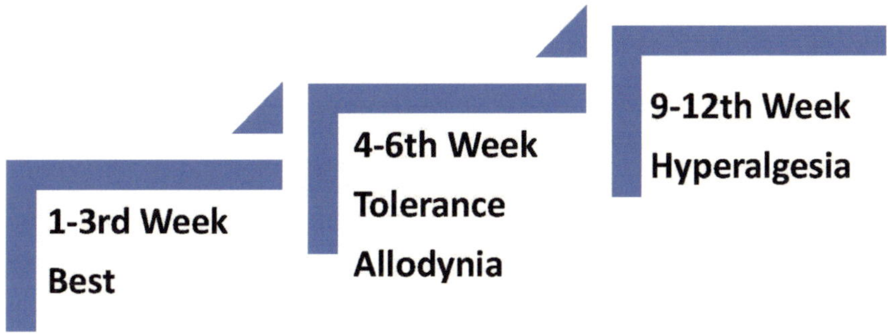

Figure 5.
Animal and clinical studies have shown Codeine, Oxycodone, Morphine, and Fentanyl when used long term, leads to neurotoxicity: Tolerance, allodynia and hyperalgesia and we need to consider better interventions to reduce pain and suffering.

Methadone is available as two racemic mixtures; R-methadone is an opioid with lower half-life and S-methadone is NMDA antagonist, Norepinephrine, and serotonin re-uptake inhibitor. Methadone has been used as harm-reduction for opioid use disorder and being used as an analgesic. Rapid titration using German, Morley Makin, Kansas, and Edmonton method in the form of stepped approach to opioid switch is possible [34, 35].

Methadone is also used when neuropathic and nociplastic pain is associated with existing opioid toxicity; twitches, jerks (myoclonus) and neurotoxicity with confusion and delirium. In such state, it is possible to use low dose twice or three times a day and ultra-low dose with slow titration is possible along with existing opioid or co-analgesics can be reduced and stopped gradually if benefit is noted [36]. Patients with mental health issues require higher dose and patients who are comfortable psychologically, pain relief and physical suffering require very low dose of methadone for cancer, acute or chronic kidney disease (**Tables 4–6**).

3.6.3 Adverse effects associated with the use of opioids

Nausea, minor hallucinations, and somnolence are common at the start of opioids, if the dose remains the same in a few days often such symptoms fade or require lower dose of opioid or therapeutic intervention for the symptom.

Glia and Immune cells release neuroexcitatory, pain enhancing substances
Arachidonic acid and prostaglandins
Excitatory amino acids (glutamate)
Pro-inflammatory cytokines/chemokines
Nerve growth factors
Reactive oxygen and nitrogen species

Table 4.
Neuroexcitatory chemicals enhance pain and the present and future research has a value to improve pain and suffering.

Opioid pharmacokinetics and use as an analgesic				
Opioid	Half-Life	Active metabolites	Excretion	Start dose
Codeine	3–4 hrs	Morphine	Renal	30 mg Q4h
Oxycodone	2–6 hrs	Oxymorphone	Renal	5 mg Q4h
Morphine	2–4 hrs	M6G, M3G	Renal	1 mg Q4h
Hydromorphone	2–4 hrs	H6G, H3G	Renal	1 mg Q4h
Fentanyl patch	17 hrs	Norfentanyl	Renal	12 mcg/h
Methadone	6–150 hrs	None known	Hepatic	1 mg? Q8h
Buprenorphine patch	37 hrs	B3G, NorB3G	Hepatic	5 mcg/h, Q7days

Opioid use as an analgesic, "start low and go slow" for pain management. Once pain is stable, same long acting opioid can be used to reduce tolerance. Medications Fentanyl patch, Methadone and Buprenorphine patch are long acting, and dose need to be adjusted, taking half-life into consideration.

Table 5.
Opioid use as an analgesic and "start low and go slow" for pain management.

Cancer clinic internal protocol methadone—Calgary					
1–7 days	**7–14 days**	**14–21 days**	**21–28 days**	**28–35 days**	**35–42 days**
1 mg daily	1 mg Q12h	1 mg Q8h	2 mg Q8h	3 mg q8h	5 mg Q8h
2.5 mg daily	2.5 mg Q12h	2.5 mg Q8h	5 mg Q8h	7.5 mg Q8h	10 mg Q8h

At the Tom Baker Cancer Centre, Pain Clinic in Calgary, Canada an Internal Protocol was applied to patients with opioids and pain has not improved. Evidence relating to neurotoxicity, tolerance, allodynia, and hyperalgesia methadone has been used at ultra-low dose and slow titration to relieve pain.

Table 6.
Opioid use as an analgesic and "start low and go slow" for pain management.

Dry mouth and constipation are common and require water sipping and laxatives, respectively.

Respiratory depression can occur with high doses of opioids.

Reduction androgen/testosterone can occur due to long-term use of opioids.

Neurotoxicity can occur associated with infection, renal insufficiency, and other medications; consists of hallucinations, delirium, twitching, jerks (myoclonus) and seizures. Such symptoms require reducing existing opioid, opioid switch, or adjunct medications.

Methadone and other substrates with enzyme interactions can lead to serotonin syndrome and QT/QTc prolongation.

3.6.4 Use of assessment tools

- Brief pain inventory (BPI) [37].
- The DN4 questionnaire [38, 39].
- Edmonton symptom assessment system revised (ESAS-R) [40].
- Opioid risk tool (ORT) [18].
- Pain disability index (PDI) [41].
- Roland Morris scale [42].

3.6.5 Malignant bowel obstruction (MBO)

Carcinomatosis can occur with cancer, intra-abdominal organs and results in bowel obstruction with pain and cramps. If it is localized surgery is helpful. If the obstruction can be seen by gastrointestinal endoscopy a stent can be inserted with pain and obstruction relief. However, if the obstruction on the bowel being multiple sites dexamethasone and somatostatin analogue is used subcutaneously. Initially injectable opioids are used for pain relief, and if obstruction is relived can reduce and stop opioids but somatostatin analogue may continue [43, 44].

4. Opioids, pain and substance use disorder

Chronic pain in patients with cancer, noncancer injury related, organ failure renal insufficiency, and trauma related individuals if they are at the end of life pain and have substance use disorder (SUD), we need to consider "comfort care" as goals and assist as best as we can.

However, similar patients engaged in survivorship, SUD need to be assessed and mental health/addiction services, need to be collaborated. Some of the patients with SUD or opioid use disorder (OUD) require Mu-agonist therapy using methadone or suboxone.

5. Potential future treatments for pain

We need to consider further research to improve care for individual patient. Chronic pain is considered as an illness with suffering. Several organizations have been working and care providers need to engage in raising questions and proceeding with research investigation.

Investigations and research in relation to genetics, non-opioids like; ion channels, alpha-2-agonists, glia, and immune cells along with non-pharmacological approach physical, psychological, social, spiritual rehabilitation and research in nutrition is worthwhile.

6. Conclusion

Palliative care consists of patients with illness in the early phase and advanced end of life care. Patient's wishes, worries, goals of care, and shared decisions along with subjective symptom like pain need to be considered.

Chronic pain is an illness and remains as a subjective symptom for an individual. Biopsychosocial, spiritual, and medical approach can benefit patient, family, and community. As care providers we ought to be up to date, evidence supported approach to relieve suffering of patient and family. Animal experiments and human clinical research have given care providers knowledge, and application of pain management can be better.

Acute pain often heals within days to weeks, but when the pain persists from an injury for more than three months chronic pain is considered. Central excitatory chemicals in the central nervous system can increase pain expression. Such change allows anxiety, frustration, and mental health issues.

Interventions like interventional, psychological, physical, pharmacological and nutrition have a value to reduce the chronic pain illness, suffering and improve function in an individual.

In the future, a2–Adrenergic agonists, ion-channel modifiers, and nanotechnology using nanoparticles to transport pharmaceuticals to reduce adverse effects and improve efficiency have a value in pain management and being investigated.

Thus, consider individual patient despite common diagnosis, require self-management skills, and endure or improve symptoms using appropriate therapies.

Education of care providers, patients and families is important; avoid stigmatizing an individual with chronic pain, substance use disorder, poor quality of life and mental health issues.

Acknowledgements

I wish to acknowledge and thank Dr. Neil Hagen, Dr. Alexander (John) Clark and Dr. Christopher Spanswick with whom I did learn and practice pain management in Calgary, Alberta, Canada. Thanks to Dr. Pippa Hawley, she allowed me to use the "Bow Tie Model" figure, in this chapter.

I wish to thank International Association for the Study of Pain, Canadian Pain Society, American Academy of Hospice and Palliative Care, Canadian Society of Palliative Care Physicians, and Pallium Foundation of Canada.

Conflict of interest

I do not have any conflict of interest and grateful to continue to work and assist patients, families, and my colleagues. The tables and figures were prepared by me and visual information was created through information from peer-reviewed publications.

Author details

Srini Chary
Cumming School of Medicine, University of Calgary, Alberta Health Services, Calgary, Alberta, Canada

*Address all correspondence to: srini.chary@ahs.ca; schary@shaw.ca

References

[1] Hawley P(P). The bow tie model of 21st century palliative care. JPM; 2013;**47**(1):e2-e5. DOI: 10.1016/j.jpainsymman.2013.10.009/

[2] Thomas K et al. Prognostic Indicator Guidance (PIG). 4th ed. © The Gold Standards Framework Centre In End of Life Care CIC. England, United Kingdom; 2011 (Google Scholar)

[3] Boulanger A, Clark AJ, Squire P, Cui E, Horbay GL. Chronic pain in Canada: Have we improved our management of chronic noncancer pain? Pain Research & Management. 2007;**12**:39-47

[4] Diatchenko L et al. Genetic basis for individual variations in pain perception and development of chronic pain condition. Human Molecular Genetics. 2005;**14**(1):135-143

[5] Zorna-Lichtenwalter K, Meloto CB, Khoury S, Diatchenko L. Genetic predictors of human chronic pain conditions. Neuroscience. 2016;**338**:36-62

[6] Tennant F. A diet for patients with chronic pain. Practical Pain Management. 2012;**11**(6):1-7

[7] Lisa B, Jessica H. Evidence synthesis—The opioid crisis in Canada: A national perspective. Health Promotion and Chronic Disease Prevention in Canada. 2018;**38**(6):224-233

[8] Raja SN et al. The revised International Association for the Study of Pain definition of pain: Concepts, challenges, and compromises. Pain. 2020;**00**(00):1-7

[9] Carr DB, Goudas LC. Acute pain. Lancet. 1999;**353**:2051-2058

[10] Bush SH, Tierney S, Lawlor PG. Clinical assessment and management of delirium in the palliative care setting. Drugs. 2017;**77**:1623-1643. DOI: 10.1007/s40265-017-0804-3

[11] Caraceni A, Shkodra M. Cancer pain assessment and classification (review). Cancers. 2019;**11**:510. DOI: 10.3390/cancers11040510

[12] Davison SN. Clinical pharmacology considerations in pain management in patients with advanced kidney failure. CJASN. 2019;**14**:917-931. DOI: 10.2215/CJN.05180418

[13] Treede R-D et al. Chronic pain as a symptom or disease. The IASP classification of chronic pain for the international classification of disease (ICD-11). Pain. 2019;**160**(1):19-27

[14] Siddall PJ. Neuroplasticity and pain: What does it all mean? The Medical Journal of Australia. 2013;**198**(940):177-178

[15] Kosek E, Cohen M, Baron R, et al. Do we need a third mechanic descriptor for chronic pain states? Pain. 2016;**157**:1382-1386

[16] aan het Rot M, Mathew SJ, Charney DS. Neurobiological mechanisms in major depressive disorder. CMAJ. 2009;**180**(3):305-313

[17] Bombay A et al. The intergenerational effects of Indian residential schools: Implications for the concept of historical trauma. Transcultural Psychiatry; 2013;**51**(3):320-338

[18] Webster LR, Webster RM. Predicting aberrant behaviors in opioid-treated patients: Preliminary validation of the opioid risk tool. Pain Medicine. 2005;**6**(6):432-442

[19] Mittinty MM, Vanlint S, Nigel Stocks MN, Mittinty GLM. Exploring

effect of pain education on chronic pain patients' expectation of recovery and pain intensity. Scandinavian Journal of Pain. 2018;**18**(2):211-219

[20] Assendelft WJ et al. Spinal manipulative therapy for low back pain. A meta-analysis of effectiveness relative to other therapies. Annals of Internal Medicine. 2003;**138**:871-881

[21] Moffett J, McLean S. The role of physiotherapy in the management of non-specific back pain and neck pain. Rheumatology (Oxford). 2006;**45**:371-378

[22] Turk DC, Swanson KS, Tunks ER. Psychological approaches in the treatment of chronic pain patients—When pills, scalpels and needles are not enough. Canadian Journal of Psychiatry. 2008;**53**(4):213-223

[23] Farrell SM, Green A, Aziz T. The current state of deep brain stimulation for chronic pain and its context in other forms of neuromodulation. Brain Sciences. 2018;**8**:158. DOI: 10.3390/brainsci8080158

[24] Sierko E, Zuzda DHK, Wojtukiewicz MZ. Personalized radiation therapy in cancer pain management. Cancers. 2019;**11**:390. DOI: 10.3390/cancers11030390

[25] Bittman RW et al. Global approach to the patient with pain in interventional radiology. Seminars in Interventional Radiology. 2018;**35**(4):342-349

[26] Smyth CE, Jarvis V, Poulin P. Brief review: Neuraxial analgesia in refractory malignant pain. Canadian Journal of Anesthesia. 2013;**61**(2):1-13

[27] Lynch ME, Watson CP. The pharmacotherapy of chronic pain: A review. Pain. 2006;**11**:11-38

[28] Finnerup NB et al. An evidence-based algorithm for the treatment of neuropathic pain. MedGenMed. 2007;**9**(2):36

[29] Chou R, Clark E, Helfand M. Comparative efficacy and safety of long-acting oral opioids for chronic non-cancer pain: A systematic review. Journal of Pain and Symptom Management. 2003;**26**(5). DOI: 10.1016/j.jpainsymman.2003.03.003/

[30] Lacagnina M, Watkins LR, Grace PM. Toll-like receptors and their role in persistent pain. Pharmacology & Therapeutics. 2018;**184**:145-158

[31] Grace PM, Strand KA, Galer EL, Maier SF, Watkins LR. MicroRNA-124 and microRNA-146a both attenuate persistent neuropathic pains induced by morphine in male rats. Brain Research. 2018;**1692**:9-11

[32] Zhuo M. Ionotropic glutamate receptors contribute to pain transmission and chronic pain. Neuropharmacology. 2017;**112**:228-234

[33] Devulder J, Jacobs A, Richarz U, Wiggett H. Impact of opioid rescue medication for breakthrough pain on the efficacy and tolerability of long-acting opioids in patients with chronic non-malignant pain. British Journal of Anaesthesia. 2009;**103**(4):576-585

[34] Fisher K, Coderre TJ, Hagen N. Targeting the N-methyl-d-aspartate receptor for chronic pain management. JPSM. 2000;**20**(5):358-373

[35] Morley JS, Makin M. The use of methadone in cancer pain poorly responsive to other opioids. Pain Reviews. 1998;**5**:51-58

[36] Chary S, Abdul-Razzak A, Galloway L. Ultralow-dose adjunctive methadone with slow titration, considering long half-life for outpatients with cancer-related pain. Palliative Medicine Reports. 2020;**1**(1):119-123

[37] Cleeland CS, Ryan KM. Pain assessment: Global us of the brief pain inventory. Annals of the Academy of Medicine, Singapore. 1994;**23**(2):129-138

[38] Perez C, Galvez R, Huelbes S, et al. Validity and reliability of the Spanish version of the DN4 (Douleur Neuropathique 4 questions) questionnaire for differential diagnosis of pain syndromes associated to a neuropathic or somatic component. Health and Quality of Life Outcomes. 2007;**5**:66. DOI: 10.1186/1477-7525-5-66

[39] Timmerman H et al. Investigating the validity of DN4 in a consecutive population of patients with chronic pain. PLoS One. 2017;**12**(11):e0187961. DOI: 10.1371/journal.pone.0187961

[40] Hui D, Bruera E. The Edmonton symptom assessment system 25 years later: Past, present and future developments. Journal of Pain and Symptom Management. 2017;**53**(3):630-643. DOI: 10.1016/j.jpainsymman.2016.10.370

[41] Pollard CA. Preliminary validity study of the pain disability index. Perceptual and Motor Skills. 1984;**59**:974

[42] Morris R. A study of the natural history of back pain, part 1: Development of a reliable sensitive measurement of disability in low back pain. Spine; 1983;**8**:141-144

[43] Aaron J et al. Management of malignant bowel obstruction associated with GI cancers. JCO Oncology Practice. 2017;**13**(7):435-437

[44] Matulonis UA et al. JPSM. 2005;**30**(6):563-569. DOI: 10.1016/j.jpainsymman.2005.05.018

Chapter 2

Regenerative Medicine

Armen Haroutunian, Tennison Malcolm and Thomas Zouki

Abstract

Chronic pain is a debilitating condition that affects millions of people world-wide, leading to physical incapacitation and financial strain. Common methods for treatment include physical therapy, oral medications, injections, surgery, and neuromodulation. Injectates with steroids and local anesthetics can be a temporizing measure with intolerable side effects. The use of autologous biologic injectates (e.g., platelet rich plasma, bone marrow aspirate concentrate, tissue grafts, and stem cells) is growing in therapeutic potential and enthusiasm, giving hope to a subset of patients that have either failed conventional therapy or are not candidates for traditional steroid injections. In this chapter, we will describe different cases in which regenerative medicine can help in painful conditions as well as neuro-degenerative conditions. Regenerative medicine can be the new frontier in providing long lasting relief through changes in cell-signaling cascades, however further trials are needed to validate their use.

Keywords: platelet rich plasma (PRP), stem cell therapy, bone marrow aspirate concentrate (BMAC), adipose tissue grafts, exosomes, mesenchymal stem cells, hematopoetic stem cells (HCC's), pain management, regenerative medicine

1. Introduction

Chronic pain is a public health issue, affecting nearly a quarter of our population, and takes different forms such as neuropathic, cancer-related or inflammatory pain [1]. This condition limits patients in their daily activities leading to despair and significant loss in quality of life. The most common methods of treatment include physical therapy, oral medications, injections, surgery and neuromodulation. The injectates that are the most commonly used include local anesthetics and steroids. The use of autologous biologic injectates (e.g., platelet rich plasma, bone marrow aspirate concentrate, tissue grafts, and stem cells) is growing in therapeutic potential and enthusiasm, giving hope to a subset of patients that have either failed conventional therapy or are not candidates for traditional steroid injections. Continued clinical trials are needed to further validate their use and help expand their application in the field of medicine. The theory of using these therapies for painful conditions stems from their cytoprotective properties, as well as their regenerative potential.

2. Terminology, history, and background

The most common types of regenerative medicine therapies include platelet rich plasma (PRP), stem cell therapy from bone marrow aspirate concentrate (BMAC) and adipose tissue grafts, and exosomes. Regenerative therapies are growing worldwide

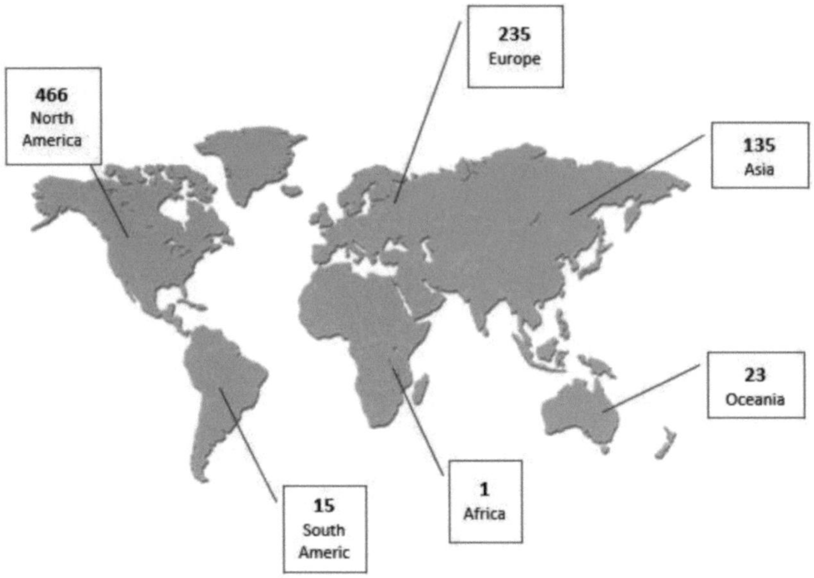

Figure 1.
An atlas of regenerative medicine therapies worldwide. Adapted from alliance for regenerative medicine.

(**Figure 1**). They are increasing from 164% in 1 year with a total of 4.1 billion dollars in total global funding [2]. These therapies can be used in conjunction or individually, and there is no set algorithm or protocol that dictates superiority [3]. Stem cell therapy in this article will refer to adult stem cells, which are multipotent and have no ethical concerns related to their use, as opposed to embryonic stem cells [4]. Typically, candidates include patients with chronic peripheral joint pain that have not responded to steroid injections, or cannot tolerate the medication due to side effects, including but not limited to hyperglycemia, hypertension, ineffective wound healing, or adrenal gland suppression. Although there is no set protocol, some studies recommend implementing a series of three injections for PRP [5]. However, some physicians may grade progress and response to the initial injection as a rationale for a repeat injection.

2.1 Platelet rich plasma

PRP is the most common and readily available treatment option. It is the plasma fraction of blood with a high platelet concentration, as well as clotting factors, growth factors, chemokines, cytokines, and other plasma proteins [6]. This therapy helps promote stem cell migration as well as healing [7]. Commonly injected into joints and tendons for repair, PRP was first coined in the 1970's and used to describe the platelet count in peripheral blood, used to transfuse patients with thrombocytopenia [6]. PRP is obtained from blood after centrifuge, which helps separate components based on density gradients (**Figure 2**). Devices used to simplify the preparation of PRP are said to amplify the concentration of PRP 2–5 times the baseline [7]. Despite the limited clinical evidence that exists, PRP has been used to initiate healing for a variety of cases, most commonly including osteoarthritis (OA), lateral epicondylitis, rotator cuff tears, ligament and tendon injuries [7]. Recent randomized control trials actually demonstrate benefit in tendinopathy [7]. It has also been suggested that PRP can play a role in elimination neuropathic pain, thought to be secondary to a cascade of inflammation followed by repair via axon and tissue regeneration [8]. PRP has also been used as an intervertebral disc injection for low

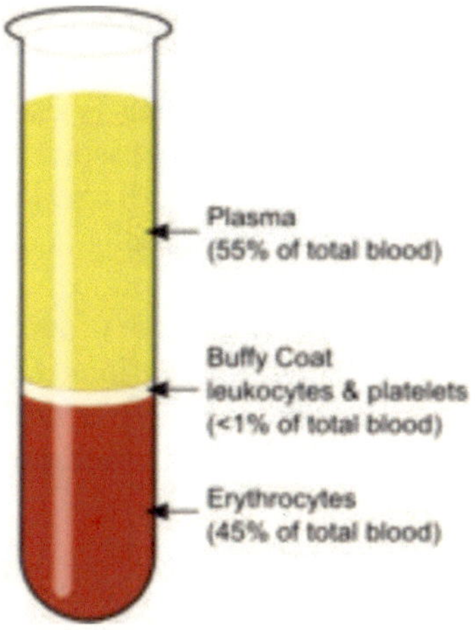

Figure 2.
Blood components after centrifugation.

back pain with promising clinical results, however more randomized controlled trials are needed [3]. Success of this therapy will ultimately depend on the preparation and composition of the injectate, location, and type and extent of injury.

2.2 Adipose tissue grafts

Stem cell therapy uses non-embryonic adult stem cells described as multipotent stem cells, and in the clinical setting refers to therapy with mesenchymal (often from adipose tissue) and hematopoietic stem cells (often from bone marrow aspirate) [3]. These cells are present in a variety of tissues (adipocytes, chondrocytes, myocytes) and are thought to play a role in immune modulation [3]. The most common source of mesenchymal stem cells (MSC) are found in adipose tissue, first discovered in 1964 by Rodell [2]. There are approximately 500 to 2500× times more MSC's when compared to bone marrow [3]. Adipose derived stem cells (ASC's) are the most promising stem cells identified in humans, since adipose tissue is easily obtained in large quantities with small donor site discomfort [4]. Sites of harvest include the abdomen, upper arm, thigh, and trochanteric fat deposits. Common mechanisms to obtain fat include liposuction or lipectomy, followed by homogenization and enzymatic digestions. Traditional cosmetic liposuction can remove large volume (>4 kg) or small volume (<4 kg) adipose tissue, however for purposes of adipose tissue grafting only 100–200 mL may be needed [9]. The resultant material is then centrifuged. Each gram of adipose tissue yields 5 × 10^3 stem cells, significantly greater than bone marrow [4]. It is important to note that stem cell harvesting is more invasive that a simple blood draw for PRP, and could thus lead to an increase risk for infection or complication for patients undergoing MSC harvesting [10]. If performed under local or tumescent anesthesia, there is minimal to no recovery time. To date, hundreds of trials are listed on the United States National Institutes of Health website (NIH) for the use of ASC's. Examples of applications include soft tissue regeneration, skeletal tissue repair, myocardial infarction, immune disorders such as lupus, multiple sclerosis, Crohn's disease, diabetes.

2.3 Bone marrow aspirate concentrate

Bone marrow aspiration is a procedure in which bone marrow is collected, usually from the pelvic iliac crest [11]. The procedure is very similar to PRP, in which the product is centrifuged. The final product is called bone marrow aspirate concentrate, or BMAC, which contains mostly hematopoetic stem cells (HCC's), and a much smaller concentration of MSCs [3]. Like MSC's, HSC's also contain growth factors and immunomodulating enzymes [11]. Unlike adipose aspiration, the concentration of MSC's in bone marrow dramatically decreases with age. Like ASCs, BMAC is also used to treat various conditions affecting tendons, ligaments, and musculoskeletal injuries. Approximately 60 mL of aspirate can produce 10 mL of BMAC after centrifuge [11]. Again, efficacy is determined by location of injection as well as extent of tissue injury. Sites include shoulders, knees, hips, various tendons, and sometimes spinal facet joints. Current literature demonstrates benefit in utilizing BMAC as an adjunct in cartilage healing, faster time to bony union, and lower rates of tendon re-rupture [11].

2.4 Exosomes

Exosomes are endocytic vesicles released by various cells including T-cells, B-cells, reticulocytes, mast cells, platelets, tumor cells as well as MSCs [12]. They are membrane-enclosed particles surrounded by a phospholipid layer and are enriched with micro-RNAs (miRNAs) which are believed to regulate gene expression in a post-transcriptional matter and, by that matter, play a role in tissue repair and regeneration [13, 14]. They are defined as nanosized membrane vesicles with a diameter of 30–100 nm that originate from multivesicular bodies (MVB's) and are released by cells into extracellular environment (**Figure 3**) [12]. They are cholesterol-rich phospholipid vesicles. There are multiple contents that are found in exosomes including cytokines, proteins, lipids, mRNAs, miRNAs and ribosomal RNAs [15, 16]. Current recommendations for extraction of exosomes suggest ultracentrifugation at high speeds which removes cells and microvesicles. It is time consuming, labor intensive, and has therefore lead to commercially available kits, such as Exoquick ©, Invitrogen ©, and Exo-Spin ©, which reliably reduce operating time to 2 hours. Exosomes ultimately have the capacity to execute specific targeted therapy due to their ability to envelope a wide range of specific contents, including lipids, RNA's, and specific protein-signaling molecules [17]. This makes them a promising tool in nanomedicine; however, like PRP and MSC's, classification and purification needs to be standardized to ensure appropriate randomized and multicenter studies.

2.5 Mechanism of action and biology

The mechanism by which these injections treat pain is still unknown and remains mainly theoretical [15]. Platelets, also called thrombocytes, contain several secretory

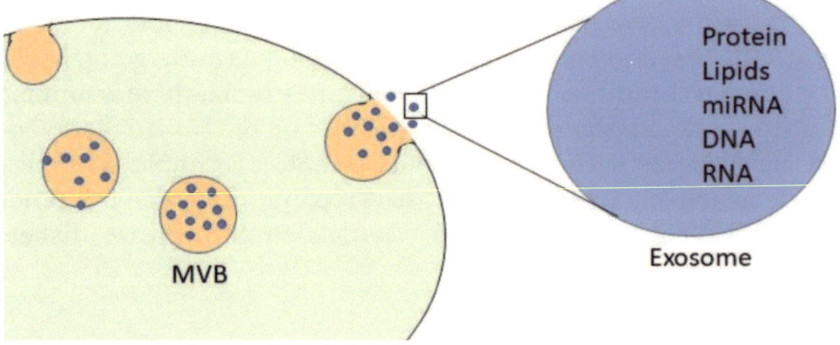

Figure 3.
Multivesicular bodies (MVB's) releasing exosomes.

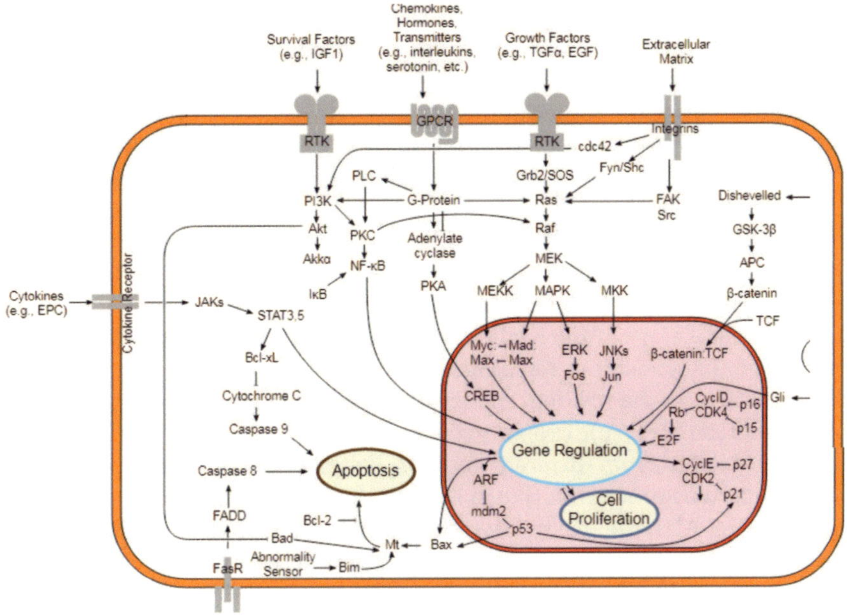

Figure 4.
Signal transduction pathways.

granules crucial to platelet function. Platelets are primarily responsible for aggregation and contribute to hemostasis through adhesion, activation, and aggregation. In recent years, research has demonstrated that platelets not only have a function in hemostasis, but also carry an abundance of growth factors and cytokines that affect inflammation, stem cell migration, and proliferation [8]. Upon activation of platelets in PRP, important growth factors, namely endothelial growth factor, fibroblast growth factor, platelet derived growth factor, epidermal growth factor, hepatocyte growth factor, matrix metalloproteinases, and interleukin 8 are released and modify the local tissue through a complex cell signaling cascade (**Figure 4**) [6].

There is increasing surfacing evidence suggesting that MSC's secrete functional paracrine factors which promote tissue regeneration, protection and repair [18–21]. Recent studies revealed that factors are released through particles known as exosomes. There is now strong belief that these exosomes secreted by MSCs are responsible for the tissue regeneration and repair rather that the ability of MSCs to trans-differentiate. They are suggested as central mediators of intercellular communication by transferring proteins, mRNAs and miRNAs to adjacent cells leading to coordinative function in organisms. Those, depending on the medium in which they are collected can halt breast cancer metastasis, regulate angiogenesis, remodel neurites and promote neurogenesis [22, 23].

Exosomes aggressively participate in the inhibition of the inflammation process. This known property of exosomes is now being considered as a novel therapeutic approach to many disease processes affecting different organ systems. Indeed, the benefits of the anti-inflammatory properties of exosomes has not only been demonstrated in various painful conditions, but also in cardiovascular and pulmonary diseases as well. MSCs-secreting exosomes lead to a reduction of white blood cell count and reduced inflammation in hearts after ischemia-reperfusion injury, which in turn decrease infarct size and enhance cardiac function. Protective properties have also been shown in the lungs for relieving symptoms of pulmonary hypertension [24, 25]. MSCs are adult multipotent cells with the ability to self-renew and differentiate into mesenchymal lineage such as osteoblasts, chondrocytes and adipocytes [26]. MSCs were originally isolated from bone marrow, they have been isolated from other adult tissues such as adipose tissue, dental pulp, placenta, amniotic fluid, umbilical cord blood and Wharton's jelly, and even in the brain [27]. The MSCs differentiation potential for tissue repair has been studied extensively but the pattern of MSC mediated regeneration is now shifting toward secretome-based paracrine activity. The matter by which miRNAs play an essential role in physiological and pathological conditions is by regulating gene expression at the post-transcription level [28]. The pre-miRNA goes through an extensive biological process prior to maturation but an exosome can contain miRNA of different maturation stages and their release is a controlled process dependent on the source and developmental stage of derived cells rather than a random process [12]. It has been suggested that exosomes released by MSCs contain miRNA that control the microenvironment in the resident niches through a balance between proliferation and differentiation [29]. Additionally, tissue-specific responses have been described for exosomes isolated from different sources. For example, adipose tissue-derived exosomes seem to be more effective in halting the central nervous system degeneration caused by Alzheimer's disease when compared to bone marrow derived MSCs-derived exosomes [30]. But neurite outgrowth seems to be more responsive to exosomes released by menstrual fluid derived MSCs when compared to umbilical cord, chorion and bone marrow. Evidence of neurite outgrowth has also been shown in a middle cerebral artery occlusion model. MSCs exposed to ischemic cerebral extracts secreted exosomes containing mi-RNA that were transferred to neurons and astrocytes via exosomes and promoted neurite outgrowth and functional recovery. The same authors reported the use of cell free MSC-generated exosomes administered intravenously in a subject that had suffered a stroke lead to improved neurite remodeling, neurogenesis and angiogenesis which in turn significantly improved the functional recovery of the subject [31]. A similar experiment in which intravenous administration of MSCs-generated exosomes enhanced angiogenesis and neurogenesis reduced the inflammation, improved spatial learning and sensory/motor function in a traumatic brain injury model [32].

2.6 Clinical applications

At present, the use of autologous biologic injectates in the treatment of most acute and chronic conditions resulting in pain is considered investigational. There are currently 977 regenerative medicine trials worldwide, including gene therapy, cell therapy, and tissue engineering [2]. Of those, there at 51 and 66 clinical trials in the categories of musculoskeletal system and central nervous system, respectively. While a myriad of sources has reported positive results following the use of autologous biologic injectate, these reports are, overall, too heterogenous and underpowered to change the clinical practice of most. The absence of well-powered, level-1 data is demonstrating the efficacy of autologous biologic injectates may simply reflect the infancy of this field. Conditions recently studied for the use of autologous blood injectates include Complex Regional Pain syndrome (formerly called Reflex Sympathetic Dystrophy or RSD), OA, joint arthropathy including facet arthropathy and sacroiliitis, tendinopathies, degenerative disc disease, Multiple Sclerosis, headaches, migraines, and peripheral neuropathy. In this chapter we will discuss autologous biologic injectates in the treatment of OA, spondylosis, and tendon and ligament injury.

2.7 Osteoarthritis

Osteoarthritis (OA) is the most common joint disorder in the United States, and is estimated to 25% of people over 18-years old [33, 34]. OA is a progressive disease affecting the joints and is characterized by perturbed immune responses to cellular injury resulting in cartilage degeneration, synovitis, bony remodeling, and chronic pain. Current treatment includes NSAIDs, opiate medications, topical analgesics, physical therapy, lifestyle modification, intraarticular steroid injections, intra-articular hyaluronic acid (HA) injection, and surgery. Non-steroidal anti-inflammatory drugs (NSAIDs), opiates, and intra-articular steroid injections are primarily limited negative side-effects that accompany escalations in medication dose and frequency. Exogenous HA has been used as a treatment modality given observed decreases in endogenous HA exhibited in OA joints. However, due to a lack of consistent evidence, HA is not recommended by the American Academy of Orthopedic Surgeons in treatment of patients with symptomatic OA of the knee [35]. At present, the therapeutic value of PRP in treating OA is a topic of debate and investigation. Available studies suggest its clinical benefit compared with HA in treating OA of the knee [36–40]. Several authors have reported meta-analyses demonstrating improved pain and function following intra-articular injection of PRP in the knee versus HA [36–38]. In a meta-analysis of 26 randomized controlled trials involving 2430 patients, Tan et al. found better Western Ontario and McMaster Universities Osteoarthritis Index (WOMAC) total scores, WOMAC physical function, and Visual Acuity (VAS) Scores at 3, 6, and 12 months following PRP injection compared to HA [38]. Evidence supporting the use of PRP in hip OA is still lacking [39]. There is still much work to be done in understanding the therapeutic role of PRP in treating OA. It is an infrequently used treatment modality, a likely reflection of limited reimbursement. Presently, the Centers for Medicare and Medicaid Services (CMS) only cover PRP use when used for the treatment of chronic non-healing diabetic, pressure, or venous wounds in patients enrolled in clinical studies [41]. Despite growing public interest, available evidence does not support use of autologous stem cells in treatment of OA [42, 43]. In a meta-analysis of nine studies, evaluating 339 patients Huang et al. found most outcome measures similar between stem cell recipients and controls [43]. VAS was found to be statistically improved among stem cell patients; but, it is unclear whether the modest differences described were clinically relevant [43].

A new 5 year study published in 2019 demonstrates better outcomes and lower pain scores in patients who underwent knee arthroscopy for osteochondral knee injuries with and without preoperative intra-articular PRP injections. This research was the first study which used clinical data more than 5 years and demonstrates that cell therapy can promote the regeneration of articular cartilage in a lasting way [44].

2.8 Spondylosis

Cervical and lumbar spondylosis represent the constellation of degenerative changes found in the cervical and lumbar spine that progressively occur in most people with aging. 25% of people under 40 years of age, 50% of people over 40 years of age, and 85% of people over 60 years of age are estimated to have cervical spondylosis [45]. Pathologically, the same degenerative processes that characterize OA extend to the vertebral joints and result in spondylosis often characterized by disc degeneration, uncinate spurring and facet arthrosis, ligamentous thickening and infolding, and deformity. Radiculopathy, myelopathy, discogenic pain, facet pain are the clinical manifestations of vertebral joint degeneration. Regenerative techniques for the treatment of cervical and lumbar spondylosis has been previously investigated with promising results. Further studies are needed to weigh safety profiles against efficacy. In an RCT of PRP vs. contrast for discogenic pain, Tuakli-Wosornu et al., reported significant improvements in pain and function at

8-week follow-up [46]. Pettine et al. reported significant reductions in pain following BMAC use for patients with discogenic pain [47]. The principle caveat of these results is the scarcity of similar results demonstrated in the literature [48].

2.9 Tendon and ligament healing

Tendon and ligament injuries are a very common cause of pain and disability, among both the very active and the elderly. Lateral epicondylitis is significantly more common among working-age patients with physical workloads [49]. As much as 80% of patients over 80 years of age are estimated to have a rotator cuff tear [50]. The use of PRP for tendon and ligament healing has mixed reviews but is considered by many a viable treatment modality given low risks of severe associated complications and numerous positive results promulgated throughout the literature. In a meta-analysis of 21 studies comparing PRP to control (betamethasone with lignocaine, saline, corticosteroid, bupivacaine, and whole blood), Chen et al. found PRP significantly associated with short-term (2–6.5 months) improvements in VAS scores among patients with rotator cuff injuries ($p < 0.01$) and lateral epicondylitis ($p < 0.01$) and long-term pain control among patients with rotator cuff injuries ($p = 0.02$), lateral epicondylitis ($p = 0.01$), and tendinopathy ($p < 0.01$) [40]. Evidence describing the clinical utility of MSCs and BMACs a in tendon and ligament injuries is lacking and mostly limited to *in vitro* and *in vivo* studies [51, 52].

2.10 Future therapy

Many experimental trials continue to assess the role of these injectates in tissue repair of the central nervous system (CNS), cardiovascular system, hepatic, renal as well as musculoskeletal system [2]. Some studies demonstrate exosomal induced neural cell growth while others have explored with success the use of exosomes as a promising potential treatment option for Alzheimer's disease and other neurodegenerative pathologies. Others demonstrate the ability of exosomes to differentiate into bone tissue and promote skeletal regeneration [53].

Additionally, regenerative therapies such as PRP have shown a lot of promise in dermatology including prevention of hair loss, the treatment of scars and post procedure recovery, skin rejuvenation, dermal augmentation, and the treatment of striae distensae [54, 55]. Despite the lack of insurance coverage, these therapeutic modalities show much promise in the innovative world of medicine and esthetics.

3. Conclusion

These various injectates present a novel and promising treatment for many degenerative conditions including neurological and musculoskeletal diseases. Not only can biologics relieve symptoms in painful conditions, but also they can halt the degeneration of tissues, regenerate tissue and prolong their lifespan. PRP, MSC's, and exosomes have made considerable progress and will therefore undoubtedly offer new and exciting prospects for a variety of musculoskeletal and nervous system conditions. Their utility in conditions such as osteoarthritis, spondylosis, and tendon and ligamentous injuries are gaining popularity with emerging clinical reports of their efficacy.

The thought that tissue repair and regeneration was a function of the MSCs themselves is now shifting toward the thinking that, exosomes, secreted by MSCs have a more direct role in the process. These exosomes can have a different effect depending on the differentiation state of the tissue from which they are extracted.

They exert their function by communicating in a paracrine fashion with the surrounding tissue and initiate a process of cellular differentiation and proliferation, playing an important role in tissue repair. The use of exosomes shows promising results in disease processes that have no current available treatment. The use of biologic injectates for painful conditions deserves further consideration. Large, well-constructed studies are needed to better understand their applications and extents of their roles in degenerative conditions.

Author details

Armen Haroutunian[1]*, Tennison Malcolm[2] and Thomas Zouki[3]

1 University of California Los Angeles, Los Angeles, CA, USA

2 Brigham and Women's Hospital, Boston, MA, USA

3 Texas Tech University Health Sciences Center, Lubbock, Texas, USA

*Address all correspondence to: armenh12@gmail.com

References

[1] Dahlhamer J, Lucas J, Zelaya C, et al. Prevalence of chronic pain and high-impact chronic pain among adults - United States, 2016. MMWR. Morbidity and Mortality Weekly Report. 2018;**67**(36):1001-1006. DOI: 10.15585/mmwr.mm6736a2

[2] Q2 2018 Data Report - Alliance for Regenerative Medicine. Available from: https://alliancerm.org/publication/q2-2018-data-report/ [Accessed: 23 August 2020]

[3] Chen H, Purita J, Nguyen M. Regenerative medicine for pain management. In: Yong RJ, Nguyen M, Nelson E, Urman RD, editors. Pain Medicine: An Essential Review. Springer International Publishing; 2017. pp. 575-580. DOI: 10.1007/978-3-319-43133-8_153

[4] LKanth K, Sanivarapu S, Moogla S, Kutcham RS. Adipose tissue - adequate, accessible regenerative material. International Journal of Stem Cells. 2015;**8**(2):121-127. DOI: 10.15283/ijsc.2015.8.2.121

[5] Smith PA. Intra-articular autologous conditioned plasma injections provide safe and efficacious treatment for knee osteoarthritis: An FDA-sanctioned, randomized, double-blind, placebo-controlled clinical trial. The American Journal of Sports Medicine. 2016;**44**(4):884-891. DOI: 10.1177/0363546515624678

[6] Alves R, Grimalt R. A review of platelet-rich plasma: History, biology, mechanism of action, and classification. Skin Appendage Disorders. 2018;**4**(1):18-24. DOI: 10.1159/000477353

[7] Akeda K, Yamada J, Linn ET, Sudo A, Masuda K. Platelet-rich plasma in the management of chronic low back pain: A critical review. Journal of Pain Research. 2019;**12**:753-767. DOI: 10.2147/JPR.S153085

[8] Knezevic NN, Candido KD, Desai R, Kaye AD. Is platelet-rich plasma a future therapy in pain management? The Medical Clinics of North America. 2016;**100**(1):199-217. DOI: 10.1016/j.mcna.2015.08.014

[9] Francesco S, Nicolò B, Michele PG, Edoardo R. From liposuction to adipose-derived stem cells: Indications and technique. Acta Bio Medica Atenei Parmensis. 2019;**90**(2):197-208. DOI: 10.23750/abm.v90i2.6619

[10] Cook CS, Smith PA. Clinical update: Why PRP should be your first choice for injection therapy in treating osteoarthritis of the knee. Current Reviews in Musculoskeletal Medicine. 2018;**11**(4):583-592. DOI: 10.1007/s12178-018-9524-x

[11] Gianakos AL, Sun L, Patel JN, Adams DM, Liporace FA. Clinical application of concentrated bone marrow aspirate in orthopaedics: A systematic review. World Journal of Orthopedics. 2017;**8**(6):491-506. DOI: 10.5312/wjo.v8.i6.491

[12] Huang L, Ma W, Ma Y, Feng D, Chen H, Cai B. Exosomes in mesenchymal stem cells, a new therapeutic strategy for cardiovascular diseases? International Journal of Biological Sciences. 2015;**11**(2):238-245. DOI: 10.7150/ijbs.10725

[13] Wen Z, Zheng S, Zhou C, Yuan W, Wang J, Wang T. Bone marrow mesenchymal stem cells for post-myocardial infarction cardiac repair: microRNAs as novel regulators. Journal of Cellular and Molecular Medicine. 2012;**16**(4):657-671. DOI: 10.1111/j.1582-4934.2011.01471.x

[14] Chen TS, Lai RC, Lee MM, Choo ABH, Lee CN, Lim SK. Mesenchymal stem cell secretes microparticles enriched in pre-microRNAs. Nucleic

Acids Research. 2010;**38**(1):215-224. DOI: 10.1093/nar/gkp857

[15] Lai RC, Chen TS, Lim SK. Mesenchymal stem cell exosome: A novel stem cell-based therapy for cardiovascular disease. Regenerative Medicine. 2011;**6**(4):481-492. DOI: 10.2217/rme.11.35

[16] Jenjaroenpun P, Kremenska Y, Nair VM, Kremenskoy M, Joseph B. Characterization of RNA in exosomes secreted by human breast cancer cell lines using next-generation sequencing. PeerJ. 2013;**1**:e201. DOI: 10.7717/peerj.201

[17] Zhang Y, Liu Y, Liu H, Tang WH. Exosomes: Biogenesis, biologic function and clinical potential. Cell & Bioscience. 2019;**9**. DOI: 10.1186/s13578-019-0282-2

[18] Tang YL, Zhao Q, Qin X, et al. Paracrine action enhances the effects of autologous mesenchymal stem cell transplantation on vascular regeneration in rat model of myocardial infarction. The Annals of Thoracic Surgery. 2005;**80**(1):229-236. DOI: 10.1016/j.athoracsur.2005.02.072

[19] Van Overstraeten-Schlögel N, Beguin Y, Gothot A. Role of stromal-derived factor-1 in the hematopoietic-supporting activity of human mesenchymal stem cells. European Journal of Haematology. 2006;**76**(6):488-493. DOI: 10.1111/j.1600-0609.2006.00633.x

[20] Tögel F, Hu Z, Weiss K, Isaac J, Lange C, Westenfelder C. Administered mesenchymal stem cells protect against ischemic acute renal failure through differentiation-independent mechanisms. American Journal of Physiology. Renal Physiology. 2005;**289**(1):F31-F42. DOI: 10.1152/ajprenal.00007.2005

[21] Haider HK, Jiang S, Idris NM, Ashraf M. IGF-1-overexpressing mesenchymal stem cells accelerate bone marrow stem cell mobilization via paracrine activation of SDF-1alpha/CXCR4 signaling to promote myocardial repair. Circulation Research. 2008;**103**(11):1300-1308. DOI: 10.1161/CIRCRESAHA.108.186742

[22] Wang M, Zhao C, Shi H, et al. Deregulated microRNAs in gastric cancer tissue-derived mesenchymal stem cells: Novel biomarkers and a mechanism for gastric cancer. British Journal of Cancer. 2014;**110**(5):1199-1210. DOI: 10.1038/bjc.2014.14

[23] Xin H, Li Y, Cui Y, Yang JJ, Zhang ZG, Chopp M. Systemic administration of exosomes released from mesenchymal stromal cells promote functional recovery and neurovascular plasticity after stroke in rats. Journal of Cerebral Blood Flow and Metabolism. 2013;**33**(11):1711-1715. DOI: 10.1038/jcbfm.2013.152

[24] Lee C, Mitsialis SA, Aslam M, et al. Exosomes mediate the cytoprotective action of mesenchymal stromal cells on hypoxia-induced pulmonary hypertension. Circulation. 2012;**126**(22):2601-2611. DOI: 10.1161/circulationaha.112.114173

[25] Arslan F, Lai RC, Smeets MB, et al. Mesenchymal stem cell-derived exosomes increase ATP levels, decrease oxidative stress and activate PI3K/Akt pathway to enhance myocardial viability and prevent adverse remodeling after myocardial ischemia/reperfusion injury. Stem Cell Research. 2013;**10**(3):301-312. DOI: 10.1016/j.scr.2013.01.002

[26] Pittenger MF, Mackay AM, Beck SC, et al. Multilineage potential of adult human mesenchymal stem cells. Science. 1999;**284**(5411):143-147. DOI: 10.1126/science.284.5411.143

[27] Teixeira FG, Carvalho MM, Sousa N, Salgado AJ. Mesenchymal stem cells secretome: A new paradigm for central nervous system regeneration? Cellular and Molecular Life Sciences: CMLS. 2013;**70**(20):3871-3882. DOI: 10.1007/s00018-013-1290-8

[28] Wang J, Greene SB, Bonilla-Claudio M, et al. Bmp signaling regulates myocardial differentiation from cardiac progenitors through a MicroRNA-mediated mechanism. Developmental Cell. 2010;**19**(6):903-912. DOI: 10.1016/j.devcel.2010.10.022

[29] Baglio SR, Rooijers K, Koppers-Lalic D, et al. Human bone marrow- and adipose-mesenchymal stem cells secrete exosomes enriched in distinctive miRNA and tRNA species. Stem Cell Research & Therapy. 2015;**6**:127. DOI: 10.1186/s13287-015-0116-z

[30] Katsuda T, Tsuchiya R, Kosaka N, et al. Human adipose tissue-derived mesenchymal stem cells secrete functional neprilysin-bound exosomes. Scientific Reports. 2013;**3**:1197. DOI: 10.1038/srep01197

[31] Xin H, Li Y, Buller B, et al. Exosome-mediated transfer of miR-133b from multipotent mesenchymal stromal cells to neural cells contributes to neurite outgrowth. Stem Cells. 2012;**30**(7):1556-1564. DOI: 10.1002/stem.1129

[32] Zhang B, Yin Y, Lai RC, Tan SS, Choo ABH, Lim SK. Mesenchymal stem cells secrete immunologically active exosomes. Stem Cells and Development. 2014;**23**(11):1233-1244. DOI: 10.1089/scd.2013.0479

[33] Zhang Y, Jordan JM. Epidemiology of osteoarthritis. Clinics in Geriatric Medicine. 2010;**26**(3):355-369. DOI: 10.1016/j.cger.2010.03.001

[34] Chen D, Shen J, Zhao W, et al. Osteoarthritis: Toward a comprehensive understanding of pathological mechanism. Bone Research. 2017;**5**: 16044. DOI: 10.1038/boneres.2016.44

[35] Guideline: Treatment of Osteoarthritis of the Knee (2nd edition). Available from: http://www.orthoguidelines.org/go/cpg/detail.cfm?id=1214 [Accessed: 03 August 2020]

[36] Han Y, Huang H, Pan J, et al. Meta-analysis comparing platelet-rich plasma vs. hyaluronic acid injection in patients with knee osteoarthritis. Pain Medicine. 2019;**20**(7):1418-1429. DOI: 10.1093/pm/pnz011

[37] Belk JW, Kraeutler MJ, Houck DA, Goodrich JA, Dragoo JL, McCarty EC. Platelet-rich plasma versus hyaluronic acid for knee osteoarthritis: A systematic review and meta-analysis of randomized controlled trials. The American Journal of Sports Medicine. 2020:363546520909397. DOI: 10.1177/0363546520909397

[38] Tan J, Chen H, Zhao L, Huang W. Platelet rich plasma versus hyaluronic acid in the treatment of knee osteoarthritis: A meta-analysis of 26 randomized controlled trials. Arthroscopy: The Journal of Arthroscopic & Related Surgery. 2020. DOI: 10.1016/j.arthro.2020.07.011

[39] Medina-Porqueres I, Ortega-Castillo M, Muriel-Garcia A. Effectiveness of platelet-rich plasma in the management of hip osteoarthritis: A systematic review and meta-analysis. Clinical Rheumatology. 2020. DOI: 10.1007/s10067-020-05241-x

[40] Chen X, Jones IA, Park C, Vangsness CT. The efficacy of platelet-rich plasma on tendon and ligament healing: A systematic review and meta-analysis with bias assessment. The American Journal of Sports Medicine. 2018;**46**(8):2020-2032. DOI: 10.1177/0363546517743746

[41] Autologous Platelet-rich Plasma | CMS. Available from: https://www.cms.gov/Medicare/Coverage/Coverage-with-Evidence-Development/Autologous-Platelet-rich-Plasma [Accessed: 04 August 2020]

[42] Strotman PK, Novicoff WM, Nelson SJ, Browne JA. Increasing public interest in stem cell injections for osteoarthritis of the hip and knee:

A google trends analysis. The Journal of Arthroplasty. 2019;**34**(6):1053-1057. DOI: 10.1016/j.arth.2019.03.002

[43] Huang R, Li W, Zhao Y, Yang F, Xu M. Clinical efficacy and safety of stem cell therapy for knee osteoarthritis: A meta-analysis. Medicine (Baltimore). 2020;**99**(11):e19434. DOI: 10.1097/MD.0000000000019434

[44] Monckeberg JE, Rafols C, Apablaza F, Gerhard P, Rosales J. Intra-articular administration of peripheral blood stem cells with platelet-rich plasma regenerated articular cartilage and improved clinical outcomes for knee chondral lesions. The Knee. 2019;**26**(4):824-831. DOI: 10.1016/j.knee.2019.05.008

[45] Kuo DT, Tadi P. Cervical Spondylosis. In: StatPearls. StatPearls Publishing; 2020. http://www.ncbi.nlm.nih.gov/books/NBK551557/ [Accessed: 04 August 2020]

[46] Tuakli-Wosornu YA, Terry A, Boachie-Adjei K, et al. Lumbar intradiskal platelet-rich plasma (PRP) injections: A prospective, double-blind, randomized controlled study. PM & R: The Journal of Injury, Function, and Rehabilitation. 2016;**8**(1):1-10. DOI: 10.1016/j.pmrj.2015.08.010

[47] Pettine KA, Murphy MB, Suzuki RK, Sand TT. Percutaneous injection of autologous bone marrow concentrate cells significantly reduces lumbar discogenic pain through 12 months. Stem Cells. 2015;**33**(1):146-156. DOI: 10.1002/stem.1845

[48] Valimahomed AK, Haffey PR, Urman RD, Kaye AD, Yong RJ. Regenerative techniques for neuraxial Back pain: A systematic review. Current Pain and Headache Reports. 2019;**23**(3):20. DOI: 10.1007/s11916-019-0758-0

[49] Shiri R, Viikari-Juntura E, Varonen H, Heliövaara M. Prevalence and determinants of lateral and medial epicondylitis: A population study. American Journal of Epidemiology. 2006;**164**(11):1065-1074. DOI: 10.1093/aje/kwj325

[50] Milgrom C, Schaffler M, Gilbert S, Van Holsbeeck M. Rotator-cuff changes in asymptomatic adults. The effect of age, hand dominance and gender. Journal of Bone and Joint Surgery. British Volume (London). 1995;**77**(2):296-298

[51] Pas HIMFL, Moen MH, Haisma HJ, Winters M. No evidence for the use of stem cell therapy for tendon disorders: A systematic review. British Journal of Sports Medicine. 2017;**51**(13):996-1002. DOI: 10.1136/bjsports-2016-096794

[52] Van den Boom NAC, Winters M, Haisma HJ, Moen MH. Efficacy of stem cell therapy for tendon disorders: A systematic review. Orthopaedic Journal of Sports Medicine. 2020;**8**(4). DOI: 10.1177/2325967120915857

[53] Narayanan R, Huang C-C, Ravindran S. Hijacking the cellular mail: Exosome mediated differentiation of mesenchymal stem cells. Stem Cells International. 2016;**2016**:3808674. DOI: 10.1155/2016/3808674

[54] Gentile P, Garcovich S. Autologous activated platelet-rich plasma (AA-PRP) and non-activated (A-PRP) in hair growth: A retrospective, blinded, randomized evaluation in androgenetic alopecia. Expert Opinion on Biological Therapy. 2020;**20**(3):327-337. DOI: 10.1080/14712598.2020.1724951

[55] Leo MS, Kumar AS, Kirit R, Konathan R, Sivamani RK. Systematic review of the use of platelet-rich plasma in aesthetic dermatology. Journal of Cosmetic Dermatology. 2015;**14**(4):315-323. DOI: 10.1111/jocd.12167

Chapter 3

Amputation Pain Management

Melinda S. Seering and Sangini Punia

Abstract

Considerable number of new amputations yearly in the United States and internationally represent considerable population experiencing pain that is not just acutely from surgical insult but chronically that is related to phantom limb pain and residual limb pain. This chronic pain can last from weeks to years in these patients and lead to other debilitation such as depression, anxiety and even opioid addiction. Early interventions help lessen long-term pain for these patients. These interventions include nerve blockade as well as multi-modal therapy. Understanding the pathophysiology of the pain experienced by these patients will better allow any provider to care for these patients effectively and help alleviate chronic pain in the long term.

Keywords: amputation, phantom pain, neuropathic pain

1. Introduction

Patients with amputations can be found living fulfilled lives. We have all seen them running marathons, in the Olympics, surfing, climbing Mount Everest and even as an MLB pitcher. However, most just want to lead normal lives and be the best parents, siblings, friends, or co-workers they can be. They want to return to their job and function in their daily lives as they did before. Recovery from an amputation is not immediate and takes significant time. Recovery time from amputation is usually prolonged. Wound healing is done in 4–8 weeks, but the prolonged mental, emotional, and physical recovery afterwards takes much longer and will be different for everyone. One of the limiting factors for recovery from an amputation is pain.

In looking at data from the Amputee Coalition, there are 185,000 in the United States every year. This means that an average of two million people is living with an amputated extremity in the United States alone [1–3]. Other data to consider is just as alarming; globally, there are 1 million amputations annually. This is an estimated 1–2 amputation per minute. Lower limb amputations are the most common, with most being due to vascular disease. 85% of lower limb amputations are preceded by a foot ulcer. About half of the people with diabetes who get a lower limb amputation will receive a second amputation [4]. African American populations are four times more likely to get an amputation than Caucasian [5]. Around a third of these patients have persistent depression and anxiety after their amputation [6]. Financially, it is noted that amputees have higher healthcare costs and if the amputation was related to vascular disease higher mortality [7].

All these factors can lead to an unknown fear for a patient undergoing an amputation. Understanding the cause of an amputation first is paramount. This can help guide a plan for better pain control in the perioperative period. The main causes of amputation are progression of disease processes such as peripheral vascular disease (82%) including ischemia and thrombosis. Diabetes and infections such as osteomyelitis and gangrene that is unresponsive to antibiotic treatment. The second major cause is trauma (16.4%). This has a high predominance in upper extremity amputations. Lower extremity amputations with trauma can also be seen with severe fractures that do not heal and frost bites as other causes. Finally, surgical removal of malignancies (0.9%) can result in amputations in upper or lower extremities depending on the location and type of the tumor and growth. Congenital malformations (0.8%) make up the final list for amputation categories [1, 2].

It is important as we consider the cause of the amputation and perioperative pain control, we also factor in the amount of time each patient had before surgery for their amputation decision. A diabetic patient that had a long time to make a decision for an amputation may have had considerable time to go through the stages of grief and accept the amputation as opposed to a trauma that did not have this time. Other things to consider are support system that the patient has at home. As discussed, wound healing is brief, but psychological healing will take longer in most and require repeated support and reminders to the patient to keep moving in a positive direction [8]. In addition to medical management, these patients will need pain-coping strategies and too many these may be a new technique for them in a life altering situation.

2. Pain classification with an emphasis on amputees

Amputation patients have a variety of different pain to consider when treating them in the perioperative setting. The broad classification of this pain is post-amputation pain. However, further classifying it in four categories helps to better understand each pain and how it originates. They are acute post-operative pain, phantom sensations, residual limb pain and phantom limb pain [2, 3].

Acute post-operative pain is the pain that most surgical patients experience after any surgery. It is the pain at the surgical incision site related to surgical trauma, swelling and tissue damage. This is usually reported as sharp and stabbing by patients due to nociceptive afferent nerve supply at the surgical site. Patient can also report muscle spasms related to the immobility of the limb or the compression dressing or brace applies to the amputation site after surgery [2, 9, 10].

Phantom sensations are the non-painful sensations arising from the amputated extremity. This is reported by 75% of patients 4 days after the amputations and higher at 6 months. This can be perceived as movement of the prior extremity or portion of the extremity (i.e. toe or finger). The patient can also note temperature changes or position changes or the missing limb. This has also been noted in mastectomies, dental extractions, and enucleations as well, and can also be seen in spinal cord injuries. Many of the phantom sensations are mild and decline but some patients have some degree persistent sensations indefinitely. There are a few patients in whom these sensations progress to severe pain and become problematic, leading to residual limb pain or phantom limb pain. There are reports of phantom sensations that do fade away and they appear to do this in a progressive fashion called telescoping. This is most common in upper extremity amputations where the phantom sensations continue to decrease such that eventually the patient is left with a sensation of the hand on the stump alone instead of distal [2].

Residual limb pain (stump pain) is the pain localized to the remained affected body segment and can be present for years. Residual limb pain can be of many different modalities as it can be described as deep tissue pain, superficial incision pain and neuropathic in nature. 75% of patients will experience a component of this chronically after surgery [11]. Neuropathic pain will be described as burning and electric in nature. Some patient may even become hyperalgesia or have allodynia on the stump site. This may lead to difficulty with prosthetic fitting for the patient. This pain is usually noted early in recovery. There are causes of increased stump pain: infection, stump neuroma, heterotopic ossification [9]. These should be assessed with prolonged or increased stump pain as these are easily treatable. Infection is not uncommon in these patients due to high prevalence of diabetes and peripheral vascular disease. This should be assessed and treated with antibiotics accordingly to prevent sepsis and wound dehiscence. Stump neuromas occur when the severed nerve at the amputation site have an inflammatory mediated immune reaction. This can cause pain, but it can also cause unmyelinated A and C fibers to form around the nerve. Neuromas develop over time and usually are characterized by point pain on the stump and sensory changes. Heterotopic ossifications usually occur later after amputation as well. These are calcium deposits that occur in the soft tissue of the stump. These ossifications occur much higher in traumatic amputations. There is some association with traumatic brain injury and the risk of this occurrence as well [2, 3, 12].

Phantom limb pain was first described in 1462 by French Surgeon, Ambrose Pare' [13]. However, it was not until 1871 that Silas Weir Mitchell, a Civil War surgeon, called this phenomenon "phantom limb" [2, 13]. Phantom limb pain is an unpleasant or painful feeling in the amputated extremity. 45–85% of patients from amputations can suffer from phantom limb pain [9]. This can have neuropathic components with burning and electrical shooting pain and nociceptive components of dull, aching, crushing and cramping pain [13]. There are two times of onset for this pain. One is usually early after amputation in the first month and the second can occur a year after amputation. The further out a patient is from amputation the less likely they will experience this. However, if a patient does begin to experience this, it can last for years. Phantom limb pain does not always have to occur alone and usually occurs with residual limb pain. While residual limb pain may be bothersome early on, phantom limb pain persists and become more bothersome later and tends to last longer. Risk factors for development or prolonging phantom limb pain are found in **Table 1** [1–3, 12, 13].

1. Female gender
2. Elevated pre-amputation pain
3. Upper extremity
4. Increasing age
5. Bilateral amputation
6. Traumatic amputation
7. Stump healing
8. Disease states such as fibromyalgia, migraines, Raynaud's, IBS, irritable bladder, depression, and anxiety
9. Poor social support
10. High expectations
11. Poor coping strategies

Table 1.
Risk factors for developing or prolonged phantom limb pain.

3. Pain signal transmission

To understand how to treat the pain from amputations, we should first take a moment to review how painful stimulation is transmitted through the body (see **Figure 1**). The human body receives signals from various inputs. If something painful happens to the body such as surgical insult, the damage is registered by nociceptors in the periphery. The distal nerve fibers coalesce and become peripheral nerves. There are pain receptors that present on the neuron and it is connected by an axon to the spinal cord. Transmission from peripheral nerve to dorsal column is obtained by different nerve fibers. These include: A-alpha fibers, the A-beta fibers, the A-delta fibers, and the C fibers. Pain travels on two different nerve fibers: A-delta and C-fibers. A-delta fibers are large myelinated fibers that carry sharp pain, whereas C-fibers are small and unmyelinated fibers that produce dull, slow spreading pain. This signal arrives to the dorsal horn and then travels up via neurotransmitters to the brain. There are a variety of neurotransmitters from the spinal cord to the thalamus. For pain, the most important to consider are Substance P which is an excitatory neurotransmitter for second order neurons in the dorsal horn. This neurotransmitter has been shown to sensitize nociceptors. In addition to pain, Substance P also related to inflammation, cell growth, vasodilation and even mood regulation. Glutamate is also a primary neurotransmitter for pain. It is the main excitatory neurotransmitter in the body. In the brain, glutamate receptors can be both pro-nociceptive as well as anti-nociceptive. This leads to many pain therapies constructed at glutamate. This is used for central sensitization in chronic pain patients [14]. Once in the dorsal horn, the second order neurons connect with thalamus and other various areas. These can include the somatosensory cortex (physical sensation), limbic system (emotion) and frontal cortex (upper level thinking). This allows a patient to feel and react with pain not just physically but emotionally as well [15].

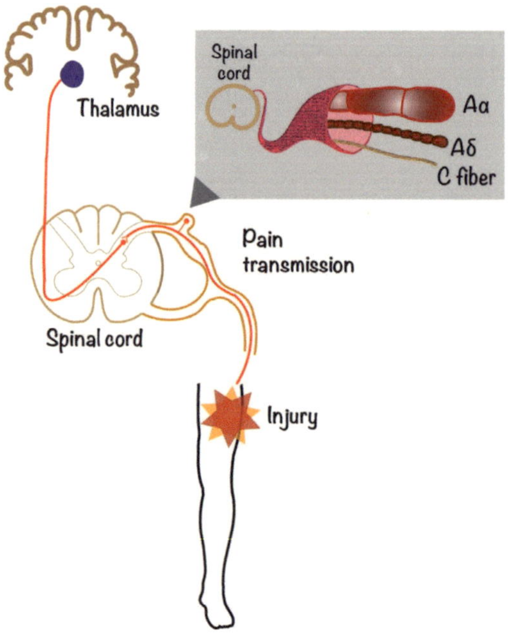

Pain Neurotransmitters

Excitatory	Inhibitory
Substance P	GABA
Glutamate	Glycine
Calcitonin Gene Related Peptide	Adenosine
ATP	Serotonin
Aspartate	Norepinephrine
	Somatostatin
	Enkephalin

Figure 1.
Path pathways.

Let us revisit how the various pain pathways are affected during amputation. Phantom pain sensations likely result from changes in the somatosensory cortex. This causes afferent nociceptive stimulation from body parts near the amputation sites (such as face for upper extremity amputation or bladder for lower extremity amputation). Due to this reorganization in the somatosensory cortex and stimulation input, the phantom sensations occur [2, 9].

Peripheral nerves likely play a large role in the phantom limb pain and residual limb pain. Damage to distal nerve endings and axons causes inflammation and alteration in neurotransmission along the usual pain pathway. The distal nerve endings will begin to regenerate but there will be non-functional axons, changes in sodium and potassium channels and different input from the spinal cord. Neuromas can form here as discussed previously. This can also result in higher pain due to more catecholamines in circulation due to increased sympathetic discharge [2, 9].

There are also spinal cord changes in the dorsal horn related to pain after amputation. The peripheral nerves are no longer able to send the usual signals along the axons to the spinal cord. The brainstem reticular areas therefore do not send inhibitory sensory transmission, so the dorsal horn receives input from this body part as high sensory feedback resulting in pain transmission [1, 2, 9].

These changes in the peripheral and spinal cord need to be considered as we are thinking about treating each patient for amputation pain.

4. Protocol for perioperative caring for amputation patients

It is well understood that effective control of acute post-amputation pain results in decreased risk of development of residual and phantom limb pain [16]. Perioperative plans need to set up within a multi-disciplinary team, ideally involving surgeon, anesthesia, in-patient acute pain teams, pharmacy, physical therapy, occupational therapy, nutrition, and social work to name a few. The pre-operative optimization is essential to control of acute post-amputation pain and help decrease the risk of development of chronic and phantom pain to help these amputation patients have the best chance for better pain control post-amputation. Thorough pre-operative evaluation is needed to look at co-medical conditions that can be optimized. The patient's nutrition should be optimized for wound healing as well. Physical therapy and occupational therapy should work with the patient before surgery to improve physical status prior to surgery and make post-operative recovery more successful. Patient should have a pre-operative discussion about post-operative pain management and expectations. This will allow goal setting and help with anxiety the patient may be experiencing.

Patients who struggle with high pain scores prior to amputation may have an elevated risk of developing chronic pain [17]. Thus, aggressive multimodal analgesic therapy instituted pre-operatively and early in the post-operative period could be beneficial in reducing the incidence of chronic pain. One study found that the presence of depressive symptoms was also a predictor of increased intensity of chronic pain in amputees [18]. Thus, it may be worthwhile to address these symptoms prior to elective amputation surgery. Patients with a complex history of chronic pain disorders and/or patients having high baseline daily opioid requirements (> 80 mg oral morphine equivalents) should be further selected to undergo a pre-operative appointment with a pain specialist. This appointment should ideally take place around 4 weeks prior to elective amputation with the goal to optimize the patient's pain regimen pre-operatively, by maximizing non-opioid modalities and reduction of daily opioid consumption if possible. This is done to improve response

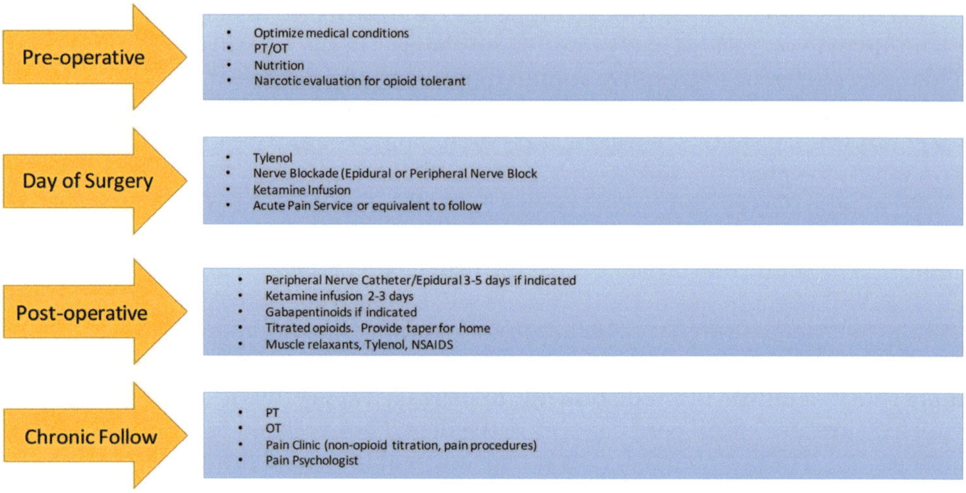

Figure 2.
Protocol for amputation pain management.

to opioid therapy in the immediate post-operative period. Thorough patient education and compassionate counseling also play a key role in developing a team relationship with the patient [19, 20]. See **Figure 2** for full protocol.

5. Nerve blockade

The current standard of care is pre-operative nerve blockade to prevent peripheral sensitization leading to future onset of phantom limb pain. Successful outcomes necessitate effective communication between the surgeon, anesthesiologist, and the various teams involved in the post-operative rehabilitation of the patient. A consultation with the Acute Pain Service or similar entity that performs peripheral nerve blockade pre-operatively and then follows the patient during their post-operative inpatient course is an important factor in the success in early prevention of acute and chronic pain for these patients.

Most patients that arrive for amputations should be evaluated to receive pre-operative peripheral nerve blocks. If this cannot be done pre-operatively, patients can be evaluated post-operatively for a nerve block. If patients do not require post-operative anti-coagulation that will preclude a continuous peripheral nerve catheter, this would be the preferred nerve block for these patients as this will help with prevention phantom limb pain and chronic post-operative pain [3]. This can be utilized for 3–5 days. Continuous nerve catheter infusions have been found to decrease post-operative morphine requirements [21]. However, in addition, there are other factors that may preclude continuous peripheral nerve catheter placement such as infection, and patient factors. If this is the case, single shot peripheral nerve blocks may be utilized. Interestingly, a systematic review and meta-analysis found no difference in pain scores at 24 hours between patients that received a nerve block and those that did not [22]. However, this study did not look at chronic pain in these patients which is the important component that these nerve blocks are used for [9].

It is important to understand the anatomy of the amputation site to have successful nerve block placement. For example, a below the knee amputation will rely heavily on a sciatic nerve blockade whereas an above the knee amputation will need blockade of both femoral and sciatic nerves for successful pain control and help with peripheral sensitization for the patient [9]. For upper extremity amputations, a forearm amputation will be lower in the brachial plexus than an above the elbow amputation or shoulder disarticulation. Tourniquet site is also paramount when planning peripheral nerve block placement. If the catheter is in the surgical site or tourniquet site, there is a risk for dislodgement. It is important to remember this with placement and keep the securement of catheter out of the surgical field. This will take good communication between anesthesia provider and surgeon to achieve this effectively.

It should be noted that epidural blockade may also be used for lower extremity amputation, especially if it will be a bilateral lower extremity amputation. There are studies that show pre-operative epidural placement in amputation patients prevent phantom limb pain due to stopping nociceptive input to the spinal cord [3]. There is no comparison of epidural to peripheral nerve catheters for lower extremity amputations, but on a practically note, peripheral nerve blockade will allow better mobilization and participation in physical therapy [3]. In addition, peripheral nerve block does not have the hemodynamic affects that epidural blockade can have [23].

6. Pharmacology

6.1 Opioids

Opioids remain a favored therapy for pain after surgery. They bind to Mu receptors in peripheral and central nerves as an agonist fashion to produce analgesia. They also can affect phantom limb pain by reducing cortical reorganization [10]. There is a wide variety to choose from post-operatively as they come in intravenous and oral formulation. Usually initially a parenteral opioid therapy with a patient-controlled analgesia (PCA) is started on post-operative day (POD) zero. Once the patient is tolerating a diet, the PCA is weaned down incrementally and oral opioid therapy is instituted. For opioid tolerant patients, we attempt to calculate their total daily morphine equivalent requirement and base our starting oral dose based on that. The goal is to wean off the PCA completely by 48 hours, coinciding with the discontinuation of other intravenous infusion [10].

6.2 N-Methyl-D-Aspartate (NMDA) Receptor Antagonists

Ketamine has been studied for post-operative pain. It has been shown that the use of this medication lowers the opioid requirements and reverses opioid tolerance needed for acute post-operative pain [24]. Ketamine is a noncompetitive NMDA receptor antagonist that targets primarily in the brain and spinal cord. The NMDA receptor is important for synaptic plasticity, central sensitization, amplification of pain signals and opioid tolerance. For amputations, it lowers the dorsal horn sensitization and stops the events that may lead to phantom limb pain and residual limb pain. Important to note, it will not prevent phantom limb pain but will reduce risks of phantom limb pain and residual limb pain [9]. Ketamine has also been shown to have anti-inflammatory properties which may be effective in the early pre-operative phase. Ketamine infusions can be started in the operating room and continued for 2–3 days post-operatively. Studies show low does ketamine infusions do reduce opioids immediately post-op but there was not a significant reduction in immediate post op pain ratings [2, 3, 10].

6.3 Gabapentinoids

Gabapentin and pregabalin are both anti-convulsant that inhibit alpha 2-delta subunit of voltage-gated calcium channels. They are structural like GABA neurotransmitter, but they are unable to bind to any GABA receptors. In addition to the use with seizures, it has been used for chronic pain, especially neuropathic in nature. Dosages must be titrated slowly, and results are not seen immediately. These doses also must be adjusted for patients with impaired renal function with the help of a pharmacist [25, 26]. However, some studies claim that its efficacy to treat phantom limb pain is inconclusive and limited by dose dependent side effects like somnolence and dizziness [2]. There are other studies more recently that show promise of administration of gabapentinoids for reducing chronic post-surgical pain and this can be exploited to amputees as well [3, 9, 10].

6.4 Acetaminophen

Acetaminophen's exact mechanism of action is not well understood, but it is thought to reduce the production of prostaglandins in the brain. Prostaglandins are chemicals that cause inflammation and swelling. Acetaminophen relieves pain by elevating the pain threshold, that is, by requiring a greater amount of pain to develop before a person feels it. Acetaminophen administration to amputation patients will help with inflammation and an adjunct to help with post-surgical nociceptive pain, which has been shown to decrease opioid requirements. Acetaminophen dosages will be lowered in patients with pre-existing liver disease [27]. This will be the most beneficial in the early pre-operative phase. It may be especially beneficially to start prior to the amputation as part of a pre-emptive analgesia. This is thought to protect the central nervous system from noxious insults which result in the patient getting hyperalgesia and allodynia [10, 28].

6.5 NSAIDs

NSAIDs work by inhibiting the activity of cyclooxygenase enzymes (COX-1 or COX-2). By blocking the Cox enzymes, many prostaglandins are not made. This means that there is less swelling and less pain. Most NSAIDs block both Cox-1 and Cox-2 enzymes. For pain, this specifically looks at enzymes that work with prostaglandins for inflammation. Like acetaminophen, these medications work well in the acute perioperative phase for nociceptive pain and reducing opioid requirements. Their use can be limited due to post-operative bleeding concerns. Usually these medications do not help with chronic post amputation pain or phantom limb pain. A short course may be suitable for some patients that have normal renal function; however, we do not advocate for chronic NSAID therapy due to the risks of gastrointestinal bleeding and renal toxicity [10, 23, 29].

6.6 Muscle relaxants

As discussed earlier, acute post-operative pain can have spasmodic pain proximal to the stump site, likely due to tissue inflammation. This can also be present with residual limb pain in some patients. There are a variety of muscle relaxants that can be tried for a short period of time [30]. If the patient is on opioids, would be cautious of adding a benzodiazepine for muscle relaxant. There is a lack of adequate literature supporting the use of muscle relaxants for post amputation pain.

6.7 Tri-cyclic antidepressants and selective norepinephrine reuptake inhibitors

Anti-depressants are commonly prescribed for chronic neuropathic pain and coexisting depression that accompanies it. These medications work by inhibiting serotonin-epinephrine uptake blockade, NMDA receptor antagonism and sodium channel blockade. These medications have not been shown to work effectively in phantom limb pain in studies. These are not usually done in the perioperative setting as they require careful titration over weeks to months which is better done as outpatient therapy. Side effects of opioids and other modalities may warrant a small dose trial in the perioperative setting to help with uncontrolled acute or phantom limb pain [9, 10, 31].

6.8 Calcitonin

Calcitonin is a hormone secreted by thyroid gland in parafollicular cells. Unlike the parathyroid hormone, its job is to reduce calcium in the blood. There are synthetic forms of this used for chronic pain syndromes. The exact pain mechanism of action is unknown. There are mixed results of phantom limb pain [10]. The greatest benefit has been shown when it is administered early in the perioperative period; usually within the first 7 days [32]. There are reports of complete resolution of phantom limb pain with its use [9].

7. Therapeutic modalities

There are many additional modalities that may be of benefit to amputee patients after the initial perioperative period to help with phantom limb pain and residual limb pain. Many of these involve experienced providers and therapists [2, 10, 12, 33–36]. These are summarized in **Table 2**.

1. Desensitization techniques
2. Mirror therapy
3. Massage
4. TENs
5. Exercise
6. Hot/cold therapy
7. Biofeedback
8. Peripheral nerve stimulation
9. Prolonged peripheral nerve blockade
10. Sympathetic nerve blocks
11. Deep brain stimulators
12. Spinal cord stimulators
13. Neurolysis

Table 2.
Therapeutic modalities for chronic amputee limb pain.

8. Conclusions

As patient's present for amputations, it is important to remember the care for these patients needs to be multi-disciplinary to prevent chronic pain. If perioperative pain plans are developed early and worked on as a team, the patient will benefit the most and have the best chance for success at not having long-term phantom limb pain and/or residual limb pain which adversely impact their quality of life.

Psychological preparation is paramount but may not always be accomplished if amputation is needed in emergent or traumatic fashion. These patients can still be cared for effectively in a modified format with high success rate if early post-operative intervention is achieved.

Author details

Melinda S. Seering* and Sangini Punia
University of Iowa, Iowa City, USA

*Address all correspondence to: melinda-seering@uiowa.edu

References

[1] Kuffler DP. Origins of phantom limb pain. *Mol Neurobiol* 2018;55:60-69.

[2] Hsu E, Cohen SP. Postamputation pain: Epidemiology, mechanisms, and treatment. *J Pain Res* 2013;6:121-136.

[3] Srivastava D. Chronic post-amputation pain: Peri-operative management - review. *Br J Pain* 2017;11:192-202.

[4] Glaser JD, Bensley RP, Hurks R et al. Fate of the contralateral limb after lower extremity amputation. *J Vasc Surg* 2013;58:1571-1577.e1.

[5] Buckenmaier CC, 3rd, Kwon KH, Howard RS et al. Double-blinded, placebo-controlled, prospective randomized trial evaluating the efficacy of paravertebral block with and without continuous paravertebral block analgesia in outpatient breast cancer surgery. *Pain Med* 2010;11:790-799.

[6] Hawamdeh ZM, Othman YS, Ibrahim AI. Assessment of anxiety and depression after lower limb amputation in jordanian patients. *Neuropsychiatr Dis Treat* 2008;4:627-633.

[7] de Mestral C, Hsu AT, Talarico R et al. End-of-life care following leg amputation in patients with peripheral artery disease or diabetes. *Br J Surg* 2020;107:64-72.

[8] McKechnie PS, John A. Anxiety and depression following traumatic limb amputation: A systematic review. *Injury* 2014;45:1859-1866.

[9] Neil M. Pain after amputation. *BJA Education* 2016;16:107-112.

[10] Kuffler DP. Coping with phantom limb pain. *Mol Neurobiol* 2018;55:70-84.

[11] Jensen TS, Krebs B, Nielsen J, Rasmussen P. Phantom limb, phantom pain and stump pain in amputees during the first 6 months following limb amputation. *Pain* 1983;17:243-256.

[12] Uustal H, Meier RH, 3rd. Pain issues and treatment of the person with an amputation. *Phys Med Rehabil Clin N Am* 2014;25:45-52.

[13] Weeks SR, Anderson-Barnes VC, Tsao JW. Phantom limb pain: Theories and therapies. *Neurologist* 2010;16:277-286.

[14] Swaran Singh TS, Wikle, J. & Rastogi, R. Multifactorial pathophysiology. In: Abd-Elsayed A. *Pain: A review guide*. Cham Switzerland: Springer Nature Switzerland, 2019.

[15] Zaky S, Zaky, C., and Abd-Elsayed, A. Anatomy of the nervous system. In: Abd-Elsayed A. *Pain: A review guide*. Cham, Switzerland: Springer Nature Switzerland, 2019.

[16] Karanikolas M, Aretha D, Tsolakis I et al. Optimized perioperative analgesia reduces chronic phantom limb pain intensity, prevalence, and frequency: A prospective, randomized, clinical trial. *Anesthesiology* 2011;114:1144-1154.

[17] Hanley MA, Jensen MP, Smith DG, Ehde DM, Edwards WT, Robinson LR. Preamputation pain and acute pain predict chronic pain after lower extremity amputation. *J Pain* 2007;8:102-109.

[18] Ephraim PL, Wegener ST, MacKenzie EJ, Dillingham TR, Pezzin LE. Phantom pain, residual limb pain, and back pain in amputees: Results of a national survey. *Arch Phys Med Rehabil* 2005;86:1910-1919.

[19] Retreived from: Https://www.Cdha.Nshealth.Ca/amputee-rehabilitation-musculoskeletal-program/patients-families-amputee-rehabilitation/coping-your-.

[20] Service UKNH. Retreived from:Https://www.Nhs.Uk/conditions/amputation/. 2020.

[21] Ayling OG, Montbriand J, Jiang J et al. Continuous regional anaesthesia provides effective pain management and reduces opioid requirement following major lower limb amputation. *Eur J Vasc Endovasc Surg* 2014;48:559-564.

[22] Bosanquet DC, Glasbey JC, Stimpson A, Williams IM, Twine CP. Systematic review and meta-analysis of the efficacy of perineural local anaesthetic catheters after major lower limb amputation. *Eur J Vasc Endovasc Surg* 2015;50:241-249.

[23] De Jong R, Shysh AJ. Development of a multimodal analgesia protocol for perioperative acute pain management for lower limb amputation. *Pain Res Manag* 2018;2018:5237040.

[24] Bell RF, Kalso EA. Ketamine for pain management. *Pain Rep* 2018;3:e674.

[25] O'Connor AB, Dworkin RH. Treatment of neuropathic pain: An overview of recent guidelines. *Am J Med* 2009;122:S22–S32.

[26] Dworkin RH, O'Connor AB, Backonja M et al. Pharmacologic management of neuropathic pain: Evidence-based recommendations. *Pain* 2007;132:237-251.

[27] Martinez V, Beloeil H, Marret E, Fletcher D, Ravaud P, Trinquart L. Non-opioid analgesics in adults after major surgery: Systematic review with network meta-analysis of randomized trials. *Br J Anaesth* 2017;118:22-31.

[28] Syal K, Goma M, Dogra RK, Ohri A, Gupta AK, Goel A. "Protective premedication": A comparative study of acetaminophen, gabapentin and combination of acetaminophen with gabapentin for post-operative analgesia. *J Anaesthesiol Clin Pharmacol* 2010;26:531-536.

[29] Melsom H, Danjoux G. Perioperative care for lower limb amputation in vascular disease. *Continuing Education in Anaesthesia Critical Care & Pain* 2011;11:162-166.

[30] Ketz AK. The experience of phantom limb pain in patients with combat-related traumatic amputations. *Arch Phys Med Rehabil* 2008;89:1127-1132.

[31] Pilowsky I, Hallett EC, Bassett DL, Thomas PG, Penhall RK. A controlled study of amitriptyline in the treatment of chronic pain. *Pain* 1982;14:169-179.

[32] Hall N, Abd-Elsayed, A, & Eldabe, S. Phantom limb pain. In: Abd-Elsayed A. *Pain: A review guide*. Cham, Switzerland: Springer Nature Switzerland, 2019.

[33] Kaur A, Guan Y. Phantom limb pain: A literature review. *Chin J Traumatol* 2018;21:366-368.

[34] Borghi B, D'Addabbo M, White PF et al. The use of prolonged peripheral neural blockade after lower extremity amputation: The effect on symptoms associated with phantom limb syndrome. *Anesth Analg* 2010;111:1308-1315.

[35] Rauck RL, Cohen SP, Gilmore CA et al. Treatment of post-amputation pain with peripheral nerve stimulation. *Neuromodulation* 2014;17:188-197.

[36] Herrador Colmenero L, Perez Marmol JM, Martí-García C et al. Effectiveness of mirror therapy, motor imagery, and virtual feedback on phantom limb pain following amputation: A systematic review. *Prosthet Orthot Int* 2018;42:288-298.

Chapter 4

Why Effective Pain Management Remains a Challenge

Nnenna Ugwu

Abstract

Pain is a subjective expression of neural impulses induced by a stimulus with a capacity to potentially damage tissues of the body. Simply put, pain is the reaction of the body to a potentially noxious or noxious stimulus, which threatens the normal homeostasis if unrelieved. Pain can be managed via pharmacological and non-pharmacological means, and pharmacological agents are the most widely accepted means, which have been shown to have variable effectiveness against pain. The barriers to effective pharmacological pain management in clinical practice are discussed in this chapter.

Keywords: analgesics, challenges, pain, pain management, pharmacological agent

1. Introduction

Despite the consistent scientific interest in pain research and pain management, pain has continued to remain an obstacle which threatens the welfare of patients. The challenging nature of pain has been extensively reported by clinicians and researchers [1–4]. Adequate pain relief is hardly achieved even when pain appears to be the most usually presented symptom by patients in the emergency department [5–8]. Pain accounts for over 40% of all the primary complaints in the emergency department [9], with a greater proportion of these patients reporting moderate to severe degree of acute pain [10]. Considering these reports, it would seem normal to assume that the institution of pain management would be prompt and effective. However, reports across all treatment settings indicate that adequate pain management is hardly achieved, and most patients continue to experience pain despite the institution of pain management strategies. For instance, nearly half of 71 patients and 74% of 842 patients presenting moderate to severe degree of acute pain complained of pain of similar intensity at discharge from the emergency department [7, 11]. The observations from the postoperative setting are also similar to that of the emergency department. Most surgical patients also reported a higher degree of intense acute pain following surgery, with over 73 million surgeries performed annually in the United States [12]. Additionally, 82% of 250 surgical patients expressed pain from the immediate postoperative period until 2 weeks post-discharge, and 86% of these patients experienced moderate to severe degree of pain [12]. Pain was also incriminated in most patient surveys and complaints to health services [13]. It is therefore clear that achieving optimal pain management is still a key issue across treatment settings even though pain is a manageable condition and effective pain management is possible as evidenced in experimental literature.

2. Concept of pain

An accurate understanding and definition of pain and related terms is fundamental to effective pain recognition, quantification, and mitigation. Pain is generally a difficult term to define. This is because pain is seen as a subjective experience with variable effects on patients [14] and as a complex phenomenon with sensory cognitive and emotional components [15]. Pain was defined by the International Association for the Study of Pain Subcommittee on Taxonomy as "an unpleasant sensory and emotional experience associated with actual or potential tissue damage" [16]. However, this definition was recently refined. Thus, the most recent definition of pain by the International Association for the Study of Pain Subcommittee on Taxonomy described pain as an unpleasant sensory and emotional experience associated with actual or potential tissue damage, or described in terms of such damage [17]. To the author's understanding, pain is a subjective expression of neural impulses induced by a stimulus with a capacity to potentially damage tissues of the body. In other words, pain is the reaction of the body to a potentially noxious or noxious stimulus and threatens the normal homeostasis if unrelieved.

2.1 The pain pathway

Essentially, the pain pathway comprises of four major steps, including transduction, transmission, projection, and perception, all working together to achieve the awareness or sensation of pain as shown in **Figure 1**. Pain begins with the stimulation of specialized nerve endings (nociceptors) by chemical, mechanical, or thermal insult in a process termed transduction, followed by the transmission of these signals to the spinal cord (dorsal horn) via afferent peripheral sensory nerves. The afferent peripheral sensory nerves are composed of two major types, the myelinated A delta and unmyelinated C fibers, whose cell bodies reside in the spinal cord. The myelinated A delta fibers are known to be localized and fast conducting, while the unmyelinated C fibers conduct slowly but are more diffuse. The resulting peripheral nerve impulses are either amplified or suppressed in a process called modulation. Following modulation, these signals are further projected through numerous pathways to the brain centers for processing into pain [18]. The perception and localization of pain are thought to occur at the level of the thalamus and in the sensory cortex, respectively. In theory, pain refers to a centralized experience resulting from nociception in the peripheral nerves [19]. The pain pathway is essentially complex and striking in the sense that there exist several junctures for intrinsic and extrinsic factors to control the nature, amplitude, location, and duration of original sensory signal [18]. As a result, pain memory is influenced by many factors including the intensity of painful events, environment, expectation of pain, and behavioral pattern of the patient [20]. The nervous system is known to be neuroplastic [20] or neuro-pliable. This denotes the change or adaptation of the biochemical and physiological functions of the nervous system in response to a stimulus [20]. The implication of this phenomenon is that response exhibited by the nervous system can be modified by an external or internal stimulus. The disadvantage of this action of the nervous system is that it could complicate the diagnosis and alleviation of pain [18]. Thus, pain is a complex neurophysiological process which can be modulated, amplified, and interrupted.

2.2 Classification of pain

There is no one unified classification of pain. Rather, there is heterogeneity in the reports classifying pain in the literature. According to Gaynor and Muir [20], it is classified based on disease such as arthritis, pancreatitis, or cancer pain; anatomy

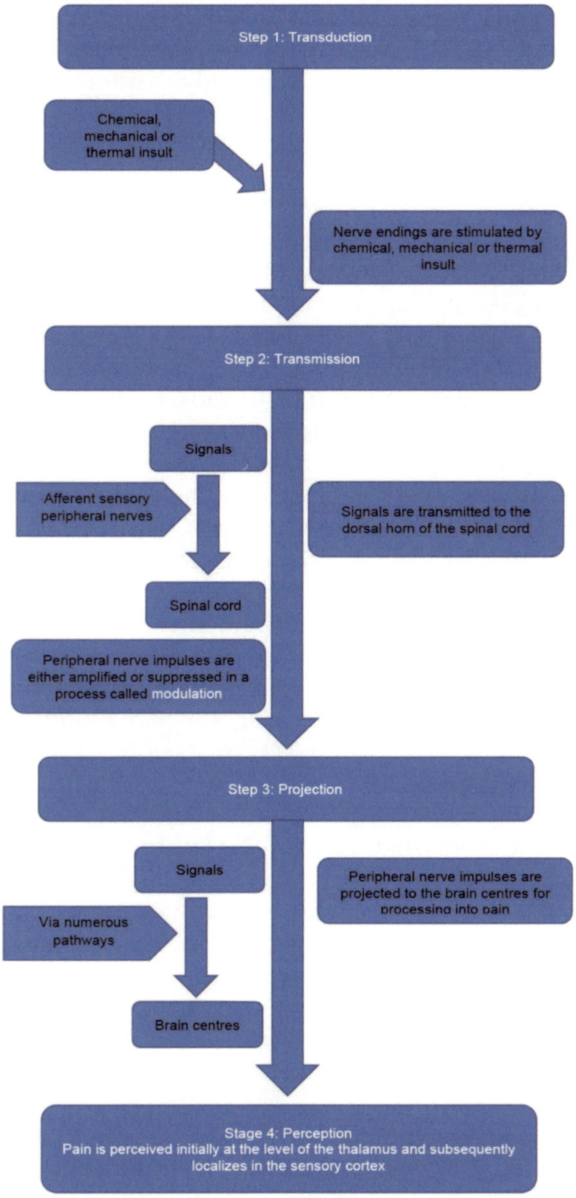

Figure 1.
A flowchart showing the pathway of pain from the point of tissue insult to perception of pain.

such as bladder, pancreatic, back, or orthopedic pain; location as in superficial, visceral, or deep pain; duration including transient, acute, or chronic pain; intensity such as mild, moderate, or severe pain; and finally, based on the response to manipulation. Pain was also classified according to the duration into acute and chronic pain [21–23] and by origin into nociceptive, pathologic, and neuropathic pain [21, 20].

Acute and chronic pain appear to be the most widely studied by researchers. Fox [24] defined acute pain as "a symptom of disease" which lasts for less than 3 months. Acute pain is said to result from injury to the body which may be self-limiting and disappears with healing [20]. Ideally, acute pain refers to pain of short duration, while chronic pain denotes pain of long duration. In practice, however, there is no clear-cut distinction between the end of acute pain and the commencement of chronic pain. It is indeed difficult to pinpoint when an acute phase of pain transcends into a chronic phase. This does not mean that every acute pain phase will gradually become chronic. However, in the absence of effective pain intervention and inability to self-limit acute pain, it is expected to assume this course.

2.3 Pain management

Pain is managed using pharmacological and non-pharmacological means. Pharmacological agents used in the management of pain include opioids, non-steroidal anti-inflammatory drugs, steroidal anti-inflammatory drugs, and local anesthetics [25]. Additionally, tranquilizers, corticosteroids, tricyclic antidepressants and antiepileptic medications (topical capsaicin, mexiletine, and N-methyl-d-aspartate receptor antagonists), serotonin norepinephrine reuptake inhibitors, calcium channel α2-δ ligands, topicals, anticonvulsants, and transdermal substances are included in the pain management regimen as adjuvants to analgesics depending on the type and severity of pain [26–29]. Non-pharmacological management of pain involves the use of suitable housing, bed rest, gentle handling and manipulation (massage, osteopathic and chiropractic), meditative movements (such as Tai Chi and yoga), and diets [30, 31]. Much recent strategies for non-pharmacological pain management were classified into sensory (massage, positioning, acupuncture, hot and cold treatment, progressive muscle relaxation, and transcutaneous electrical nerve stimulation), psychological interventions, and others including music, belief, and spirituality [31, 32]. These non-pharmacological means are thought to play a huge role in relieving postsurgical pain.

3. Challenges to effective pharmacological pain management

The challenges militating against effective pharmacological pain management strategy are categorized into five, including pain recognition and quantification error, patient factor, practitioner factor, drug factor, and gap between scientific evidence and clinical applications.

3.1 Pain recognition and quantification error

Critical to successful pain intervention is the ability to accurately recognize and quantify pain. Pain is often not given due recognition, underreported and undetected, especially in the nonverbal and patients with communication difficulties or cognitive impairment [33, 34]. In patients who can verbally communicate, pain recognition and quantification rely on the judgment of these individuals in addition to the physiological indicators of pain. On the other hand, the accurate recognition and quantification of pain in nonverbal or cognitively impaired patients is dependent on the practitioner or care provider. Some patients with communication difficulties as seen in intensive care units (ICUs) relay pain using other cues such as signaling with eyes, leg movements, guarding of painful region, and making physical contacts with the practitioner [35]. Hence, these behaviors were incorporated into pain scales for ICU patients under sedation [35]. Practitioners have also employed the use of surrogates and analgesic trials to assess pain [36]. Hence, the successful recognition of pain in these instances lies on the expertise of the practitioner. Additionally, pain recognition and quantification error could result from the patient's inability to express pain even after experiencing a potential painful episode, or from patient not displaying consistent signs of pain.

3.2 Patient factor

There are differences in patients' responses to pain and pain management strategies, thus, necessitating the need to understand the peculiarity of each patient experiencing pain. Proper examination of patient history and adequate knowledge of patient information are vital when considering the choice of pain management regimen. Several studies have reported demographics such as age [37–40], sex [38, 41, 40], and cultural differences including ethnicity [39–40, 42–43] in response to pain and these should be borne in mind. Additionally, the patient's response to pain is influenced by previous pain experience [44], nature of injury [37, 38, 45], and presence of underlying conditions which cause sensory impairment or communication difficulties [46]. These potentially complicate pharmacological pain management strategies. Therefore, understanding and treating each patient as unique is crucial for a successful alleviation of pain.

3.3 Personnel factor

Adequate understanding of pain, its physiology, myths and misconceptions, ethics, recognition, and quantification and management is essential for every pain management personnel. While this is obviously the standard, information in the literature revealed that there are extensive knowledge deficits among most pain practitioners and care providers [47–51]. In hospital settings, provision of pain management relies on trained nurses often following physician's prescriptions [49]. In nonhospital settings such as residential care homes and patients' homes, pain management is performed by the patient or a caregiver in case of morbidity and cognitive impairment. In all these instances, proper knowledge of the pharmacologic agent, its mode of action, duration of the effect, recommended dose, and adverse effects are very important but hardly achieved. Several studies have demonstrated poor pain management strategy practiced by nurses [47–51], which was attributed to education deficit, errors in pain assessment, and side effects of opioids [47].

3.4 Drug factor

The choice of a pharmacologic agent for pain management is influenced by its efficacy and cost, patient response, and practitioner's preference. Different classes of drugs are often combined to maximize pain alleviation. For instance, effective pain management is dependent on the choice of drug, its efficacy, dose, administration technique, adverse effects, time, and consistency of intervention. Pain management is often ineffective because of misuse errors resulting from underdosage, poor administration technique, and inconsistency in timing of administration.

To minimize the complications resulting from the use of a sole analgesic and to achieve balanced analgesia, different classes of agents are combined in a multimodal fashion [52–54]. Though complex, cited advantages include effective and efficient analgesia, and possibly, reduction in doses of one or more individual drugs [54]. However, if misused, they can hinder the effectiveness of analgesics and thus constitute a barrier to effective pain management.

3.5 Gap between scientific evidence and clinical applications

Even though there exist many scientifically proven analgesic regimens for pain mitigation in the literature [55], effective pain management has not been adequately achieved across treatment settings. It does appear that these evidence-based recommendations are not properly incorporated in clinical practice, thus, presenting an obvious aperture between these scientific recommendations on pain management strategies and applications in treatment settings. Supporting this claim is the study of Bennetts et al. [56] which demonstrated that the staff of the Australian emergency departments recognized the gap between recommendations and everyday practice-based pain as a barrier to effective pain management. Additionally, the report of Glajchen [57] underscored knowledge gaps as clinician's barrier to effective pain relief. This paucity in the incorporation of evidence-based findings in actual practice may be driven by lack of awareness and knowledge deficits on scientifically proven optimal pain management regimens which are constantly evolving [56, 57], hence, the need to be up-to-date. Therefore, regular training of practitioners through continued education programs and dissemination of current scientific findings in a convenient user-friendly format may help militate this challenge.

Furthermore, the lack of incorporation of scientific findings in treatment settings may also be due to the existence of abundant low-quality scientific evidence which does not meet the required standard to be incorporated into clinical guidelines for pain management [58]. This observation supports the need for high-quality research using refined methods, randomized trials, and efficient research-collaborations. Thus, this has implications for future research.

4. Conclusion

In conclusion, effective pain management is possible, though, challenges resulting from pain recognition and quantification, patients, practitioners, drugs, and gap between scientific evidence and practical applications need to be taken into proper consideration. Knowing and understanding the peculiarity of each patient would help to control the patient-induced challenges, continuous education or training of practitioners and care providers on pain recognition, and quantification methods would not only eliminate the practitioner-related challenges but will also address pain recognition and quantification errors, and possibly, bridge the gap between scientific evidence and clinical usage. Additionally, the improvement in current research methods and the incorporation of high-quality scientific evidence will also bridge the gap between research and practice. Finally, proper knowledge of pharmacology and the use of evidence-based analgesics in recommended doses and combinations will help overcome the drug-related challenges. Therefore, future research should aim at investigating the effectiveness of these recommendations.

Author details

Nnenna Ugwu[1,2]

1 Department of Veterinary Surgery, Faculty of Veterinary Medicine, University of Nigeria, Nsukka, Nigeria

2 School of Veterinary Sciences, University of Bristol, United Kingdom

*Address all correspondence to: nnenna.ugwu@unn.edu.ng

References

[1] Puntillo K, Pasero C, Li D, Mularski RA, Grap MJ, Erstad BL, et al. Evaluation of pain in ICU patients. Chest. 2009;**135**:1069-1074

[2] Watt-Watson J, Stevens B, Garfinkel P, Streiner D, Gallop R. Relationship between nurses' pain knowledge and pain management outcomes for their postoperative cardiac patients. Journal of Advanced Nursing. 2001;**36**:535-545

[3] Heikkinen K, Salantera S, Kettu M, Taittonen M. Prostatectomy patients' postoperative pain assessment in the recovery room. Journal of Advanced Nursing. 2005;**52**:592-600

[4] Wang HL, Tsai YF. Nurses' knowledge and barriers regarding pain management in intensive care units. Journal of Clinical Nursing. 2010;**19**:3188-3196. DOI: 10.1111/j.1365-2702.2010.03226.x

[5] Rupp T, Delaney KA. Inadequate analgesia in emergency medicine. Annals of Emergency Medicine. 2004;**43**:494-503

[6] Karwowski-Soulie F, Lessenot-Tcherny S, Lamarche-Vadel A, et al. Pain in an emergency department: An audit. European Journal of Emergency Medicine. 2006;**13**:218-224

[7] Todd KH, Ducharme J, Choiniere M, et al. Pain in the emergency department: Results of the pain and emergency medicine initiative (PEMI) multicenter study. The Journal of Pain. 2007;**8**:460-466

[8] Mitchell R, Kelly AM, Kerr D. Does emergency department workload adversely influence timely analgesia? Emergency Medicine Australasia. 2009;**21**:52-58

[9] Pletcher MJ, Kertesz SG, Kohn MA, Gonzales R. Trends in opioid prescribing by race/ethnicity for patients seeking care in US emergency departments. JAMA. 2008;**299**(1):70-78

[10] McCaig LF, Nawar EW. National Hospital Ambulatory Medical Care Survey: 2004 emergency department summary. Advance Data. 2006;**372**:1-29

[11] Guru V, Dubinsky I. The patient vs caregiver perception of acute pain in the emergency department. The Journal of Emergency Medicine. 2000;**18**(1):7-12

[12] Apfelbaum JL, Chen C, Mehta SS, Gan TJ. Postoperative pain experience: Results from a national survey suggest postoperative pain continues to be undermanaged. Anesthesia and Analgesia. 2003;**97**(2):534-540

[13] National Institute of Clinical Studies. National Emergency Department Collaborative Report. Melbourne: National Institute of Clinical Studies; 2004

[14] Cohen M, Quintner J, Van Rysewyk S. Reconsidering the IASP definition of pain. PAIN Reports. 2018. DOI: 10.1097/PR9.0000000000000634

[15] Vinuela-Fernandez I, Jones E, Welsh EM, Fleetwood-Walker SM. Pain mechanisms and their implication for the management of pain in farm and companion animals. Veterinary Journal. 2007;**174**:227-239

[16] Treede R, Cohen M, Quintner J, Van RS. The International Association for the Study of Pain definition of pain: As valid in 2018 as in 1979, but in need of regularly updated footnotes. PAIN Reports. 2018;**3**:3-5

[17] International Association for the Study of Pain. IASP's Proposed New Definition of Pain: Released for Comment. 2019. Available from: https://www.iasp-pain.org/PublicationsNews/NewsDetail.aspx?ItemNumber=9218 [Accessed: 16 August 2020]

[18] Woolf CJ. Central sensitization: Implications for the diagnosis and treatment of pain. Pain. 2011;**152**: S2-S15. DOI: 10.1016/j.pain.2010.09.030

[19] Hudson C, Whay H, Huxley J. Recognition and management of pain in cattle. In Practice. 2008;**30**:126-134

[20] Gaynor JS, Muir WW. Handbook of Veterinary Pain Management. 2nd ed. St. Louis, Missouri: Mosby, Elsevier; 2009

[21] Joshi SK, Gebhart GF. Visceral pain. Current Review of Pain. 2000;**4**: 499-506

[22] Lamont LA, Tranquilli WJ, Grimm KA. Physiology of pain. The Veterinary Clinics of North America. Small Animal Practice. 2000;**4**:703-728

[23] Roberston SA. Pain management in laboratory animals-are we meeting the challenge? Journal of the American Veterinary Medical Association. 2002;**221**:205-208

[24] Fox SM. Pathophysiology of osteoarthritic pain. In: Proceedings of the 1st World Orthopaedic Veterinary Congress; 5-8 September 2002; Munich, Germany: Milano: Press Point; 2002. pp. 85-87

[25] Hansen B. Analgesia and sedation in the critically ill. Journal of Veterinary Emergency and Critical Care. 2005;**15**(4):285-294

[26] Park HJ, Moon DE. Pharmacologic management of chronic pain. he Korean Journal of Pain. 2010;**23**:99-108

[27] Varrassi G, Muller-Schwefe G, Pergolizzi J, et al. Pharmacological treatment of chronic pain the need for change. Current Medical Research and Opinion. 2010;**26**(5):1231-1245

[28] Bates AJ, Sutherland MA, Chapple F, Dowling SK, Johnson AP, Saldias B, et al. A new method of administering local anesthesia for calf disbudding: Findings from a comparative on-farm study in New Zealand. Journal of Dairy Science. 2019;**102**:2492-2506. DOI: 10.3168/jds.2018-15033

[29] Rekatsina M, Paladini A, Piroli A, Zis P. Pathophysiologic approach to pain therapy for complex pain entities: A narrative review. Pain and therapy. 2020;**9**:7-21 https://doi.org/10.1007/s40122-019-00147-2

[30] Nadler SF. Nonpharmacologic management of pain. JAOA. 2004;**104**: 6-12

[31] Tick H, Nielsen A, Pelletier KR, Bonakdar R, Simmons S, Glick MPHR, et al. Evidence-based nonpharmacologic strategies for comprehensive pain care: The Consortium Pain Task Force white paper. Explore: The Journal of Science & Healing. 2018;**14**:177-211. DOI: 10.1016/j.explore.2018.02.001

[32] Geziry AE, Toble Y, Kadhi FA. Non-pharmacological pain management. In: Pain Management in Special Circumstances. Intech; 2018. DOI: 10.5772/intechopen.79689. [Accessed: 16 August 2020]

[33] Aslan FE, Badir A, Selimen D. How do intensive care nurses assess patients' pain? Nursing in Critical Care. 2003;**8**:62-67

[34] McAuliffe L, Nay R, O'donnell M, Fetherstonhaugh D. Pain assessment in older people with dementia: Literature review. Journal of Advanced Nursing. 2009;**65**:2-10. DOI: 10.1111/j.1365-2648.2008.04861.x

[35] Payen JF, Bru O, Bosson JL, Lagrasta A, Novel E, Deschaux I, et al. Assessing pain in critically ill sedated patients by using a behavioral pain scale. Critical Care Medicine. 2001;**29**: 2258-2263

[36] Puntillo KA, White C, Morris AB, Perdue ST, Stanik-Hutt J, Thompson CL, et al. Patients' perceptions and responses to procedural pain: Results from Thunder Project II. American Journal of Critical Care. 2001;**10**:238-251

[37] Brown JC, Klein EJ, Lewis CW, Johnston BD, Cummings P. Emergency department analgesia for fracture pain. Annals of Emergency Medicine. 2003;**42**:197-205

[38] Arendts G, Fry M. Factors associated with delay to opiate analgesia in emergency departments. The Journal of Pain. 2006;**7**:682-686

[39] Heins JK, Heins A, Grammas M, Costello M, Huang K, Mishra S. Disparities in analgesia and opioid prescribing practices for patients with musculoskeletal pain in the emergency department. Journal of Emergency Nursing. 2006;**32**:219-224

[40] Motov SM, Khan AN. Problems and barriers of pain management in the emergency department: Are we ever going to get better? Journal of Pain Research. 2009;**2**:5-11

[41] Chen EH, Shofer FS, Dean AJ, et al. Gender disparity in analgesic treatment of emergency department patients with acute abdominal pain. Academic Emergency Medicine. 2008;**15**:414-418

[42] Todd KH, Deaton C, D'Adamo AP, Goe L. Ethnicity and analgesic practice. Annals of Emergency Medicine. 2000;**35**:11-16

[43] Paulson M 3rd, Dekker AH. Healthcare disparities in pain management. The Journal of the American Osteopathic Association. 2005;**105**(6 Suppl 3):S14-S17

[44] Eccleston C. Role of psychology in pain management. British Journal of Anaesthesia. 2001;**87**:144-152

[45] Silka PA, Roth MM, Geiderman JM. Patterns of analgesic use in trauma patients in the ED. The American Journal of Emergency Medicine. 2002;**20**:298-302

[46] Pasero C, McCaffery M. When patients can't report pain: Assessing patients with communication difficulties. The American Journal of Nursing. 2000;**100**:22-23

[47] Lai YH, Chen ML, Tsai LY, Lo LH, Wei LL, Hong MY, et al. Are nurses prepared to manage cancer pain? A national survey of nurses' knowledge about pain control in Taiwan. Journal of Pain and Symptom Management. 2003;**26**:1016-1025

[48] Fang HE, Tsai LY, Hong ML, Wu MJ, Chen LC, Chen SC. Knowledge about cancer pain management—Comparison between nurses working in hospice and internal medicine inpatient wards. New Taipei Journal of Nursing. 2004;**6**:49-61

[49] Coulling S. Nurses' and doctors' knowledge of pain after surgery. Nursing Standard. 2005;**19**:41-49

[50] Yen HF, Chiu LW. Knowledge of and attitudes toward pain management and related factors among physicians and nurses working in critical and emergency care wards. Evidence-Based Nursing. 2005;**1**:292-301

[51] Tsai FC, Tsai YF, Chien CC, Lin CC. Emergency nurses' knowledge of perceived barriers in pain management in Taiwan. Journal of Clinical Nursing. 2007;**16**:2088-2095

[52] Joshi GP, Schug SA, Kehlet H. Procedure-specific pain management and outcome strategies. Best Practice & Research. Clinical Anaesthesiology. 2014;**28**:191-201

[53] Cascella M. Introductory chapter: The rationale for a multimodal

approach to pain treatment. In: From Conventional to Innovative Approaches for Pain Treatment. Intech; 2019. DOI: 10.5772/intechopen.85864. [Accessed: 16 August 2020]

[54] Cuomo A, Bimonte S, Forte CA, Botti G, Cascella M. Multimodal approaches and tailored therapies for pain management: The trolley analgesic model. Journal of Pain Research. 2019;**12**:711-714

[55] Australian and New Zealand College of Anaesthetists and Faculty of Pain Medicine. Acute Pain Management: Scientific Evidence. 2nd ed. Melbourne: ANZCA; 2005

[56] Bennetts S, Campbell-Brophy E, Huckson S, Doherty S. Pain management in Australian emergency departments: Current practice, enablers, barriers and future directions. EMA - Emergency Medicine Australasia. 2012;**24**:136-143. DOI: 10.1111/j.1742-6723.2011.01499.x

[57] Glajchen M. Chronic pain: Treatment barriers and strategies for clinical practice. The Journal of the American Board of Family Practice. 2001;**14**:211-218

[58] Gordon DB, de Leon-Casasola OA, Wu CL, Sluka KA, Brennan TJ, Chou R. Research gaps in practice guidelines for acute postoperative pain management in adults: Findings from a review of the evidence for an American pain society clinical practice guideline. The Journal of Pain. 2016;**17**(2):158-166

Section 2

Pain Management and Psychology

Chapter 5

Empathy for Pain

Ece Ozdemir Oktem and Seyda Cankaya

Abstract

Empathy is essential for being human for understanding and sharing other people's affective and mood, including pain. Pain empathy is a mental ability that allows one person to understand another person's pain and how to respond to that person effectively. The same neural structures as pain and empathy have recently been found to be involved in functional magnetic resonance imaging (fMRI) studies. When someone witnesses other's pain, besides the visual cortex, various parts of the nervous system activate, including the neural network of empathy. Empathy includes not only pain but also other emotions, such as anger, sadness, fear, distress. These findings raised beg the question of whether empathy for pain is unique in its neural correlates. It is essential to know for revealing empathy is a specific context or in a state of chronic pain, depression or anxiety disorders. Because of this, pain empathy has been the central focus of empathy research in social neuroscience and other related fields, highlighting the importance of empathy for pain in daily life. Considering how pain plays a crucial role in the quality of life, determining its network and neurocognitive correlations in the empathy processing may provide a novel therapeutic approach for pain management. This area, which is still under investigation, can provide new information about pain. Under the recent studies and hypothesis, we have aimed to clarify the term of pain empathy, its components, and its neural correlates.

Keywords: pain empathy, functional magnetic resonance imaging, pain, empathy

1. Introduction

1.1 Empathy for pain

Empathy is a crucial component of social interactions allowing not only understand and feel other's emotions but also promoting prosocial behaviour which is vital for our social life [1–3]. Most definitions of empathy based on empathy are about a capacity of sense of knowing another person's personal experience [4]. Empathy in the context of pain has been attracted since observing somebody in pain activates similar neurons as if the observer were feeling pain himself [5, 6]. The effect of experience and observing of pain bring an interpersonal interaction in observers.

Facing the pain of others might result from ignoring to comfort or help. Having personal pain experiences facilitate to reveal empathic responses when observing someone in pain [6]. Also, sharing emotional experiences with friends may promote empathy [7]. Personal beliefs about pain may affect the level of empathy in that person [8].

Additionally, personal identity was positively correlated with empathy in nurses, doctors, and teachers. Studies have shown successful teaching requires the link between cognitive and affective empathy [9]. Empathy promotes students' academic achievement and teachers' professional growth [10, 11]. Empathy was negatively correlated with a burnout in the nursing profession [12]. Furthermore, a 10-week empathy training experiment in nurses showed significantly improved professional identity [10].

As summed above pain empathy is influenced by several factors, such as personal identity [13, 14], gender [15], attention [15, 16], prosocial characteristics, and attitude [17]. Besides these, some neuropsychiatric disorders such as schizophrenia, psychopathy, and autism may lead to impaired empathic reactions. These individuals are less responsive to their pain and others [18, 19].

Sex differences are another affecting factor in empathy for pain. Women reported more significant empathic concern and affective distress via Empathy for Pain Scale in pain compared with men [20].

Regarding contextual influences in daily life, developing a sense of knowing another person's experience in pain has been affected by several factors, such as observer's learning experiences, shared knowledge, and observed person's pain expressions, etc. All elements contribute to more or less person's affective responses as well as behavioural responses. So, a person's reaction to what they see is not identical. Although there are different mentions on the core components of empathy, there is a consensus in the literature that empathy takes a multiple and interacting process between cognition, distinction and affective state of the person.

This pain empathy process occurs from observing the pain because of his/her sense of knowing of the other's personal experience and his/her affective response to this. In this context, empathy has divided into the three-part: firstly, cognitive/evaluative part is similar to mentalising and theory of mind, ability to identify, and understand other people's emotion [21]. Second, the distinction is distinguishing of self pain from someone else's pain. The last part is pointing that sharing of the other person's affective state (which refers to the catching and automatic mimicking of other people's emotions) [22].

Successful internal balancing of empathy parts provides increased intimacy and closeness to other's emotions. So, a mother may sense a child's pain, understand the child's feelings and may kiss the wound. In an unsuccessful situation for differentiating cognitive and affective part in empathy may cause to observer's distress and burnout [8]. Finally, it would be sensible to assume that successful regulating our own emotions provide reliably use them to assess the content and sense of others' feelings correctly.

2. Evaluation of empathy for pain

Pain is a subjective term, and individuals mostly use this term through their previous experience related to the injury. When a person receives cues that another person is in pain, neural pain networks within the brain are activated, and one observing another's pain experience embodied empathic reactions such as distress. Several cues can communicate pain to another person: visualisation of the injury causing event, the injury itself, the injured's behavioral efforts to avoid further harm, and displays of pain and distress such as facial expressions, crying, and screaming [23]. To standardise and measure the empathic responses "*Empathy for Pain Scale (EPS)*" has been developed [24]. In this questionnaire, four painful scenarios are using 12 identical items rated on a scale ranging from 1 to 5 points (1 = strongly disagree; 5 = strongly agree. The scenarios are: (1) a person undergoing a surgical procedure (e.g., on the television hospital drama); (2) a person who has a surgical procedure (e.g., with stitches or bandaged amputation stump); (3) a person who is accidentally injured (e.g., in a car accident); and (4) a person who is physically assaulted. The 12 response items are distress, discomfort, disgust, fear, restlessness, sense of compassion, sense of what it feels like, a need to get help, a desire to look away, non-painful sensations, painful sensations and visceral sensations (e.g., nausea). *Interpersonal Reaction Index (IRI)* is also used as a measurement tool for evaluating empathic reactions. The tool is self-report comprising 28-items answered on a 5-point Likert scale ranging from "Does not describe me well" to "Describes me very well" [25]. The four subscales are:

1. *Perspective Taking* – the tendency to spontaneously adopt the psychological point of view of others.

2. *Fantasy* – taps respondents' tendencies to transpose themselves imaginatively into the feelings and actions of fictitious characters in books, movies, and plays.

3. *Empathic concern* – assesses "other-oriented" feelings of sympathy and concern for unfortunate others.

4. *Personal distress* – measures "self-oriented" feelings of personal anxiety and unease intense interpersonal settings.

3. Neural network for pain empathy

With the improvements in functional brain neuroimaging, most studies have focused on activity patterns and neural networks of empathy for pain [6, 26–28].

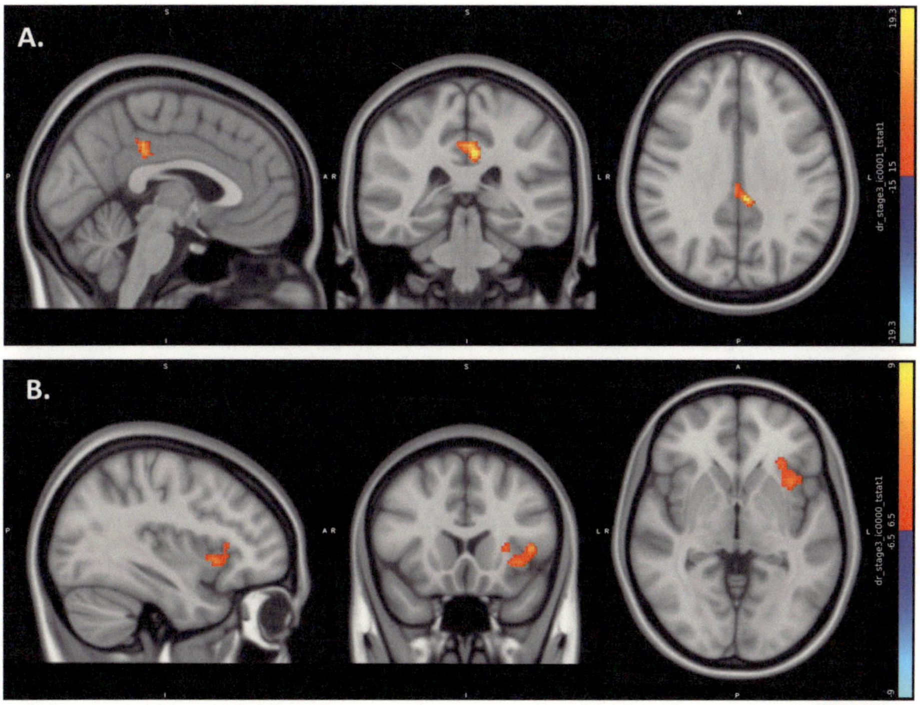

Figure 1.
(A) Mid-cingulate cortex (MMC) and (B) anterior insula (AI) are most impressed areas in empathy for pain studies.

Since early functional neuroimaging studies, the revealing of the same nervous system activation in the case of first-hand pain with responses to pain in others has prompted researchers to explore empathy for the pain core. In these studies, compared with experienced vs. observed pain, experiencing pain activates more extensive regions (with a posterior gradient) than observing pain [29]. Left mid-cingulate cortex (MMC) and left anterior insula (AI) were most impressed two regions in empathy for pain studies (**Figure 1**) [28–30], and pointed regions were also activated by the physical experience of pain [28, 31, 32]. A comprehensive study systematic search from 128 functional brain imaging studies has been confirmed neural correlates of empathy has a core network comprising AI, MCC, postcentral gyrus, inferior parietal lobe, thalamus, amygdala, and brainstem (**Table 1**) [26].

Even though there was considerable overlap in networks for pain empathy and empathy for non-pain negative affective states, empathy for pain uniquely activated bilateral mid-insula and more extensive MCC [30]. Also, activated areas of empathy network showed differentiation with the type of stimuli in the brain. While the core empathy regions evoked with painful faces and pain inflictions, acute pain inflictions also activated additional regions, including medial frontal and parietal cortex [26]. A meta-analysis of neuroimaging studies on the role of visual information indicated that individuals have different activated area response to three factors: visual cues (body parts, facial expressions), visuospatial (first-person, third-person), and cognitive (self-, stimuli-, other-oriented tasks) perspectives [33]. Body-parts distinctly activated sensorimotor processing areas (superior and inferior parietal lobules, anterior insula) while facial expression distinctly involved the inferior frontal gyrus. They have concluded that pain empathy relies on a core network which is modulated by several secondary networks [33]. This second system may contribute to process depending on the visual cues available and the observer's mental state. When we consider the pain for empathy has a quite complex mood, and network, the existing of undefined secondary structures would not be surprised.

The differentiation of activated regions has also been observed in the types of empathy. Although perceptual/affective and cognitive/evaluative parts of empathy show similar neural circuitry, cognitive/evaluative paradigms activated more left MCC regions while perceptual/affective paradigms activated more right AI (**Table 2**) [34]. The studies with paracetamol show that it might decrease psychological reactivity and alter the pain empathy in healthy human subjects [35, 36]. Paracetamol was altering specifically the affective part while keeping the cognitive part of empathy largely intact in healthy subjects. These findings mean that paracetamol reduces the emotional response to other people's negative pain experiences without affecting the pain's mentalising and internalisation. Inconsistent with this, one study suggested that paracetamol increased state empathy scores with activation of paracingulate

Anterior insula (AI)
Mid-cingulate gyrus (MCC)
Postcentral gyrus
Inferior parietal lobe
Thalamus
Amygdala
Brainstem

Table 1.
The neural correlates of empathy.

Affective-perceptual empathy	Cognitive empathy
Right ACC	Left OFC
Right DMT	Left MCC
Midbrain	Left DMT
Right AI	Left AI*
Left AI*	

Dorsal anterior cingulate cortex (dACC), anterior mid-cingulate cortex (aMCC), dorsal medial thalamus (DMT), orbital frontal cortex (OFC), anterior insula (AI).
**Region that involved in both types of empathy.*

Table 2.
The differences in regions are activated in cognitive–evaluative and affective–perceptual empathy [34].

gyrus is responsible for the processing of cognitive empathy in headache group [37]. The researchers concluded this paradigm that pain experience related adaptive brain changes might be strongly linked to the cognitive part of empathy, and targeting pain-induced empathetic neuroplasticity pathways could be a novel treatment strategy for the development of novel painkillers [37].

As we mentioned in pain empathy part, balancing of emotions provides us respond effectively and adaptively to the environmental factors. Otherwise, empathy could be destructive and unhelpful for us. Usually, individuals use to regulate their emotions with cognitive reappraisal. For example, a recent study demonstrated the exaggerated individuals' emotional pain empathy intensity, if the judgement of pain made after the participant's pain experiences as a cognitive bias. But, that bias disappeared when participants used reappraisal to regulate their empathy [38]. The emotion regulation, and mainly reappraisal-based downward regulation, is associated with executive control and limbic networks, namely the prefrontal cortex and the amygdala [39, 40]. A study compared activated region with fMRI for empathising with painful *vs* non-painful scenarios as well as for reappraising painful *vs* non-painful scenarios. Empathising with painful scenarios was associated with increased connectivity with the mid-cingulate and anterior cingulate cortex (ACC), as well as with the bilateral post-central cortex [41].

Conversely, during reappraisal of painful *vs* non-painful scenarios, increased connectivity was found between the inferior frontal gyrus (IFG) and the bilateral lateral occipital cortex, as well as with the left IFG, left posterior insula and left parahippocampal gyrus. Interestingly, different regulation strategies resulted in increased connectivity with other parts of the network. Empathic watch resulted in increased connectivity with regions involved in the processing of self-pain. In contrast, reappraisal resulted in increased connectivity with regions involved in the simulation of other pain, as well as self-pain processing [42]. Activation in the left supramarginal gyrus (SMG) and the right middle frontal gyrus (MFG) was found during empathic watch only, suggesting that these two regions play a critical role and are associated with the process of feeling empathy for the pain of others [41].

4. Conclusion

In line with getting raising numerous study, it could simplify the role of empathy for pain based on a matching of psychological states between the sufferer and the observer. This matching contributes to prosaically actions, affective sharing, emotion regulation, and provide to alleviating the pain and suffering of others.

Under the light of empathy for pain studies, it should be indicated that the neural networks of empathy for pain have not still exactly clarified yet.

Whether the underlying processing of empathy for pain/pain empathy is associated with other non-pain negative affective states still needs more investigation. This gap mentioned-above is particularly relevant for studying empathic responses in different contexts, with diverse populations (age, sex, culture, vocation, etc.) and other affective/sensory states. In the context of the crucial role of pain in the quality of life, empathy for pain deserves more experimental studies for effective pain management in people suffering intractable pain attacks. This chapter discusses not only the definition of empathy for pain, but also the importance of its brain -network correlates, and the ability to empathise with pain in others. Future studies are required for revealing the essential components of pain empathy by different pain stimuli and paradigms.

Author details

Ece Ozdemir Oktem* and Seyda Cankaya
Department of Neurology, Alaaddin Keykubat University, Alanya, Turkey

*Address all correspondence to: ece.oktem@alanya.edu.tr

References

[1] Eisenberg N, Strayer J: *Empathy and its Development.* CUP Archive; 1990.

[2] Ickes WJ. *Empathic Accuracy*. Guilford Press; 1997

[3] Rilling JK, Gutman DA, Zeh TR, Pagnoni G, Berns GS, Kilts CD. A neural basis for social cooperation. Neuron. 2002;**35**:395-405

[4] Ickes W. *Everyday Mind Reading: Understanding What Other People Think and Feel*. Prometheus Books; 2010

[5] Botvinick M, Jha AP, Bylsma LM, Fabian SA, Solomon PE, Prkachin KM. Viewing facial expressions of pain engages cortical areas involved in the direct experience of pain. NeuroImage. 2005;**25**:312-319

[6] Jackson PL, Meltzoff AN, Decety J. How do we perceive the pain of others? A window into the neural processes involved in empathy. NeuroImage. 2005;**24**:771-779

[7] Rimé B, Herbette G, Corsini S: The Social Sharing of Emotion: Illusory and Real Benefits of Talking about Emotional Experiences. 2004.

[8] Goubert L, Craig KD, Vervoort T, Morley S, Sullivan MJ. de CAC W, Cano a, Crombez G: Facing others in pain: The effects of empathy. Pain. 2005;**118**:285-288

[9] Gao J, Wang J, Zhao J. Decoupling of transportation energy consumption from transportation industry growth in China. Procedia-Social and Behavioral Sciences. 2012;**43**:33-42

[10] Wang XQ, Zhu J, He X, Hu Y-Y, Li F, Liu M-F, et al. Affective and cognitive empathy in pre-teachers with strong or weak professional identity: An ERP study. Frontiers in Human Neuroscience. 2019;**13**:175

[11] Peck NF, Maude SP, Brotherson MJ. Understanding preschool teachers' perspectives on empathy: A qualitative inquiry. Early Childhood Education Journal. 2015;**43**:169-179

[12] Yuguero O, Ramon Marsal J, Esquerda M, Vivanco L, Soler-González J. Association between low empathy and high burnout among primary care physicians and nurses in Lleida, Spain. European Journal of General Practice. 2017;**23**:4-10

[13] Singer T, Lamm C: The social neuroscience of empathy. *Annals of the New York Academy of Sciences* 2009, 1156:81-96.

[14] Singer T, Seymour B. O'doherty J, Kaube H, Dolan RJ, Frith CD: Empathy for pain involves the affective but not sensory components of pain. Science. 2004;**303**:1157-1162

[15] Han S, Fan Y, Mao L. Gender difference in empathy for pain: An electrophysiological investigation. Brain Research. 2008;**1196**:85-93

[16] Gu X, Han S. Attention and reality constraints on the neural processes of empathy for pain. NeuroImage. 2007;**36**:256-267

[17] Decety J, Yang C-Y, Cheng Y. Physicians down-regulate their pain empathy response: An event-related brain potential study. NeuroImage. 2010;**50**:1676-1682

[18] Wojakiewicz A, Januel D, Braha S, Prkachin K, Danziger N, Bouhassira D. Alteration of pain recognition in schizophrenia. European Journal of Pain. 2013;**17**:1385-1392

[19] Decety J, Chen C, Harenski C, Kiehl KA. An fMRI study of affective perspective taking in individuals with psychopathy: Imagining another in pain

does not evoke empathy. Frontiers in Human Neuroscience. 2013;**7**:489

[20] Tracy LM, Giummarra MJ. Sex differences in empathy for pain: What is the role of autonomic regulation? Psychophysiology. 2017;**54**:1549-1558

[21] Leslie AM, Friedman O, German TP. Core mechanisms in 'theory of mind. Trends in Cognitive Sciences. 2004;**8**:528-533

[22] Hatfield E, Cacioppo JT, Rapson RL. Emotional contagion. Current Directions in Psychological Science. 1993;**2**:96-100

[23] Cacioppo JT, Norris CJ, Decety J, Monteleone G, Nusbaum H. In the eye of the beholder: Individual differences in perceived social isolation predict regional brain activation to social stimuli. Journal of Cognitive Neuroscience. 2009;**21**:83-92

[24] Giummarra MJ, Fitzgibbon B, Georgiou-Karistianis N, Beukelman M, Verdejo-Garcia A, Blumberg Z, et al. Affective, sensory and empathic sharing of another's pain: The E mpathy for P Ain S cale. European Journal of Pain. 2015;**19**:807-816

[25] Davis MH. Measuring individual differences in empathy: Evidence for a multidimensional approach. Journal of Personality and Social Psychology. 1983;**44**:113

[26] Timmers I, Park AL, Fischer MD, Kronman CA, Heathcote LC, Hernandez JM, et al. Is empathy for pain unique in its neural correlates? A meta-analysis of neuroimaging studies of empathy. Frontiers in Behavioral Neuroscience. 2018;**12**:289

[27] Jackson PL, Rainville P, Decety J. To what extent do we share the pain of others? Insight from the neural bases of pain empathy. Pain. 2006;**125**:5-9

[28] Zaki J, Wager TD, Singer T: The anatomy of suffering: Understanding the [15_TD $ DIFF] relationship between nociceptive and empathic pain. *Pain* 2016, 20:21.

[29] Lamm C, Decety J, Singer T. Meta-analytic evidence for common and distinct neural networks associated with directly experienced pain and empathy for pain. NeuroImage. 2011;**54**:2492-2502

[30] Corradi-Dell'Acqua C, Hofstetter C, Vuilleumier P. Felt and seen pain evoke the same local patterns of cortical activity in insular and cingulate cortex. Journal of Neuroscience. 2011;**31**:17996-18006

[31] Peyron R, Laurent B, Garcia-Larrea L. Functional imaging of brain responses to pain. A review and meta-analysis (2000). Neurophysiologie Clinique/Clinical Neurophysiology. 2000;**30**:263-288

[32] Wager TD, Atlas LY, Lindquist MA, Roy M, Woo C-W, Kross E. An fMRI-based neurologic signature of physical pain. New England Journal of Medicine. 2013;**368**:1388-1397

[33] Jauniaux J, Khatibi A, Rainville P, Jackson PL. A meta-analysis of neuroimaging studies on pain empathy: Investigating the role of visual information and observers' perspective. Social Cognitive and Affective Neuroscience. 2019;**14**:789-813

[34] Fan Y, Duncan NW, de Greck M, Northoff G. Is there a core neural network in empathy? An fMRI based quantitative meta-analysis. Neuroscience and Biobehavioral Reviews. 2011;**35**:903-911

[35] Mischkowski D, Crocker J, Way BM. From painkiller to empathy killer: Acetaminophen (paracetamol) reduces empathy for pain. Social

Cognitive and Affective Neuroscience. 2016;**11**:1345-1353

[36] DeWall CN, MacDonald G, Webster GD, Masten CL, Baumeister RF, Powell C, et al. Acetaminophen reduces social pain: Behavioral and neural evidence. Psychological Science. 2010;**21**:931-937

[37] Cankaya S, Oktem EO, Saatci O, Velioglu HA, Uygur AB, Ozsimsek A, et al. Paracetamol alters empathy scores in healthy and headache subjects: Functional MRI correlates. Journal of Clinical Neuroscience. 2020

[38] Naor N, Shamay-Tsoory SG, Sheppes G, Okon-Singer H. The impact of empathy and reappraisal on emotional intensity recognition. Cognition and Emotion. 2018;**32**:972-987

[39] Menon V, Uddin LQ. Saliency, switching, attention and control: A network model of insula function. Brain Structure and Function. 2010;**214**:655-667

[40] Seeley WW, Allman JM, Carlin DA, Crawford RK, Macedo MN, Greicius MD, et al. Divergent social functioning in behavioral variant frontotemporal dementia and Alzheimer disease: Reciprocal networks and neuronal evolution. Alzheimer Disease and Associated Disorders. 2007;**21**:S50-S57

[41] Naor N, Rohr C, Schaare LH, Limbachia C, Shamay-Tsoory S, Okon-Singer H. The neural networks underlying reappraisal of empathy for pain. Social Cognitive and Affective Neuroscience. 2020;**15**:733-744

[42] Shamay-Tsoory SG. The neural bases for empathy. The Neuroscientist. 2011;**17**:18-24

Chapter 6

Review of Psychological Interventions in the Management of Arthritic Pain: The Case of Africa

Ann Ukachi Madukwe

Abstract

This chapter reviewed the scientific reports of the prevalence of arthritis pain and the potential of applying various psychological techniques in arthritis pain management among Africans. It initially reviewed the publications on arthritic disease-types, causes and prevalence among Africans and the current status of arthritic treatment options in Africa, cognitive, emotional, and behavioral components of arthritic pain experience, and then later focused on potential application of psychotherapies as part of comprehensive pain management protocol in African clinics and hospitals. The chapter discussed psychological explanations of pain and theoretical bases for pain management. It provided information on chronic arthritic pain assessment from a psychological perspective, beneficial psychotherapies and techniques applicable to this health condition. In general, the chapter explained the importance of incorporating psychological interventions as part of a comprehensive treatment plan to help improve the health outcome of arthritic patients presenting at hospitals in Africa. Psychological interventions are recommended to achieve better treatment outcomes for arthritis patients in African nations.

Keywords: Africa, arthritis pain, pain management, psychological intervention

1. Introduction

A 2015 research report stated that 90% of the global burden of disease lies in Low- and Mid- Income Countries [1]. A different report in the same year stated that over 24% of global disease burden lies in Africa, has access to only 3% health workers and less than 1% of the world's financial resources [2–4]. Healthcare system in Africa has estimated medical personnel (physician) to patient ratio of 2.7:10,000 compared to 5.9 South East Asia, 12.7 Eastern Mediterranean, 15.5 Western Pacific, 21.5 Americas, and 32.1 European region [3]. Generally, Africa is heavily burdened by non-infectious diseases and health conditions (e.g., diabetes, cancer, cardiovascular disease, pregnancy and childbirth related problems, musculoskeletal diseases, road accidents, etc.) and these are also the major causes of mortality and disability in the African population [3, 5–7]. Arthritis belongs to this category and is a major reason for adult disability in the continent. Rheumatoid arthritis was reported to have worldwide prevalence of 1%, while between 1990 and 2010 prevalence in Africa seem to have increased from 0.36 to 0.42% [8]. In a more recent review, the prevalence of Rheumatoid arthritis was recorded as follows: 0.40% in South Asia, 0.37% in Eastern Mediterranean, 0.62% in Europe, 1.25% in America and 0.42% in Western Pacific, no information was provided on the African burden of Rheumatoid arthritis [7]. However, a study reported a 0.13% prevalence of Rheumatoid Arthritis in urban Barika Algeria, North Africa in 2013 with an estimated 0.15% prevalence for the general population [9].

Major challenges to arthritis management in Africa include the fact that its' economic/health import is downplayed in favor of communicable or infectious diseases. Consequently, research in this area is minimal with small sample population & clinic-based studies that are not representative of the true situation of arthritis disease (prevalence, treatment burden and resulting disability) in the African population. Also, little is known about causes and types of arthritis disease; and the psychosocial challenges patients face especially with regards to gender, ethnic or tribal dichotomies in the continent. However, these issues are beyond the scope of this chapter. This paper is focused on providing information about the state of psychological interventions in the management of arthritis pain in Africa and what can be done to improve the situation so as to offer more effective pain management protocols to arthritis patients. This review covers the use of psychological interventions in arthritis treatment in general drawing from clinical practices and studies conducted across gender and outside Africa.

2. Arthritis disease: Types, symptoms and prevalence

Arthritis is widely recognized as a leading cause of pain and disability among the aged (adults 50 years and above) across the globe. Its burden is well noted in developed nations like the United States and measures are taken to care for sufferers. The case is different in African countries, starting with under-diagnosis due to little or no presentation of cases at orthodox hospitals, misconceptions about the disease, poverty, expensive (unaffordable) medical care, inadequate medical facility and distractions by heavy burden of infectious diseases in the health sectors, as such little attention is given to arthritis disease in these countries. South Africa with on 85 rheumatologists is reported to have the largest number of rheumatologists in Africa [3].

Arthritic disease has been described as a chronic inflammatory disorder that affects joints of the body [10]. It has painful, debilitating and detrimental [5, 11] effects on the health and well-being of those affected. While it is assumed to be more common among the elderly (65+ years), it afflicts people of all age brackets including children, male and female alike. Over a hundred type of arthritis have been recorded [11, 12] overtime and across the globe. Studies in Africa have noted the existence of seven types of arthritis- 1) Rheumatoid arthritis 2) Osteoarthritis (Mseleni Joint Disease) 3) Ankylosing Spondylitis 4) juvenile idiopathic arthritis 5) juvenile chronic arthritis 6) psoriatic arthritis 7) Gout 8) Osteoarthritis. Literature showed that most studies on arthritis were conducted with non-African populations. Majority of the studies conducted in African Nations were centered on Rheumatoid Arthritis (RA) a few on osteo arthritis. Some meta-analytic reviews were on the prevalence of various types of arthritis in Africa. Both genetic and environment have been reported to contribute to the onset or arthritic conditions (e.g. aging, obesity, injury). The arthritis conditions identified among Africans will be briefly discussed.

Rheumatoid Arthritis (RA): RA is described as an autoimmune disease in which the immune system attacks the lining of joints and connected tissues [8, 7] causing inflammation of small joints of the hand, wrist, knee and feet. It is a chronic condition that if left untreated leads to extensive erosion on cartilage causing deformity and disability [13]. Its symptoms include daily pain, morning stiffness, fatigue, swelling of joints, generalized weakness, loss of weight, and low-grade fever. This is the most studied arthritic condition in Africa [6]. Generally, RA is reported to have 1–2% prevalence in western world and 1% worldwide [14]. Another report showed an increasing incidence of RA across African Nations including Uganda, Kenya, Nigeria and South Africa [6]. Report reveals a prevalence rate range of 0.1% to 2.5% in various urban and rural settings of Democratic Republic of the Congo (DRC), Lesotho and South Africa [10]. RA is most prevalent in South Africa with a prevalence ratio of 2:3 for men to women [8]. The report on Nigeria and Liberia with the next highest occurrences of RA showed greater incidence in men with a prevalence range of 3:1 for men to women. However, two studies that used the American College of Rheumatology (ACR) 1987 rheumatic arthritis criteria for diagnosis found no incidence of RA in Botswana and Nigeria.

Osteoarthritis (OA): Osteoarthritis occurs among older people of 65+ years. It is described as a

> *Degenerative joint disease that can affect any bodily joint but typically affects the hands, hips, kneel and spine. OA causes degradation of articular cartilage overtime resulting in bones rubbing up against one another leading to pain, joint swelling, tenderness and limited mobility ([12], p. 5-6).*

It has also been affirmed that the degenerative nature of osteoarthritis affects cartilage and its surrounding tissues, remodels the subarticular bone, causes osteophyte formation, ligamentous laxity, weakening of particular muscles and at times synovial inflammation [13]. Mseleni Joint Disease is a type of osteoarthritis common among people in Northern Kwazulu Natal province of South Africa and locally known as unyonga, meaning a disease of the joints [15]. It affects large joints in mid childhood. Some symptoms include joint pain, morning stiffness and stiffness on resumption of activity, limited mobility, bone enlargement, joint instability and severe physical disability. OA disease progresses slowly, and knee OA is reported as the most prevalent compared to hand and hip OA. People who are above age 50, obese, inactive, who smoke and who have joint injury are at greater risk of developing OA. The incidence of OA increases with age and it is reported more in women than males aged over 50 years. Osteoarthritis is recorded as the most prevalent form of arthritis in Africa with a prevalence range of 55.1% to 82.7% in urban and rural South Africa respectively [10]. However, it is not as extensively studied as RA.

Juvenile Arthritis: This includes Juvenile Idiopathic Arthritis (JIA) and Juvenile Chronic Arthritis (JCA) among others that afflict children of 15 years and younger. Juvenile arthritis is a progressive inflammatory autoimmune disease that may affect multiple joints (e.g., knee, hand, elbow, ankle, wrists, etc.) in the body by the time the child becomes an adult resulting in restricted mobility [12]. The symptoms include swelling, joint pains and stiffness. JIA is reported as the most prevalent arthritis in this class [10]. Reported records of the prevalence of JIA among African children (10–15 years) are as follows: 0.003–0.33% prevalence in Egypt and 00.1% in Cameroun.

Psoriatic Arthritis: It is described as a chronic inflammatory join disease with negative test for rheumatoid factors and cutaneous psoriasis [16]. The symptoms include morning stiffness, joint pain, skin flaking, intermittent swelling, fatigue and itching. This type of arthritis has also been noted to be incident in Africa with a 4.4% prevalence rate in urban South Africa, 1% & 0.1% in Uganda and Cameroun respectively. In Africa records of its incidence is linked to HIV infection.

Gout: This particular type of arthritis is considered to have significant genetic underlining as it is found to run in families [12]. Its symptoms include acute joint pain, swelling in the knees, foot and big toe. It is more prevalent in males than females. The prevalence of gout is reported as 0.70% among white South African and 0.30% among HIV-infected population in Burkina Faso.

Ankylosing Spondylitis: It is a chronic, progressive arthritic condition that leads to severe disability. It occurs in early adulthood with symptoms like pain in the mid and lower back, heel, eyes, shoulder, ankle, and knee, reduced flexibility in the spine, sleep disorder, inflammatory bowel disease, and abnormal bone formation. Some occurrences of this type of arthritis are recorded in South Africa, Cameroun and Egypt [10, 17].

2.1 Arthritis pain experience

Pain often contributes to dramatic reduction in a patient's quality of life. Like every other pain, arthritis pain is multidimensional [18]. It has physical, social, psychological and economic dimensions and how each person perceives these dimensions influences their treatment outcome. Despite the obvious, treatment of pain and arthritis pain in particular is usually and largely based on the biomedical procedures like medication, surgery and physical therapy. Traditionally, arthritis disease known as a musculoskeletal disorder is classified as a biological and physiological condition. As such, its epidemiology, pathogenesis as well as treatment efforts have been majorly focused on and drawn from the biomedical field. This has largely served to under-prioritize the potential contributions of other approaches especially psychological approaches to the treatment and care of arthritis patients. It has also indirectly suppressed the understanding of pain, in this context arthritic pain, as a psychological experience with cognitive, emotional and behavioral components.

Pain is described as an unpleasant experience signaled by behavioral expressions such as crying, screaming, withdrawal, change in posture, gait or facial expression [19] which limits, hinders or alters the bearer's behavior. Pain was defined as an unpleasant sensory and emotional experience associated with actual or potential tissue damage or described in terms of such damage [14]. The relationship between the incidence of pain and possible cell damage or existence of disease provides clear evidence or support for the biomedical understanding of pain. Nevertheless, this connection is not able to explain why two individuals with the same level of cell damage or disease activity would have varying degrees of pain. The biomedical perspective is considered as being weak due to its inability to explain the differentials in pain responses of patients with similar disease activity [20], neither is it able to address psychological factors in the experience of pain. Again, the biomedical drug treatment approach to the management of arthritis in Africa with recourse to non-pharmacological or surgical treatments may have increased the likelihood for self-medication among sufferers. This is most likely because of the problems of inaccessible, unavailable or expensive healthcare services in Africa (especially among rural women dwellers). A situation that may explain the seemingly low prevalence rates arthritis disease reported by studies originating from Africa. Therefore, the argument that pain sensation is not merely a biological process but mostly a psychological experience forms the basis for this call to fully adapt psychological techniques in the management of arthritis pain among Africans and all people in general. The importance of this call for the use of psychological techniques in the treatment of arthritis pain, relates to the bio-psychosocial model of [21] which postulated that no particular factor can account for health outcome. Rather, that health outcome depends on the synergistic and reciprocal interactions of various factors that relates to a patient's disease experience. In this paper, it is argued that because the perception of pain depends on a lot of factors including but not limited to age, sex, wellbeing, cognition, belief, learning, emotional stability, culture, economic status, etc., The insistence or rigidity that sustains the biomedical model of pain management has to be revaluated in light of new knowledge and best practices across the globe. When adopted, psychological methods [21–23], would mostly enhance patients' health outcome by:

a. Improving patients' understanding of perceived illness

b. Improving patients' adherence to treatment protocols and life style changes

c. Improving level of acceptance of the illness

d. Addressing ethno-cultural factors contributing to illness experience and illness sustenance

e. Addressing issues of interpersonal relationship, communication, and social support relating to patient care.

f. Addressing gendered issues that may be hindering positive health outcome or hinder access to health services.

g. Assessing and treating pre- or co-morbid psychological problems like drug misuse/abuse, depression, anxiety, sleep problems, etc.

h. Teaching patients effective selfcare and pain management protocols.

2.2 Arthritis pain treatment options in Africa

There is a clear challenge of limited empirical studies on arthritis in Africa. A report [10] showed that between 1975 and 2014, about fifty studies relating to arthritis were published across Africa. However, none of those studies and none that was found in the course of writing this chapter were focused on African women or arthritis treatment. Instead, most were on prevalence and the remaining, either studied risk factors or are meta-analytic reviews of others. Meanwhile, information on women experience of arthritis pain and its treatment is lacking. Studies from other parts of the world including United States of America, United Kingdom and France point to the use of non-drug treatments in the management of arthritis pain. A meta-analytic study that assessed the efficacy of psychosocial interventions in the management of arthritic pain in the United States, reported that patients who received psychosocial interventions displayed significantly lower post-treatment anxiety, depression and psychological disability [23, 24]. Reported the use of non-pharmacological treatments as depending on disease progression, personality, environment and objectives of the patient [25]. Some identified non-pharmacological treatments include physiotherapy, balneotherapy, spa therapy, psychological interventions, therapeutic patient education, dietetics and acupuncture.

3. Psychological theories on pain and pain management

Attempts to explain pain and human experience of pain dates back to the time of Descartes in the 17th century, with pain described and understood as a sensory experience. Later theories like the pattern theory also derived from the biomedical models, till mid-20th century when Melzack and Wall in 1965 propounded the gate control theory of pain. Unlike the biomedical models before it, the gate control theory expanded the understanding of pain perception and experience to include psychological factors like stress, emotions, motivations, past experience, context and their impact on pain processing in the brain. This new understanding of pain opened doors for the use of psychological therapies in the control and management of pain. The understanding that not all kinds of pain can be explained by disease activity or tissue damage that are responded to by peripheral nerves gave room for a potentially better explanation of pain [26]. Consequently, the gate control theory proposed that higher neural mechanisms in the brain make meaning of a pain experience by incorporating other individualized factors including cognition, emotion, and motivation.

This theory contributed to a better understanding of pain so that it is scientifically understood and clinically practical that pain is dependent on a reciprocal relationship between ascending nociceptive input from peripheral nerves (pathophysiology) and feedback from higher brain activities (psychological factors) see **Figure 1**.

Psychological theories that form the bases for pain management psychotherapies include the behavioral, cognitive and humanistic models and modern models like the psychological flexibility model. Behavioral theories like operant conditioning of BF Skinner and classical conditioning of IvanPavlov explain behavior as an outcome of learning and as such a learned behavior can also be unlearned [27]. Therapies that generate from these theories like behavior modification techniques (e.g., token economy) cause behavioral change, either by decreasing unwanted behavior or increasing wanted behavior [28]. In the instance of chronic pain, these patients are taught new coping skills that would help them reduce or eliminate aversive or problematic pain behaviors. On the other hand, cognitive theories of psychology like Albert Ellis rational emotive behavior and Beck's cognitive theory would address a patient's thoughts, feelings and actions in relation to their pain experience [28]. These theories and therapies generating from them would explain problems like depression, pain catastrophizing, pain avoidance behaviors, feelings of helplessness, etc., that commonly accompany chronic pain conditions. The humanistic theories of psychology would explain pain experience in its social, economic, cultural, etc., contexts. How these factors could be contributing to the experience and sustenance of pain or how they can help alleviate the problem. Therapies developed from this

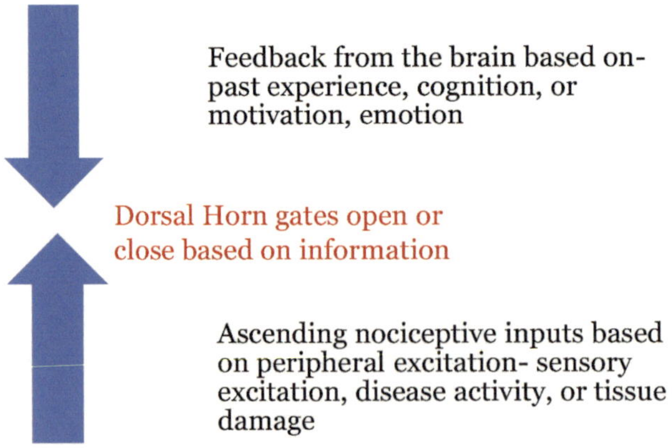

Figure 1.
An illustration of how activities in the higher brain areas and inputs from nociceptive neurons influence gate opening or closing in the dorsal horn to elicit a pain experience. Pain is experienced when the combined activities results in the opening of the gate.

theoretical background would focus on providing emotional support while encouraging social support and selfcare strategies with a goal of reducing the psychological distress experienced by the patient. Finally, the *psychological flexibility model for chronic pain management* is a recently developed understanding that is attracting the attention of researchers and practitioners in recent times. The model refers to "the capacity to persist or to change behaviour in a way that (a) includes conscious and open contact with thoughts and feelings, (b) appreciates what the situation affords and (c) is guided by one's goals and values". This model integrates both cognitive and environmental influences in describing and understanding behavior [29]. It focuses on such processes like acceptance, cognitive defusion, flexible present-focused attention, self-as-observer, values, and committed action; of these, acceptance has risen in popularity among psychotherapist and in treatment of chronic conditions.

Effective pain management protocols are therefore expected to also cover the psychological (cognition, emotional, behavioral) aspect of pain experience. Pain management especially management of chronic pain (like arthritis pain) that is based on biomedical approach is apparently deficient of the psychological intervention protocol and would most likely result in poor health outcome. This is true and supports or explains the extensive acceptance and inclusion of psychological interventions in comprehensive wholistic pain management approaches used in developed nations like France.

Across the globe but especially in Africa, the use of psychological interventions in the management of pain is quite minimal. Psychological interventions are mostly present in the management of cancer patients, hence, the development of Psycho-Oncology; but lacking in the management of other chronic conditions particularly arthritis. This is despite the established knowledge that arthritis disease onset, progression, severity and treatment outcome affects and can be affected by a person's life style, psychological and social circumstances [24]. It has therefore become imperative to reawaken psychologists and other health care professionals in Africa to the need to provide better healthcare service to arthritis patients by incorporating psychological interventions that could improve treatment outcome, quality of life, and adjustment skill for the patient. This can be done by referring arthritis patients presenting in the hospitals and clinics to psychologists for pain management psychological therapies. Such referral can be made when chronic arthritis pain results in or is as a result of the following:

1. Depression

2. Disability

3. Low self-efficacy for pain control

4. Pain catastrophizing

5. Inadequate social support (informational, behavioral and emotional)

6. Stress

7. Insomnia (Sleep disorder)

8. Emotional distress

9. Anxiety [24].

3.1 Psychological focus in clinical pain assessment

Assessment of chronic pain condition for which psychological intervention is required should be characterized by the following;

3.1.1 Pain sensation must have been on for at least six months and more to qualify as chronic pain

3.1.2 Full history of the pain must be taken

a. Circumstances surrounding the pain; where and when it occurs

b. Duration; how long does the pain last at each episode – chronic, intermittent or remitting.

c. Severity of the pain from the beginning

d. Which joint(s) of the body does the pain sensation occur and how often in a day, week, or month.

e. What triggers the pain sensation and what makes it better or brings relief

f. Use visual analogue scale to rate severity of pain experience at initial clinical assessment. An example is using a scale of 0–10, with zero as no pain and ten as severe pain

g. Client's beliefs and thoughts about the pain; is pain seen as unacceptable, a punishment or beyond their control. This relates to pain catastrophizing.

h. Client's feelings about and perception of the pain and the circumstances surrounding it. This relates to pain locus of control

i. Client's lifestyle and coping strategies being used to cope with the pain; also assess client's activity level

j. Client's belief about their ability to control the pain experience. This relates to pain self-efficacy

k. Social context and stress level of patient suffering arthritis pain

l. Addiction to drugs (including misuse or abuse of prescription drugs for pain management)

m. Anxiety disorder

n. Sleep disorder

o. Depression

There are also evidence-based pain assessment instruments developed to measure various pain related concern like coping and self-efficacy. Some commonly used ones are pain self-efficacy questionnaire, coping strategies questionnaire, brief COPE inventory, and chronic pain coping inventory. The scale a therapist chooses to use depends on their interest. Generally, the scales are developed to measure behavioral and or cognitive aspects of pain experience or pain coping. A therapist can select a scale if they want to have a more objective assessment of how well a patient uses a particular coping skill when experiencing pain. The following are some coping skills assessed with the scales; diverting attention, reinterpreting pain sensation, guarding, resting, asking for assistance, coping self-statement, ignoring pain, praying and hoping, relaxation, task persistence, exercise, increasing behavioral activities, catastrophizing, stretching and seeking social support [30].

3.1.3 Treatment Planning

This will involve clinical decision about required or further investigation to help decide the nature of pain as well as the treatment protocol of choice. Assessment of personality variables, lifestyle, thinking pattern and social network are also important. And the results of biomedical investigations like laboratory, radiological and physical examinations should also be considered. Though arthritis pain is the general concern, psychotherapy should be tailored to suit the personal needs and circumstances of each arthritis patient. Patients, therefore, work with therapists in a collaborative manner during assessment and treatment planning stages, to design the best interventions possible to achieve their treatment goals in the shortest time possible or help them function better with minimal pain and psychological distress.

3.2 Psychological techniques in treatment or management of pain

A. Cognitive restructuring aimed at changing existing beliefs about pain and creating new ways to think about it and resolve it.

B. Relaxation techniques to help deal with anxiety induced by the painful condition

C. Stress management, this is important as painful conditions can be stressful or worsened by other stressors (e.g., work related stress)

D. Psychoeducation about possible psychological symptoms

E. Assertiveness skills to help with pain communication between patients, their caregivers and other support network

F. Hypnosis and Distraction techniques

3.3 Psychotherapies in arthritis pain management

Treatment approach can be either group or individual or both as the case may be. Therapy can be as short as 8 sessions; however, the length of psychotherapy depends on the severity of the problem. Common therapies applied to arthritis patients include:

a. Cognitive-behavioral therapy: This is used especially when client is presenting with comorbid depression and or anxiety disorder. Techniques used here would address the affect, cognition and behavior of a patient in relation to pain experience. Some applicable techniques are relaxation, cognitive restructuring, problem solving, *in vivo* desensitization, sleep hygiene, etc., [28].

b. Behavioral therapy: This is aimed at changing existing unhelpful pain behaviors, lifestyle, diet and to get the client to adopt new, more adaptive and pain relieving behaviors that will encourage continuous participation in work and recreational activities (habit reversal techniques). Some applicable techniques include assertions, exercise, deep muscle relaxation, token economy, etc.

c. Psychosocial counseling: The goal here is to help the patient clarify, calibrate, differentiate and understand their various concerns. It is common that the practical problems like pain, reduced physical activity and low income would have accompanying emotional distress. Therapies using this model would help patients separate the two and address the practical problems and the emotional distress sequentially. It is supposed that once the emotional distress is resolved client would be more capable to perform tasks that could help resolve the practical problems. Some applicable techniques are supportive counseling, problem solving, psychoeducation for adaptive coping skills, etc.

d. Other psychotherapies that could address issues like depression, catastrophizing, anxiety, fear of pain and other accompanying psychological problems can also be applied. However, psychological interventions for chronic pain management are best when applied as a multicomponent therapy that would address the various psychosocial dimensions of pain experience.

4. Conclusion

Treatment of arthritis is largely done using drugs and surgery, however, the use of other non-pharmacological and psychosocial approaches have been widely noted in other parts of the world aside Africa. There is no clear and reliable evidence of the reality of arthritis disease burden in Africa. Hence, the seemingly misleading conclusion that arthritis is less prevalent in African nations compared to the developed and industrialized nations of the world. Rather, poverty, inadequate healthcare facility, expensive healthcare service as well as reliance on traditional remedies might explain the seeming lack of hospital presentations or low diagnosis of arthritis in Africa. Psychological interventions have been proven to be beneficial in other nations. The chapter highlighted various psychological interventions and their positive impacts on the existing arthritis treatment protocols.

Author details

Ann Ukachi Madukwe
Department of Psychology, Faculty of Social Sciences, Imo State University, Owerri, Nigeria

*Address all correspondence to: annemichael2002@yahoo.com; anna.madukwe@imsu.edu.ng

References

[1] Adebayo EF, Uthman OA, Wiysonge CS, et al. A systematic review of factors that affect uptake of community-based health insurance in low-income and middle-income countries. BMC Health Services Research. 2015;**15**:543

[2] Africa Renewal. Healthcare systems: Time for a rethink [Internet]. 2017. Available from: https://www.un.org/africarenewal [Accessed: August 13, 2020]

[3] Mody GM. Rheumatology in Africa-challenges and opportunities. Arthritis Research and Therapy. 2017;**19**(49):1-3. DOI: 10.1186/s13075-017-1259-3

[4] Nortjé N, Albertyn R. The cultural language of pain: A south African study. South African Family Practice. 2015;**57**(1):24-27. DOI: 10.1080/20786190.2014.977034

[5] Brennan-Olsen SL, Cook S, Leech MT, Bowe SJ, Kowal P, Naidoo N, et al. Prevalence of arthritis according to age, sex, socioeconomic status in low- and middle-income countries: Analysis of data from the World Health Organization study on global aging and adult health (SAGE). Wave 1. BMC Musculoskeletal Disorders. 2017;**18**(217):1-12. DOI: 10.1186/s12891-017-1624-z

[6] McGill P. Rheumatoid arthritis in sub-Saharan Africa. Annals of the Rheumatoid Disease. 1991;**50**:965-966

[7] Rudan I, Sidhu S, Papana A, Meng S, Xin-Wei Y, Wang W, et al. Prevalence of rheumatoid arthritis in low-and middle-income countries: A systematic review and analysis. Journal of Global Health. 2015;**5**(1):1-10. DOI: 10.7189/jogh.05.010409

[8] Dowman B, Campbell RM, Zgaga L, Adeloye D, Chan KY. Estimating the burden of rheumatoid arthritis in Africa: A systematic analysis. Journal of Global Health. 2012;**2**(2):1-9. DOI: 10.7189/jogh.02.020406

[9] Slimani S, Ladjouze-Rezig A. Prevalence of rheumatoid arthritis in an urban population of Algeria: A prospective study. Rheumatology. 2014;**53**:571-573. DOI: 10.1093/rheumatology/ket446

[10] Usenbo A, Kramer V, Young T, Musekiwa A. Prevalence of arthritis in Africa: A systematic review and meta-analysis. PLOS One. 2015;**10**(8):1-19. DOI: 10.1371/journal.pone.0133858

[11] Raychaudhuri SP, Moriyama H, Bagchi D. Arthritis, aging society, exercise, nutrition, & other precautionary measures. In: Bagchi D, Moriyama H, Raychaudhuri SP, editors. Arthritis Pathophysiology, Prevention and Therapeutics. New York: Taylor & Francis; 2011. pp. 559-561

[12] Sumner LA, Nicassio PM. The importance of the biopsychosocial model for understanding the adjustment of arthritis. In: Nicassio PM, editor. Psychosocial Factors in Arthritis: Perspectives on Adjustment and Management. New York: Springer; 2016. pp. 1-11. DOI: 10.1007/978-3-319-22858-7

[13] Litwic A, Edwards MH, Dimension EM, Cooper C. Epidemiology and burden of osteoarthritis. British Medical Bulletin. 2013;**105**:185-199. DOI: 10.1093/bmb/lds038

[14] Pengel HM, Maher CG, Refshauge KM. Systematic review of conservative interventions for subacute low back pain. Clinical Rehabilitation. 2002;**16**(18):811-820

[15] Dinkele ES, Ballo R, Fredlund V, Ramesar R, Gibbon V. Mseleni

joint disease: An endemic arthritis of unknown cause. The Lancet Rheumatology. 2020;**2**(1):e8-e9. DOI: 10.1016/S2665-9913(19)30104-3

[16] Ouédraogo D, Meyer O. Psoriatic arthritis in sub-Saharan Africa. Joint, Bone, Spine. 2012;**79**:17-19. DOI: 10.1016/j.jbspin.2011.06.007

[17] Singwe-Ngandeu M, Meli J, Ntsiba H, Nouedoui C, Yollo AV, Sida MB, et al. Rheumatic diseases in patients attending a clinic at a referral hospital in Yaounde, Cameroon. East African Medical Journal. 2007;**84**(9):404-409. Epub 2007/12/14. PMID: 18074958

[18] Hadjistavropoulos T, Craig KD. An introduction to pain: Psychological perspectives. In: Hadjistavropoulos T, Craig KD, editors. Pain: Psychological Perspectives. New Jersey: Lawrence Erlbaum Associates Publishers; 2004. pp. 13-34

[19] Madukwe A. Understanding Psychobiology and Behaviour. Gabtony Prints Ltd: Owerri; 2016

[20] Keefe FJ, Somers TJ. Psychological approaches to understanding and treating arthritis pain. Nature Reviews Rheumatology. 2010;**6**:210-216. DOI: 10.1038/nrrheum.2010.22

[21] Engel G. The need for a new medical model: A challenge for biomedicine. Science. 1977;**196**:129-136

[22] Size M, Soyannow OA, Justins DM. Pain management in developing countries. Anaesthesia. 2007;**62** (Suppl. 1):38-43

[23] Dixon KE, Keefe FJ, Scipio CD, Perri LM, Abernethy AP. Psychological interventions for arthritis pain and management in adults: A meta-analysis. Health Psychology. 2007;**26**(3):241-250

[24] Mohiuddin AK. Non-drug pain management: Opportunities to explore. American Journal of Biomedical Science and Research. 2019:1-36

[25] Forestier R, André-Vert J, Guillez P, Coudeyre E, Lefevre-Colau M, Comber B, et al. Non-drug treatment (excluding surgery) in rheumatoid arthritis: Clinical practice guidelines. Joint, Bone, Spine. 2009;**76**:691-698. DOI: 10.1016/j.jbspin.2009.01.017

[26] Melzack R, Katz J. The gate control theory; reaching the brain. In: Hadjistavropoulos T, Craig KD, editors. Pain: Psychological Perspectives. New Jersey: Lawrence Erlbaum Associates Publishers; 2004. pp. 13-34

[27] Schultz DP, Schultz SE. Theories of Personality. Thomson Wadsworth: USA; 2005

[28] Prochaska JO, Norcross JC. System of Psychotherapy: A Transtheoretical Analysis. Thomson Brooks/Cole: Belmont; 2007

[29] McCracken LM, Morley SJ. The psychological flexibility model: A basis for integration and progress in psychological approaches to chronic pain management. The Journal of Pain. 2014;**15**(3):221-234. DOI: 10.1016/j.jpain.2013.10.014

[30] Somers TJ, Kelleher SA, Shelby RA, Fisher HM. Understanding and enhancing pain coping in patients with arthritis pain. In: Nicassio PM, editor. Psychosocial Factors in Arthritis: Perspectives on Adjustment and Management. Cham: Springer; 2016. pp. 35-52. DOI: 10.1007/978-3-319-22858-7

Chapter 7

Clinical Insights into the Importance of Scars and Scar Release in Paediatric Chronic Myofascial Pain

Gillian Lauder and Nicholas West

"Scars have the strange power to remind us that the past is real".

Cormac McCarthy, All the Pretty Horses.

Abstract

Humans exhibit biotensegrity, whereby the whole body is a three-dimensional visco-elastic vehicle whatever position it adopts: bones form non-contact compression struts embedded in a networked and tensioned myofascial matrix; each part of the organism combines with the mechanical system to create an integrated functional movement unit and contributes to the stability of the whole system. When tissue at/below the dermis is breached by surgery/injury, healing leads to scar tissue formation. Scars can cause local and distant effects that are not purely cutaneous. Restriction of normal movement of underlying tissues from defective fascial sliding generates anomalous tension that affects the fascial continuum leading to distorted biomechanics, altered biotensegrity and chronic pain. Scars are common in children and significant contributors to chronic pain presentations. Scars can be released (soft tissue mobilization and/or needling) to sustainably improve pain, flexibility and range of motion. This chapter outlines the importance of skin and fascia in the biotensegrity model. Emphasis is placed on the fundamental need to assess scar history and scar characteristics to determine if scars should be treated as a component of multidisciplinary chronic pain management. Case studies outline some key clinical observations. Appropriately controlled research studies are required to fully demonstrate the highlighted benefits.

Keywords: chronic pain, paediatric pain, myofascial pain, scars, scar release, treatment approaches, fascia, biotensegrity

IntechOpen

1. Introduction

1.1 Skin

> *"Our skin mediates the most important transactions of our lives, Skin is key to our biology, our sensory experience, our information gathering, and our relationships with others......although rarely appreciated, it is one of the most remarkable and highly versatile parts of the human body."*
>
> *Nina Jablonski, Skin – A Natural History [1]*

The skin is the largest organ in the body. It provides a crucial interface between the body and its environment. It has very diverse functions, which include: a defensive barrier against toxic agents and micro-organisms, a multidimensional sensor between the body and the external environment, a protective shield from sunlight, a harnesser of sunlight to begin the process of Vitamin D production in the body, and host to a large part of our microbiome [1, 2]. The skin is thinnest at the eyelids and thickest on the soles of the feet. Skin consists of the epidermis and the dermis, which differ markedly in their structure and function.

The epidermis, the outermost layer is a stratified keratinizing epithelium, approximately 1 mm thick, which is in constant turnover. It maintains a shield against environmental toxins, resists water and protects against heat. The main types of cell found in the epidermis are the keratinocytes, but there are also melanocytes, Langerhans cells, T-lymphocytes and Merkel cells.

Basal keratinocytes are known to differentiate and flatten out to create the stratum corneum. The balance of proliferation and differentiation of the basal keratinocytes is essential for epidermal integrity and ongoing epidermal tissue renewal. Keratinocytes are in close physical contact with free sensory afferent nerve endings and therefore involved in nociceptive responses [3]. Keratinocytes also have some specialised functions, such as: synthesis of keratin, neuropeptides, neurotransmitters, endogenous opioids and autacoids; involvement in local inflammatory responses; as well as expression of multiple different receptors [3]. Tactile stimulation is known to induce peripheral oxytocin release from keratinocytes to mediate local, peripheral oxytocin mediated analgesia [4]. In addition, keratinocytes play a fundamental role in the pathogenesis of neuropathic pain and central sensitization [3, 5–8]. Keratinocytes play a significant role in skin tissue repair, but an abnormal balance of proliferation and differentiation of keratinocytes may lead to generation of pathological scars [9].

Melanocytes are responsible for the primary pigment colour of the skin and the production of melanin. Melanin content is the differentiator for skin colour. Lighter skin or depigmented skin has less melanin, associated with living in more northern climates, where the lighter skin can synthesise more Vitamin D from exposure to sunlight. Merkel corpuscles are skin mechanoreceptors, whereas Langerhans cells and the T-lymphocytes have immunomodulatory properties.

The dermis is a thick layer of connective tissue, which is elastic, pliable, and has substantial tensile strength. The dermis is split into the upper papillary dermis, and the lower reticular dermis. The reticular dermis is characterised by dense irregularly packed collagen, elastin, and reticulin, from which it derives its name. It will be seen later that the duration and intensity of the inflammatory process within the reticular dermis, following surgery or injury, has an impact in the development of pathological scars. The dermis houses other essential organs of the skin including hair follicles, sebaceous glands, endocrine glands and apocrine glands which are absent in scarred skin.

Whereas the primary cells of the epidermis are the keratinocytes, the primary cells of the dermis are the fibroblasts. The dermis gets its strength from a combination of collagen and elastin fibres. The fibroblast is a connective tissue cell that secretes collagen, elastin and other elements of the extracellular matrix. Collagen bundles in healthy normal skin are organised in a three-dimensional basket-weave pattern [10], whereas collagen bundles in scarred skin are organised in parallel to the epithelial surface [11]. Fibroblasts are critical in all phases of wound healing, wound contraction, and remodelling of scars. There are multiple distinct subpopulations of dermal fibroblasts. Fibroblasts with abnormal phenotypes (altered proliferation profile and different patterns of cytokine release) are associated with the development of pathological scars [12].

There are different receptors within the skin, which include: Meissner's corpuscles for light touch; Merkel's discs for constant pressure; Pacinian corpuscles for deep pressure or vibration sense; and Ruffini corpuscles for skin stretch and temperature sensation. The skin is also a primary site of small fibre nociceptive endings [13]. Underneath the dermis is the subcutaneous layer, which contains fat that insulates us to prevent heat loss, and fascial layers that give the skin mobility relative to the muscles, tendons and bones.

Adipose tissue has long been considered just a means of fat storage. However, it has important metabolic and endocrine functions. Regulation of whole-body energy metabolism occurs through its storage function in white, brown or beige adipocytes. Its endocrine function occurs through production of adipocytokines, including leptin and adiponectin. Neurons of the sympathetic nervous system innervate different fat deposits to create communication with adipocytes. Leptin is hormone secreted from white adipose tissue to alter the sympathetic outflow centrally. This leptin-dependent neuro-adipose tissue connection plays an important part in regulating lipolysis and thermogenesis [14]. Leptin also acts on the hypothalamus to regulate food intake [15]. Adiponectin, also a protein hormone produced by adipocytes, has organ protective functions that result from the binding of adiponectin to receptor sites on many organs to activate exosome formation and release for cellular haemostasis [16]. Adiponectin and adipocytes are key players in skin health and disease [17].

The skin is electrically active and contains many nerve elements for interaction with the nervous system [18], the autonomic nervous system [18, 19], and the locomotor apparatus [20]. There is continual nervous activity, in afferent and efferent mode, between the skin and central nervous system to maintain normal physiological and biomechanical homeostasis [18, 21]. There is an independent central emotional connection, principally between the anterior cingulate cortex and the skin, whereby a sympathetic electrical signal can be detected in the skin in response to viewing emotionally charged images [22].

1.2 Touch

Information from skin sensors is relayed via A-delta and C-tactile fibres to the spinal cord and from there to the thalamus, then to specific regions in the primary somatosensory cortex and further on to higher somatosensory areas. The somatosensory maps are not represented in direct proportion or alignment to the body. Certain regions are magnified in response to the density of mechanoreceptors in the associated skin; for example, fingers and lips. The brain receives converging input from numerous nerves innervating adjacent regions of the skin to enable recognition of a specific touch sensation. Neuroplastic adaptive changes occur in the somatosensory map related both to increased repetitive activity and to disuse. Although the primary somatosensory cortex responds appropriately to touch information, the brain's higher centres are more strongly influenced by cognitive factors, such as expectations, context, and attention.

Wide dynamic range neurones integrate afferent pain and touch information. Others converge afferent viscero-somatic information into the spinal cord [23, 24]. Integration of these pathways can sometimes lead to sensory illusions. For example, referred pain is exemplified by shoulder pain from irritation of air under the diaphragm, or left arm pain in association with angina. Conversely, convergence of efferent sensory and sympathetic innervation to skin vasculature may explain sympathetic involvement in conditions such as complex regional pain syndrome and fibromyalgia [25, 26].

It is clear that the skin is a versatile and important organ, but it cannot be considered in isolation from its underlying fascia when considering the impact of scars.

1.3 Fascia

> *"The unsung hero of spine biomechanics."*
>
> *M. Driscoll [27]*

Fascia has long been thought of as the annoying tissue that has to be dissected off to get to the underlying anatomy. This traditional view of fascia has now been surpassed. The most up to date definition describes fascia as a sheath, a sheet or any number of dissectible aggregations of connective tissue that forms beneath the skin [28]. However, this definition is too simplistic, and it is the definition of the fascial system that highlights the importance of fascia in biomechanical regulation:

> *"The fascial system consists of the three-dimensional continuum of soft, collagen containing loose and dense fibrous connective tissues that permeate the body. It incorporates elements such as adipose tissue, adventitiae and neurovascular sheaths, aponeuroses, deep and superficial fasciae, epineurium, joint capsules, ligaments, membranes, meninges, myofascial expansions, periostea, retinacula, septa, tendons, visceral fasciae, and all the intramuscular and intermuscular connective tissues including endo-/peri-/epimysium. The fascial system surrounds, interweaves between, and interpenetrates all organs, muscles, bones and nerve fibres, endowing the body with a functional structure, and providing an environment that enables all body systems to operate in an integrated manner."*
>
> *Adstrum et al. [29], Stecco et al. [30] in Adstrum and Nicholson [28]*

Fascia is multi-layered and has both loose and hard fibrous connective tissue components. Loose fascia functions to help slide and glide between structures and dense fascia exerts a tensile strength in tissues like tendons. Fascia and muscle tissue have a complex interplay to achieve skeletal balance, co-ordination, posture, and locomotion.

Fascia contains cells (fibroblasts, fasciacytes, myofibroblasts, and telocytes), an **extracellular matrix (ECM)**, nerve elements (proprioceptors, interoceptors, and nociceptors), and a system of vascular micro-channels (the primo vascular system) [30, 31]. The fasciacytes produce hyaluronan in response to shear stresses [32]. Hyaluronan (formerly known as hyaluronic acid or hyaluronate) is a glycosaminoglycan of the ECM. Hyaluronan exists between fascia and muscle and promotes sliding and gliding between fascia, muscle, blood vessels, nerves, and lymph channels. It is one of the most important determinants of the viscoelastic properties of a tissue [32–35]. The fascial fibroblasts produce collagen in response to load and stretching. Both acute and chronic fascial loading stimulate collagen

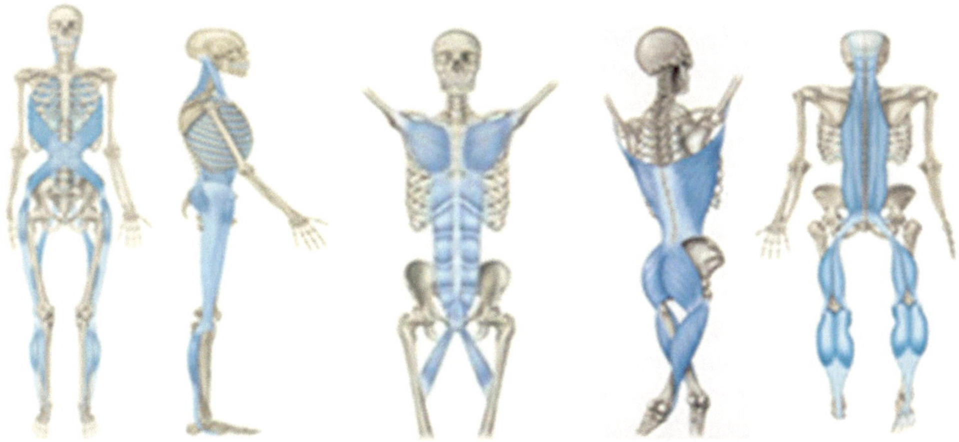

Figure 1.
Myofascial chains, from left to right: spiral line, lateral line, front functional line, back functional line, and superficial back line (adapted from Wilke et al. [36], with permission from Elsevier).

re-modelling [37]. Myofibroblasts within large sheets of fascia are considered to exert clinically significant change in fascial tension in response to sustained mechanical tension, cytokines, low pH, oxytocin, and other agents such as nitric oxide. The myofibroblasts' contractile properties may contribute to spasms, dysfunction, and pain [18, 38]. Telocytes are probably important in regeneration [39]. Fascial tissue has highly variable density, stiffness, humeral action, and metabolic activity, depending on its location and purpose [23].

As the fascia envelops every structure within the body, it creates structural continuity that provides form and function to every tissue and organ. Fascia is one of the essential biological structures that combines with muscles, tendons and bones to create the tensioned and compressed parts that create the **biotensegrity** properties of the human body [40]. Fascia has active mechanical, proprioceptive, nociceptive, and biomechanical and biotensegral properties [30, 36, 41]. Fascia is essential for physiological and metabolic haemostasis as well as healing and repair [30, 31]. Fascia conveys mechanical forces directly or indirectly: directly through muscles at the attachments to bones [42]; or indirectly, as extramuscular fascial chains [43]. There is evidence to support the existence of five myofascial chains (**superficial back line**, **back functional line**, **front functional line**, **lateral line** and **spiral line**, see **Figure 1**) [36], which work within the biotensegrity model [44]. These chains have opposing chains mirrored on either side of the body to achieve balance within the musculoskeletal system. This emphasises the complex nature of human movement and why range of motion at one peripheral articulation is dependent on the positioning of the entire myofascial chain system of the body [45]. Like the skin, fascia is also innervated by the autonomic nervous system and afferent free nerve endings [23, 46] and can be considered as a sensory organ of human biomechanics [23, 46–48]. Fascial tissue homeostasis is a complex, inadequately elucidated, interaction which depends upon active communication between cellular components of the fascia and the related ECM [43, 49].

1.4 The extracellular matrix

> *"The Organ of Form"*
>
> *Varela and Frenk [50]*

The extracellular matrix (ECM) is defined by Grey's Anatomy as "*the extra cellular components of connective and supporting tissues. Essentially, it consists of a system of insoluble protein fibres, adhesive glycoproteins and soluble complexes composed of carbohydrate polymers linked to protein molecules (proteoglycans and glycosaminoglycans), which bind water. The ECM distributes the mechanical stresses on tissues and also provides the structural environment of the cells embedded in it, forming a framework to which they adhere and on which they can move. It provides a highly hydrated medium, through which metabolites, gases and nutrients can diffuse freely between cells and the blood vessels traversing it*" [51].

The ECM is present within every tissue of the body to provide fundamental physical scaffolding for the cellular constituents and orchestrate vital biochemical and biomechanical functions required for morphogenesis, differentiation, and homeostasis. The ECM is basically composed of water, salts, and macromolecules consisting of fibrous proteins (collagen, elastin), adhesive glycoproteins (laminin, fibronectin, tenascin, integrin), and carbohydrate polymers (proteoglycans and glycosaminoglycans). Collagen is the most abundant ECM fibrous protein. However, each individual tissue has a heterogeneous ECM composition providing highly variable but unique biochemical, protective, organisational and biomechanical ECM properties, which differ from one tissue to another. This composition is primarily dependant on that tissue's particular function [52]. The ECM is a highly dynamic structure, constantly being remodelled with its molecular components subject to a multitude of modifications.

Morphological organisation and physiological function of the ECM is orchestrated by binding growth factors and interacting with cell-surface receptors to elicit signal transduction and regulate gene transcription. Enzymes released from fascial cells degrade the ECM, such as cathepsins, heparinase, hyaluronidases, and metalloproteases, to maintain normal tissue turnover.

Matrix metalloproteinases (MMPs) are key in ECM remodelling as they degrade matrix components. MMPs are classified according to substrate specificity; for example, collagenases or gelatinases [52]. It will be seen later that the ratio of MMPs to MMP-inhibitors is of importance in the development of atrophic scars.

2. Scars

2.1 The healing of wounds and scar creation

Any breach of the dermal layer will result in a scar. When the dermis is breached by surgery or injury, a healing process occurs that leads to the formation of scar tissue [53]. There are two main types of healing: primary intention and secondary intention. Healing by primary intention occurs in wounds with dermal edges in close proximity; for example, a surgical incision. Healing by secondary intention occurs when there is unavoidable tissue loss with abnormal tension, infection or necrosis, creating a large deficit where the sides of the wound are not opposed or too big to heal by primary intention; therefore, healing must occur from the bottom of the wound upwards. For both primary and secondary intention healing, there are three overlapping stages to healing after haemostasis is achieved; inflammation, proliferation, and remodelling [54]. This extremely complex and co-ordinated process is guided by cytokines plus chemokines secreted by platelets, macrophages, endothelial cells, keratinocytes, fibroblasts, and adipocytes [2, 12, 17, 18, 55, 56].

Wound healing and scar maturation can take years to complete, but depend on the size and nature of the initial wound. During remodelling, type 3 collagen is replaced by a stronger type 1 collagen, but not in an ordered manner. Scar tissue is therefore strong, but not as elastic or flexible as normal tissue [38, 54]. Normal scars first appear as a red line, but maturation results in a slightly broadened white line, in the same plane with the surrounding skin, known as a normotrophic scar. Normotrophic mature scars are less innervated than the surrounding normal skin [57, 58]. Scar tissue, therefore, has different properties to the tissue it replaced prior to injury. Skin healing is not just dependent on the size and site of the wound, but is also influenced by bacterial contamination, nutrition, comorbid medical conditions, as well as genetic and epigenetic factors [56, 57]. Once normotrophic scars are established, they are often forgotten and ignored unless they constitute a cosmetic embarrassment.

2.2 Scar morphology

If the healing process is interrupted by tissue disruption, infection or a comorbid disease process, then a pathological scar may occur, which may be atrophic, hypertrophic, tethered, or keloid in nature. Development of pathological scars may be related to genetics, as well as differences in the duration, and intensity of the inflammatory process in the reticular dermis [56, 59–61]. Excessive scar tissue movement, scar rubbing, scar scratching or abnormal tension related to surgery or injury may also induce an enhanced neurogenic inflammatory response [18, 62–65]. This may be an important consideration when reflecting on what constitutes a significant scar in terms of myofascial dysfunction later.

Atrophic scars are concave indentations resulting from tissue loss (including collagen) associated with relative shift in the ratio of MMPs to tissue inhibitors of MMPs that favours a lytic process and the development of an atrophic scar [66]. Chicken pox scars are atrophic, which can occur in up to 20% of children following chicken pox infection [67, 68]. Acne scars are a common problem in developed countries, occurring in 80% of 11–30 years old and 5% of adults aged over 30 years [69]. Acne scars are usually atrophic, subdivided into rolling, boxcar, or ice-pick. However, acne scars can also present in hypertrophic or keloid morphology. Hypertrophic scars and keloid scars have excess deposition of collagen. Hypertrophic scars form early within the time frame of injury and remain within the boundaries of the inciting injury. Keloid scars have excess thickened hyalinized collagen. Keloid scars may have a delayed onset of formation and extend beyond the boundaries of the original scar. Keloid scars are more likely to occur in dark-skinned individuals, between ages 10–30, at times of peak hormones (puberty, pregnancy), with a positive family history, and in association with hyperimmunoglobulinemia E, or blood type A [70].

2.3 Scar assessment

Clinical documentation of scar size, thickness, and treatment effects are usually performed with the use of serial photographs, scar scales (such as the **Vancouver Scar Scale, VSS**), and validated questionnaires, such as the **Patient and Observer Scar Assessment Scale (POSAS)** or Dermatology Life Quality Index (DLQI). There are few reliable, objective non-invasive tools to measure scar characteristics. Ultrasonography and high-definition optical coherence tomography (HD-OCT) have also been reported for objective measurement of scars [71–73]. Scar pliability (mechanical property of the skin's stiffness, extensibility, and adherence) is measured using adheremeters, cutometers, and ultrasonography [74]. Viscoelastic properties of scars and connective tissue around scars are measured using sonoelastography [75–78]. Scar colour can be assessed using narrow-band reflectance spectrophotometry colour analysis or Tristimulus colour systems [79], and scar perfusion can be measured with Laser Doppler Flowmetry [79].

2.4 Scar management

Scar optimization and mitigation are key principles that are vitally important in medical practice, but beyond the scope of this article. Readers are directed to algorithms of management that exist for both the adult and paediatric populations [70, 80–83].

2.5 Asymptomatic or symptomatic scars

Diverse symptoms can occur in up to 70% of patients with scars [74]. Symptoms can occur at random timing and even at long intervals after wound healing. Some of these symptoms are highlighted in **Figure 2**.

Scars may be intrinsically painful or play a role in pain located at an anatomically distant site. Scars may present as painful or itchy at the site of the healed scar. One potential cause of intrinsic pain in a healed scar is a neuroma, derived from a regenerating nerve trapped in the fibrotic scar tissue. This is usually associated with numbness in the innervated area of the injured nerve and a positive percussion test. In the absence of a neuroma, the estimated prevalence of painful scars is 2%, but increases in the burn population to 30–68% [57]. Intrinsic scar pain occurs in 7–18% of patients following lower segment Caesarean section [84–86]. Pathological and intrinsically painful scars have been shown to have an in imbalance between non-peptidergic unmyelinated c-fibres and peptidergic c-fibres, but not necessarily in total nerve fibre density [57]. There is also an increased abundance of neuropeptides, and nociceptors in pathological scars, especially hypertrophic scars [18, 87].

It is clear that what is happening underneath a scar is critical to whether it subsequently creates symptoms. Scar tissue can adhere to fascia, underlying muscles, organs, blood vessels and nerves, and recognition has been given to scars as an etiological factor in post-surgical visceral dysfunction [88, 89], nerve entrapment syndromes [90], and symptoms related to obvious contractures. However, very little is documented for the role of scars in locomotor dysfunction [91–95] or chronic myofascial pain [38, 95–97].

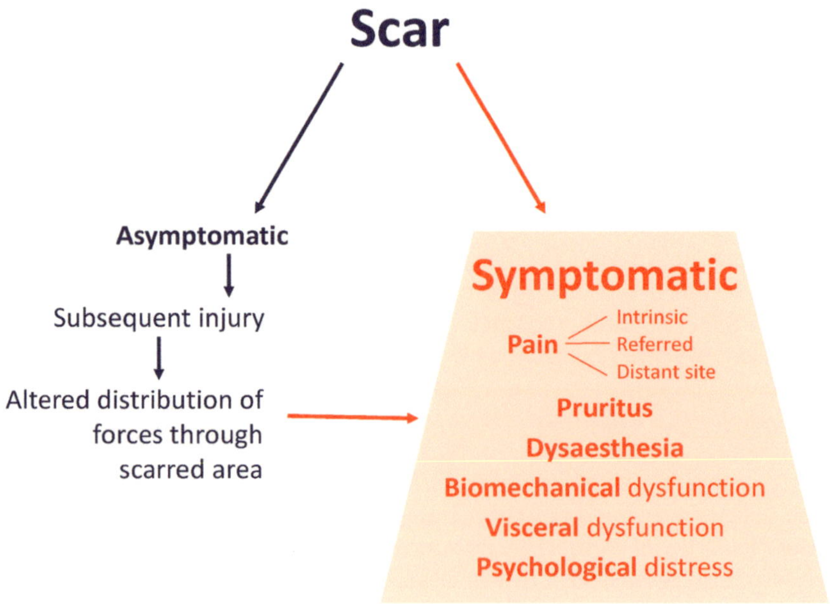

Figure 2.
Symptoms related to scars.

In patients asked to move actively, electrical activity from a scarred area is higher than that from normal tissue in the same patient doing the same movement [93]. Mechanoreceptors and mechanosensitive nociceptors in scarred areas may sense an alteration in tension from normal and send non-physiological signals creating a pathological reflex arc [18], inducing neurogenic inflammation and worsening scar formation and pain [18, 63].

2.6 How scars impact fascia, muscles and movement

> *"Any skin injury, like a scar, even if small, affects the organism and constitutes an active obstacle to its normal functioning"*
>
> *Alvira-Lechuz et al. [98]*

Scars can limit normal movement and the flexibility of skin, the underlying fascia, and its associated muscles. It is clear that any scar that restricts fascial or muscular movement will also have an impact on whole body movement related to the myofascial chains discussed in the fascia section above [18, 99]. The fascia is recognised as a significant contributor to chronic pain [100–102]. Other factors that may play a role include alterations in fascial density. Changes in hyaluronan may lead to fascial densification that restricts fascial sliding and gliding, aggravating fascial dysfunction associated with musculoskeletal disorders and chronic pain [32, 103–109]. Injury reduces the flexibility of fascia; for example, a compound fracture may be associated with periosteal tethering to the skin during healing. The subsequent defective fascial sliding generates anomalous tension, which affects the fascial continuum leading to musculoskeletal pathology, pain and progressive immobility [18, 32, 103, 110–112]. Fascial injury also leads to fascial dysfunction as well as significant loss of sports performance [18, 21, 113, 114]. Symptoms may not necessarily just occur at the site of injury, but also at a distant site related to referred pain and impacts through myofascial chains. Reduced fascial mobility, related to movement restriction secondary to injury, worsens over time, but may persist even when movement is subsequently restored [110]. This was demonstrated with ultrasound imaging of adults with chronic low back pain with increased thickness and reduced mobility of the thoracolumbar fascia [102, 110, 115]. Sonoelastography has been used to measure viscoelastic properties of the connective tissue around scars: it superimposes a parametric image, in a range of colours, over the ultrasound anatomical scan image to semi-quantitatively correlate images with that tissue's elasticity. Sonoelastography has been used to show the changes in post-surgical scars following manual therapy [75, 76].

Fascial trauma or injury may also irritate primary afferent nociceptive fibres leading to spinal cord wind up and central sensitization as another mechanism of ongoing pain [35, 96].

Myofascial pain is characterised by the presence of myofascial trigger points. Myofascial trigger points develop in response to many different insults such as: trauma, injury, surgery, repetitive microtrauma, poor posture, muscle overuse or overload. Myofascial trigger points that cause pain can originate in scars, skeletal muscle, and/or fascia. **myoActivation®** [116] is an innovative structured assessment and therapeutic process targeting release of fascia (including scars) and muscles in sustained contraction.

myoActivation is unique in focusing on aspects of the immediate and past trauma history (often overlooked in a classical medical history) and relating this to the current chronic pain presentation. The **timeline of lifetime trauma (TiLT)** inventory explores all injuries, especially those occurring at a young age, mechanisms of injuries, healing processes, and the perceived physical impact of

Features in the past medical history and timeline of lifetime trauma (TiLT) inventory	Scars incurred at a young age, especially the first or earliest scar in childhood
	Ongoing pain occurring in the immediate timeframe of a surgical procedure which is unexplained and resistant to other forms of therapy
	History of poor wound healing, wound infection or wound dehiscence
	Painful/itchy scars
	Scars incurred at a time of intense emotional turmoil or trauma.
	History of mood disorders may indicate any chin scars will be significant
	History of anxiety may indicate any chest wall scars will be significant
	History of "brain fog" (confused, disorganised, find it hard to focus or put thoughts into words) may indicate a face/chin/sternal or midline abdominal scars will be significant
	History of injury in the presence of an asymptomatic scar (injury may be months or years after scar acquisition), which results in pain in the region of this previously asymptomatic scar
Type of scars	Scars related to chicken pox infection, surgery and especially surgical drain scars, burns and animal (or human) bites
Site of scar	Over bony prominences, e.g. anterior chest, in feet, scar in region of main pain complaint, on the same side as a unilateral pain complaint
	At sites of periosteal tethering
Scar characteristics	Painful scars, purple discolouration, widened scar, palpable densities within or around the scar, scar dysesthesia, adherent/tethered scars
myoActivation examination BASE test [116]	If scar is situated in region of most painful or restricted BASE test on myoActivation examination, even if it looks like a normal scar and/or reported as asymptomatic
Response to dry needling release	Enhanced "biting" sensation when scar is released with dry needling even with appropriate use of topical anaesthesia and/or vapo-coolant spray
	Reported pain decreased or moved immediately following scar release
	Improvement in ROM and flexibility immediately following scar release
	Decreased irritability of other palpable pain points in region of and distant to area of scar release
Size of scar	Size of scar does **not** seem to play a factor as tiny epidural needle scars or chicken pox scars can be as significant as large surgical wounds.
Less significant scars	Some scars seem to be less significant in terms of myofascial dysfunction and chronic pain, e.g.
	• Superficial self-harm scars
	• Tattoos (although they may be hiding another significant scar)
	• Stretch marks

Table 1.
Clinical factors indicating a scar may have potential for myofascial dysfunction and chronic pain.

those injuries to that person. Assessment involves the use of a series of **systematic movement tests (BASE tests)** [116], postural observations and examination of tissues to find palpable pain points and determine if there are important myofascial sources of perceived pain. A key principle in myoActivation is that the site of perceived pain is often not the true source of pain. The most painful or restricted movement on BASE tests identifies the most important tissues to treat first. Careful inspection and palpation of these tissues localises the myofascial source of pain. Treatment entails refined trigger point injections to restore anatomic integrity to injured tissues. Fine gauge hypodermic needles are inserted into trigger points that compromise function of muscle, ligament, tendon, subcutaneous fascia, scar tissue, and the peripheral nerves of the skin. After each individual myofascial area is treated, BASE movement tests are repeated to demonstrate immediate change and direct the clinician to the next most important target area. Several cycles occur during each myoActivation session to unravel multiple sources of myofascial dysfunction in a structured way, to help resolve chronic myofascial pain. Immediate treatment responses occur, which include reduction in pain, increased flexibility, and improved fluidity of movement. This process often reduces or resolves pain sufficiently to enable the subsequent weaning of prescription and over-the-counter analgesia medications [117]. myoActivation is not effective in all patients because pain perception is a complex biopsychosocial phenomenon, but determination of those who will respond rests with the TiLT inventory, clinical history and the series of BASE tests on examination.

Clinical experience with myoActivation [116] reveals that a scar can play a very significant role in chronic myofascial dysfunction and pain even if that scar has the appearance of a normotrophic scar and is reported to be asymptomatic. An ankle scar may alter the gait dynamics through maldistribution of myofascial loads [18] and may also present with ongoing pain at a distant site on the ipsilateral side. Patients with scars in the abdominal region, such as a Caesarean section scar or an abdominoplasty scar, may present with low lumbar back pain related to impaired mobility of the soft tissues of the abdomen, which then puts stretch on the lumbar muscles, thoracolumbar fascia, and the posterior myofascial chain [92, 93, 112]. Scars may also have an impact on the distribution of forces that pass through the body at the time of an injury, such as during a motor vehicle accident [18], causing a previously asymptomatic scar to be the inciting event for myofascial impairment and pain.

2.7 Significance for myofascial dysfunction and chronic pain

Classic scar assessment techniques such as use of adheremeters, cutometers, ultrasonography, and rating scales (POSAS or VSS) [74] were not designed to determine a scar's relevance to myofascial dysfunction and pain. A scar may be significant in terms of myofascial dysfunction and chronic pain, but not be characterised as a pathological scar in current "classical" medical terminology. Clinical experience with myoActivation therapy has found some features, outlined in **Table 1**, that indicate a scar may cause significant myofascial dysfunction and/or chronic pain. These observations will have to be researched to determine which ones are the more common and substantial factors in myofascial pain and dysfunction.

3. Scar release

Non-surgical scar release can be achieved with soft tissue mobilisation techniques, subcision or dry needling [84, 93, 118–121]. Subcision, or microneedling, also known as percutaneous collagen induction therapy, is a minimally invasive minor surgical procedure used for treating depressed cutaneous scars and wrinkles. A simple hypodermic needle or a dermaroller are the tools used to effect subcision [122]. Subcision was first described in 1995 [123]. It is a safe and effective microneedling technique used as an aesthetic treatment for several different dermatological conditions including scars, rhytids, and striae [122, 124, 125]. Histological changes have been demonstrated with this technique [126]. It is hypothesised that microneedling stimulates the body's own regenerative mechanisms through collagen bundle break down and new collagen formation (neocollagenesis), stimulation of the release of platelet and neutrophil derived growth factors and cytokines (FGF, TGFα, TGFβ, VEGF, FGF-76, EGF, platelet derived growth factor, connective tissue growth factor, and connective tissue activating protein), resulting in increased production of collagen, elastin and glycosaminoglycans [122, 127–132]. Up-regulation of TGF-β3 (which prevents aberrant scarring) in excess of TGF-β1 and TGF-β2 may be responsible for the benefits seen with microneedling [129, 133].

The other physiological effects of dry needling are not yet fully elucidated, but may include local, hormonal, neuronal, and placebo effects [134]. Neuronal effects include: modulation of the peripheral nervous system; gate control mechanisms; and central pain modulation, such as activation of the diffuse noxious inhibitory control systems [135]. Dry-needling stimulation of skin nociceptive nerve fibres may release endogenous opioids to activate enkephalinergic inhibitory dorsal horn interneurons and oxytocin to mediate peripheral inhibition of c-fibre discharge [4].

For the release of scars, the myoActivation needling technique involves the sequential insertion of 30 g hollow bore needle in the line of the scar and in any areas of densification around the scar performing multiple perforations approximately 3 mm apart. Clinical experience reveals that a patient report of a "biting sensation" with needling is characteristic of a myofascially significant scar. This biting occurs even if the scar has been treated with appropriately timed topical anaesthetic or pre-needling vapocoolant spray.

The release of scars with micro-needling techniques has been shown to produce relief of chronic pain [116, 136]. Currently, the immediate relief of chronic pain following needling of surgical scars is limited to case reports [116, 120, 136], and to date there is insufficient evidence to advise on the right time to treat scars after injury or surgery. It has been suggested that the skin can keep a memory of trauma [118, 137]. It is clinically important to consider this and be cognizant of events which were associated with creation of a scar. Scars inflicted at a time of severe emotional distress or at the time of a traumatic event can be associated with flashbacks or emotional release at the time of, or a number of hours after, treatment whether the therapy was with a needling procedure or manual manipulation [138].

3.1 Effects of scar release

As all structures of the human body are intricately connected through skin and the myofascial system, scar and myofascial release (often at a distant site) can result in immediate improvement of pain, flexibility and range of motion [116] (**Table 2**), but it is imperative that this is combined in a multidisciplinary approach to address the whole biopsychosocial aspects of pain especially in the paediatric population [136]. It is absolutely essential to prevent needle-related pain in paediatric patients; the practitioner should employ a variety of non-pharmacological techniques including distraction, breathing techniques, music, virtual reality or mobile devices. Pharmacological modalities can be added when non-pharmacological methods are considered insufficient to address the patient's anxiety and needle-related pain. Topical anaesthetic cream can be applied to target sites (especially scars) an

Immediate effects	Decreased pain or pain which has shifted to a new location
	Increased flexibility and range of movement in myoActivation BASE tests
	Altered weight distribution on feet
	Emotional release
	Reports of feeling lighter or "walking on a cloud"
	Sympathetic response
	Vasovagal response
	Bruising
	Post treatment pain at site of needle insertions lasting minutes to hours
	Exacerbation of muscle spasms (requires additional needle insertions to resolve)
	Adverse events (Injury to adjacent structures e.g. pneumothorax when needling around lung fields)
Long-term effects	Improved pain
	Improved flexibility
	Improved mood
	Improved sleep
	Maturation to a normotrophic scars

Table 2.
Effects of scar release.

Absolute	New scars in process of normal healing and remodelling
	At sites of active infection
Relative	Near indwelling metalwork/hardware to minimise risk of hardware infection.
	Near indwelling mesh to minimise risk of infection.
	Where it is considered to be too painful (especially foot scars)
	When patient has needle aversion or needle phobia

Table 3.
Relative and absolute contra-indications to needling scars.

hour before the appointment to minimise needle pain. Oral benzodiazepines can be useful for anxiolysis. If the above methods are not adequate, IV sedation with appropriate anaesthetic monitoring and care may have to be utilised.

Over and above these considerations there are some relative and absolute contra-indications to needling of scars (**Table 3**).

4. Case based discussion of important points

Chronic myofascial pain is common in the paediatric population and its prevalence has increased since the 1980s [139]. Musculoskeletal pain is a common cause of pain in adolescents, with incidence ranging from 30 to 65% [140–144], and is a leading cause of years lived with disability among children and adolescents [145]; 4% of all primary care consults represent musculoskeletal issues in children aged up to 15. Between 4 and 40% of adolescents report limb pain and 14–24% complain of low back pain [146]. The prevalence of paediatric chronic myofascial pain increases with increasing age [139, 147–150] and is more common in females [146, 151]. Young children are not immune with a 10% prevalence of musculoskeletal pain in 6-year-old children. A staggering one-third of this six-year-old population has chronic musculoskeletal pain and 44.6% of them report that pain is multisite in nature [152].

Despite its prevalence, reported musculoskeletal pain is often under-diagnosed in adolescents [153, 154]. Healthcare providers may be unfamiliar or not trained to diagnose chronic pain, muscle trigger points, palpable pain points, and fascia in tension [155–158]. Presenting symptoms such as neck pain, shoulder pain, abdominal pain and headaches do not immediately direct a physician to look for a myofascial component to pain. Myofascial pain can also imitate other pathologies; for example, a trigger point in the quadratus lumborum muscle can mimic the symptoms of appendicitis on the ipsilateral side, or fascial tension in the peri-coccygeal soft tissues may present as neck pain. System, practice and time pressures may also limit the ability to undertake a full history and physical examination [159, 160].

Experience dictates that dysfunctions in muscles, fascia and scars are common in the paediatric population and are significant contributors to paediatric chronic pain [116, 136]. The following cases highlight the importance of scars in paediatric myofascial pain presentations. It must be emphasised that scars are not treated in isolation, but as one element of myoActivation, which is one component of multidisciplinary care.

The children described in these case studies were referred to the **Complex Pain Service (CPS)** at BC Children's Hospital in Vancouver, Canada, and were treated within a program of multidisciplinary care based on the "**3P**" principle (*P***harmacology,** *P***hysiotherapy,** *P***sychology**). The data for these case studies were collected with the approval of the University of British Columba/Children's and Women's Research Ethics Board (H20-01862).

4.1 Case 1: standard myoActivation assessment finding unreported scars

A 13-year-old, 54 kg female was referred to the CPS for management of multi-site chronic pain of 3 years duration with a diagnosis of "pain syndrome" focused mainly on the left knee, but also affecting the low back and neck. The low back pain of 3 years was reported to be secondary to a fall 3 years previously. She had been involved in a motor vehicle accident (MVA) 2 years after that when she was struck on the left side whilst walking across a road. She was admitted by ambulance to the local emergency room (ER) and discharged later that day with a diagnosis of bruising to her left knee and ribs after normal imaging. She initially mobilised with crutches and gradually regained physical functioning, but with ongoing pain.

She described her current pain as dull and achy with stabbing pain elements. Pain was aggravated by walking long distances or any physical activities or exercise. She stated that she had some irritability and sadness related to her pain. She complained about some inability to concentrate due to pain and had been absent from school for 21 days in the previous 3 months. She reported that pain also affected her ability to fall and stay asleep. Her TiLT inventory revealed no other injuries. She reported that she had no scars. She had been using acetaminophen and ibuprofen or naproxen for analgesia as required. She was otherwise healthy and her family history was unremarkable.

She was assessed by her orthopaedic surgeon and family doctor. Previous classical examination, imaging (X-rays and MRI) and bloodwork revealed no remedial cause of her pain.

myoActivation examination revealed unreported scars on the left knee and the right upper back, fascia in tension and multiple muscles in sustained contraction.

A myofascial component to her pain was diagnosed. She was enrolled in the 3P care plan. She was started on Magnesium Bisglycinate, Vit K2 and Vit D (MgBis/K2/D3). Written information about myoActivation was given to the family. One month later, there was a reduction in pain with improved fluidity of movements. Her family also reported improved mood and sleep.

4.1.1 myoActivation session 1

It was deemed appropriate to proceed with myoActivation at this one month follow up based on her stoical character. Written consent was obtained. Distraction techniques, vapocoolant spray and topical anaesthetic for scars were used to minimise procedural pain. All needling was done using sterile technique.

The right thoracic paraspinal, right gluteus medius, right gluteus maximus and left iliopsoas were sequentially activated based on the repeat cycles of assessment to determine the most restrictive and painful BASE tests [116]. The three left knee scars and upper back scar were in regions of worst BASE tests so they were considered significant and released. Scar release consisted of sequential perforation needling of the scar using a 30 g hollow bore needle. After this first myoActivation session the patient experienced immediate improvement in pain and flexibility.

4.1.2 myoActivation session 2

Five days after her first myoActivation session the patient reported that her low back pain no longer bothered her. She reported that the left knee pain felt less tight and tense and she was able to move "more freely", but going up and down stairs was still a problem. The left lumbar paraspinal, left rectus femoris, left vastus lateralis and left pubic fascia were sequentially activated based on the repeat cycles of assessment to determine the most restrictive and painful BASE tests [116].

4.1.3 myoActivation session 3

At the next myoActivation session, 1 day later, the patient reported that her pain had moved to the medial aspect of her left knee overnight. Repeat myoActivation examination revealed marked improvement in all core BASE tests with no pain except mild limitation of squats with arms down and arms up. The left vastus medialis was activated with improvement in squat with the arms down. A left shin scar was noted and released with improvement in squats with the arms up. The patient reported no pain at the end of this session.

4.1.4 myoActivation session 4

One month later, the patient again reported that her low back pain no longer bothered her. She reported that the left knee pain returned on stopping MgBis/K2/D3, so she restarted them. Based on the repeat cycles of assessment to determine the most restrictive and painful BASE tests [116], the right lumbar paraspinal, right hamstring, left gluteus medius and left iliopsoas were sequentially activated. Based on core BASE tests, the left knee scars were also re-released.

Four months after initial assessment, she only had minimal left knee pain with long walks, was sleeping, and was attending school full time with no absences. She required no prescribed or over-the-counter analgesia medications. On examination, she had normal movements in all core BASE tests with no pain. She was discharged from CPS care and advised to slowly wean MgBis/K2/D3.

4.1.5 Key points

- During examination, it is important to view as much skin as possible to find scars that patients do not remember or acknowledge are present.

- Scar found in the region of most restrictive or painful myoActivation BASE test should be released even if they are small, look normotrophic and are reported as asymptomatic.

- Scars may have to be re-released on subsequent myoActivation sessions.

- myoActivation is unique in enabling the unravelling of multiple contributors to pain, as in this case with low back and left knee pains.

- The patient-physician relationship is enhanced by hands-on examination and demonstration of change with sequential examinations.

- In children and adolescents, it is important to utilise techniques to minimise procedural needling pain.

- As a component of multidisciplinary care, myoActivation enhances recovery, even in patients with a history of years in pain.

4.2 Case 2: non-verbal patient

An 18-year old, 46 kg, non-verbal, wheelchair bound male with cerebral palsy (Gross Motor Function Classification System V), global developmental delay and seizures, was referred to the CPS. His paediatrician requested that the CPS determine if a series of myoActivation sessions might help with ongoing management of worsening bilateral leg spasms and pain. The patient had multi-physician paediatric care of his condition and was optimised on multiple medications (analgesic, antiepileptic, and antispasmodic).

His carer believed that his pain was focused to his legs and was worsened with touching his legs or changing his diaper. It would take him 30–45 minutes to settle and seem calm after diaper changes or turns. Benzodiazepine rescue medication was used to help with spasms at these times. There was no specific pain pattern, with the pain occurring daily and restricting ability to move him and change diapers. There were no changes in skin colour or temperature and no oedema. Each night he is moved every 2 hours as he is unable to move himself; however, his carer felt that sleep was further disturbed by pain. He could not tolerate lying prone.

Multiple surgeries in the past included: posterior spinal instrumentation and fusion T3-Pelvis; right femoral head excision and subtrochanteric valgus osteotomy; circumferential release of capsule right hip; right and left pelvic osteotomy; left femoral osteotomy; and bilateral leg soft tissue releases and Botox injections. His imaging confirmed normal healing and no complications related to his multiple surgeries.

A complete myoActivation assessment examination could not be performed given his non-verbal and wheelchair-bound status. Lying flat multiple bilateral scars were noted from the listed surgeries. His right leg was shortened and externally rotated. There was a torso shift to the right and the pelvis was lower on the right. The right knee was hyper-flexed. The left iliopsoas, rectus femoris and vastus medialis appeared to be in sustained contraction. He was started on MgBis/K2/D3 supplements. One month after initial assessment, scar release was performed under anaesthesia to release all the right-sided leg scars. Scar release consisted of sequential perforation needling of the scar using a 30 g hollow bore needle, using sterile technique.

Two months after initial assessment, myoActivation scar release was done to release all the left sided leg scars and activate the left iliopsoas, left rectus femoris and left vastus medialis under anaesthesia.

At follow up 1 month later, 3 months after initial assessment, his caregiver reported that he was much happier with no further episodes of crying out in pain with movement or diaper changes. He was also able to lie on his front without any issues.

4.2.1 Key points

- It is difficult to assess pain in a non-verbal patient.

- Children and adolescents with developmental delay may not be able to participate in a structured myoActivation examination; therefore, the pain physician will have to rely on parent or carer observations (most painful movements or triggers of pain, most comfortable positions when awake and during sleep).

- In a non-verbal patient, clinical experience and acumen determine if there is a myofascial component to the patient's pain and help direct therapy to the most likely sources of myofascial pain.

- As in developmentally normal children, techniques to minimise procedural needling pain are essential, as in this case where multiple scars were released utilising procedural sedation.

4.3 Case 3: patient requiring general anaesthetic for release of foot scar, distant from pain site

A 14-year old, 57 kg male was referred to the CPS for management of chronic left shoulder pain of 7 months duration. His pain was severe, graded as 8/10 on a visual analogue scale, localised to the left shoulder with no radiation. There was no inciting event to his pain. The pain was exacerbated by any movement of his shoulder. He had mild left sided hemiplegia secondary to removal of a thalamic astrocytoma at age 6. He had undergone a left ankle tendon transfer at age 13. He reported that pain significantly affected his ability to fall and stay asleep. His TiLT inventory revealed he had had a fractured left ankle, but no MVAs. He had scars related to the above surgeries as well as scars from his right sided venous access device, which was inserted at the time of diagnosis of his astrocytoma and removed a year later upon successful treatment of his oncological presentation. He was otherwise healthy, and his family history was unremarkable.

He was assessed by his orthopaedic surgeon, neurologist and oncologist. Previous classical examination, imaging (X-rays, CT and MRI) and bloodwork revealed no remedial cause of his pain and no recurrence of his astrocytoma. Prior to referral to CPS, he was already integrated with regular physiotherapy and intermittent massage therapy. Medications at initial assessment were as required tramadol, acetaminophen, and ibuprofen. myoActivation examination revealed a myofascial component to his pain. In view of distressing pain symptoms, it was agreed that myoActivation should be performed at the initial assessment to help relieve his pain. Written consent was obtained and myoActivation information given to the family. Distraction techniques and vapocoolant spray were used to minimise procedural pain.

The left external oblique, left subscapularis, left platysma were released based on structured regional tests for the shoulder [116]. After this first myoActivation session, the patient experienced immediate improvement in range of motion of the left shoulder and decreased pain. Eight days after this myoActivation session the patient reported that his left shoulder pain was "way better than before" and his mum reported that he was complaining less about his shoulder and was able to sleep better. He had some ongoing left shoulder pain. Repeat myoActivation was performed at one-month intervals using BASE tests and regional test for shoulder function. On the fourth and final myoActivation session his left foot scars were released. As foot scars can be painful, even with appropriately applied topical anaesthetic and vapocoolant spray, it was agreed to release these scars with procedural sedation using standard anaesthetic monitoring and care.

At the time of discharge, 3 months after initial assessment, he had no pain, he was able to function physically within the restrictions of his existing hemiplegia, but with no pain, and was attending school full time. He was discharged from CPS care and advised to slowly wean MgBis/K2/D3. Fourteen months after discharge he remains pain free.

4.3.1 Key points

- In the presentation of severe ongoing pain, it is sometimes important to address regional tests, like the shoulder in this case before addressing potential myofascial triggers in BASE tests.

- For some children and adolescents, there is a need for a general anaesthetic to perform needling of scars or trigger points: for example, in anxiety/mood disorder, young age, non-verbal patients, or where it will be considered too painful (e.g., foot scars) as in this case.

- Distant site same-side scars can be clinically important with respect to the tension they create through myofascial chains and biotensegrity principles described above. For example, left foot scar release to resolve left shoulder pain as outlined in this case.

4.4 Case 4: standard myoActivation assessment and treatment of multisite pain

A 15-year-old, 57 kg female was referred to the CPS by her orthopaedic physician for management of right knee pain of 3 years duration with a diagnosis of "possible tendonitis or tendinosis of medial hamstring" with normal blood work and imaging (X-rays and MRI). Her main hobby was horse riding and she had sustained multiple injuries related to her recreational activities. She related her knee pain to one of these injuries, 3 years ago, when she was bucked off her horse and then the horse stood on her right knee. Immediately after this injury, she attended the local ER and was discharged after normal imaging. She initially mobilised with crutches and gradually regained physical functioning over the course of the subsequent 2 months.

She described her current pain as dull and achy with stabbing pain elements radiating up her leg and down into her calf. Pain was aggravated by running, horse riding, doing squats, or any other physical activities or exercise. She had to wear a knee brace and only used the left stirrup when riding her horse as use of the right stirrup aggravated her right knee pain. She reported no effect on mood related to her pain. She had not been absent from school in the previous 3 months. She reported that pain sometimes affected her ability to fall asleep. Her TiLT inventory revealed multiple horse-riding related injuries. She reported that she had scars from a recent laparoscopic appendicectomy and scars on her right knee from a wire penetrating injury when she was aged 6. She had been using over-the-counter simple analgesia as required. She was otherwise healthy and her family history was unremarkable.

myoActivation examination revealed unreported scars on the right knee and the abdomen, fascia in tension, and multiple muscles in sustained contraction. A myofascial component to her pain was diagnosed. She was enrolled in the 3P care plan. She was started on MgBis/K2/D3. Written information about myoActivation was given to the family.

4.4.1 myoActivation session 1

Five weeks later she reported feeling better and stronger, but no real change in her knee pain. It was deemed appropriate to proceed with myoActivation at this time. Written consent was obtained. Distraction techniques, vapocoolant spray and topical anaesthetic for scars were used to minimise procedural pain. All needling was done using sterile technique.

The right thoracic paraspinal, and right gluteus medius were sequentially activated based on the repeat cycles of assessment to determine the most restrictive and painful BASE tests [116]. The three appendicectomy scars and right knee scar were in regions of worst BASE tests so they were considered significant and released. After this first myoActivation session, the patient experienced immediate improvement in pain and range of motion in all BASE tests.

4.4.2 myoActivation session 2

Three weeks after her first myoActivation session, the patient reported that her right knee pain had moved down to the inner aspect of the right calf. The pain felt was less than on initial assessment. She reported that she could sit in saddle, horse riding for longer, but found eversion of her ankles painful. The left iliopsoas and left rectus abdominis were sequentially activated based on the repeat cycles of assessment to determine the most restrictive and painful BASE tests [116]. The three appendicectomy scars were again in regions of worst BASE tests so they were considered significant and re-released. After this myoActivation session, the patient experienced immediate improvement in pain and range of motion in all BASE tests.

Three months after initial assessment, she reported she could move better, had less pain, was horse riding for much longer with both feet in the stirrups. She required no over-the-counter analgesia medications. On examination, she had normal movements in all core BASE tests with no pain. She was discharged from CPS care and advised to slowly wean MgBis/K2/D3.

4.4.3 Key points

- The site of pain may not be the true source of pain. The right hamstrings were never activated, even though they were the initial site of pain.

- Release of a scar from the youngest age in the region of most restrictive or painful myoActivation BASE test can make clinically substantial change, as was the case for this girl.

- Scars acquired after onset of pain may also play an important role in a myofascial pain presentation.

- This case again illustrates that myoActivation, as a component of multidisciplinary care, enhances recovery even in patients with a history of years in pain and multiple injuries.

4.5 Case 5: standard myoActivation assessment and treatment of chronic multi-site pain secondary to trauma related pelvic and femoral fractures

A 16-year old, 57 kg, female was referred to the CPS for management of multisite pain related to injuries sustained when hit by a car whilst crossing a road. She was referred by her orthopaedic surgeon, 1 year following injury, when ongoing recovery of physical functioning was hampered by multisite pain. She had been fit and healthy prior to this accident.

She was a pedestrian who was struck on the right side and knocked down sustaining multiple pelvic ring fractures and a left femoral fracture. She sustained no other injuries. She required external fixators and an intramedullary femoral rod to stabilise her fractures and control blood loss at the time of admission. She was an inpatient in hospital for a month and then transferred for inpatient rehabilitation at a local rehabilitation centre. The external fixator was removed 2 months after application. She was discharged from the rehabilitation centre 5 months after the date of her presenting injury. She continued with ongoing outpatient physiotherapy, kinesiology, daily exercises and regular counselling but had recently stopped seeing a physiotherapist due to lack of financial support. Imaging confirmed normal healing and no complications related to the surgical sites.

The pain was multisite, affecting the upper, mid and low back, left knee, bilateral thighs, and bilateral ankles with no radiation and no motor or sensory deficits. Her pain was variable and intermittent, but aggravated by exercise. She had been absent from school for 5 days in the previous 3 months due to pain. She reported that pain also affected her ability to fall and stay asleep. Her lifetime trauma history revealed no other injuries. She took ibuprofen as required. She was otherwise healthy and her family history was unremarkable.

myoActivation examination revealed a myofascial component to her pain. Scars were noted from the external fixator and at the site of the left intramedullary nail. There were also abrasion scars from the injury on the left thigh and hip. She was enrolled in the 3P care plan and was started on MgBis/K2/D3. Written myoActivation information was given to the family.

One month later, there was a reduction in pain with improved fluidity of movements just with the addition of MgBis/K2/D3 and re-engagement with physiotherapy. It was deemed appropriate to proceed with myoActivation at this one-month follow-up visit, based on her very stoical character. Written consent was obtained. Distraction techniques and vapocoolant spray were used to minimise procedural pain. Fascial densification, muscles in sustained contraction and the scars in areas of most significant BASE tests [116] were released. Release of the surgical scars and the scars related to the injury made a clinically significant change in pain and range of motion during these sessions.

With such significant injuries and multiple areas required to be treated, she required nine myoActivation session in the course of the following year whilst integrated with the CPS. At the time of discharge, 16 months after initial assessment, she was able to function physically with no restrictions and minimal pain. She was sleeping well and successfully graduated from school with good marks. She noted that her scars were paler, flatter and less obvious than at the start of therapy. She was discharged from CPS care and advised to slowly wean MgBis/K2/D3.

4.5.1 Key points

- Patient reported change in function, just related to institution of the 3P approach, massage, and MgBis/K2/D3, helps to confirm a myofascial component to pain.
- This approach, with the addition of myoActivation, can have a substantial impact even in the presence of such devastating previous injuries.
- Release of the surgical scars and the scars related to the injury made clinically significant change for this patient.

The cases cited above have provided a view of how scars have made a substantial impact in pain presentation. Scar release (using a needling technique) helped make meaningful change for these patients, often when all other avenues of classic medical care for pain aetiology and resolution had been exhausted. Not only is this rewarding for the patients and their families, but also the CPS team who are helping them in their journey to recovery.

5. Conclusion

Humans exhibit biotensegrity, where each individual part of the organism combines with the mechanical system to create an integrated functional movement unit. All structures of the human body are intricately connected through skin and the myofascial system, they are in a continual process of change dependant on and adapting to the forces acting on and within them. When tissue is breached by surgery or injury, the healing process leads to the formation of scar tissue. Scars can limit normal movement of underlying and remote tissues. Defective fascial sliding, secondary to scars, generates anomalous tension that affects the fascial continuum and may lead to distorted biomechanics and chronic pain.

Scars are common in the paediatric population and are significant contributory factors to chronic pain. Many years, even decades, may pass between scar acquisition and the development of biomechanical dysfunction or myofascial pain. A subsequent trauma may be the inciting event as force transmission throughout the body is changed by a scar. Hence, it is important to assess the TiLT inventory, and characteristics of all scars, even when they appear to look "normal".

There are many characteristics of a scar that disrupt the myofascial system, which have been highlighted in the cases discussed. When scars are deemed significant, scar release should be considered as one component in a multidisciplinary approach to address the whole biopsychosocial aspects of chronic pain [136]. Scar and myofascial release, with soft tissue mobilisation or needling techniques, can result in immediate and sustainable improvements in pain, flexibility, and range of motion [116]. When contemplating scar release, consideration should be given to minimising procedural pain and to ensure support for any emotional reactions that may occur immediately or within the hours following scar release.

Research is required to ascertain the exact characteristics of a scar that determine whether it will have a significant contribution to myofascial dysfunction and chronic pain. The cases presented above illustrate that these investigations must recognise the multiple and complex biopsychosocial factors that contribute to a myofascial chronic pain presentation.

Whilst definitive answers are awaited, we need to think beyond scars as just being innocuous mementos of the past. Clinical experience indicates that they may be restrictive barriers, exerting pervasive biomechanical and nociceptive effects in the present. Left untreated, that "*strange power*" *of a scar* may go on to have substantial impact in the future as well.

Acknowledgements

The authors would like to thank Dr. Doug Courtemanche and Dr. Greg Siren for their insightful comments on a draft of this chapter.

Conflict of interest

The authors have no conflicts of interest to declare.

Author details

Gillian Lauder[1*] and Nicholas West[2]

1 Pediatric Anesthesiologist and Pediatric Complex Pain Physician, BC Children's Hospital, Vancouver, BC, Canada

2 Clinical Research Coordinator, University of British Columbia, Vancouver, BC, Canada

*Address all correspondence to: glauder@cw.bc.ca

References

[1] Jablonski NG. Skin: A Natural History. Berkeley, CA: University of California Press; 2006

[2] Virador GM, de Marcos L, Virador VM. Skin wound healing: Refractory wounds and novel solutions. In: Turksen K, editor. Skin Stem Cells: Methods and Protocols. Totowa, NJ: Humana Press; 2018. pp. 221-241

[3] Keppel Hesselink J, Kopsky D, Bhaskar A. Skin matters! The role of keratinocytes in nociception: A rational argument for the development of topical analgesics. Journal of Pain Research. 2016;**10**:1-8

[4] González-Hernández A, Manzano-García A, Martínez-Lorenzana G, Tello-García IA, Carranza M, Arámburo C, et al. Peripheral oxytocin receptors inhibit the nociceptive input signal to spinal dorsal horn wide-dynamic-range neurons. Pain. 2017;**158**(11):2117-2128

[5] Cunha TM, Verri WA, Silva JS, Poole S, Cunha FQ, Ferreira SH. A cascade of cytokines mediates mechanical inflammatory hypernociception in mice. Proceedings of the National Academy of Sciences. 2005;**102**(5):1755-1760

[6] Manjavachi MN, Costa R, Quintão NL, Calixto JB. The role of keratinocyte-derived chemokine (KC) on hyperalgesia caused by peripheral nerve injury in mice. Neuropharmacology. 2014;**79**:17-27

[7] Pang Z, Sakamoto T, Tiwari V, Kim Y-S, Yang F, Dong X, et al. Selective keratinocyte stimulation is sufficient to evoke nociception in mice. Pain. 2015;**156**(4):656-665

[8] Drummond PD, Dawson LF, Finch PM, Drummond ES, Wood FM, Fear MW. Up-regulation of cutaneous α1-adrenoceptors after a burn. Burns. 2015;**41**(6):1227-1234

[9] Yang S, Sun Y, Geng Z, Ma K, Sun X, Fu X. Abnormalities in the basement membrane structure promote basal keratinocytes in the epidermis of hypertrophic scars to adopt a proliferative phenotype. International Journal of Molecular Medicine. 2016;**37**(5):1263-1273

[10] de Vries HJC, Enomoto DNH, van Marle J, van Zuijlen PPM, Mekkes JR, Bos JD. Dermal organization in Scleroderma: The fast Fourier transform and the laser scatter method objectify fibrosis in nonlesional as well as lesional skin. Laboratory Investigation. 2000;**80**(8):1281-1289

[11] Verhaegen PDHM, van Zuijlen PPM, Pennings NM, van Marle J, Niessen FB, van der Horst CMAM, et al. Differences in collagen architecture between keloid, hypertrophic scar, normotrophic scar, and normal skin: An objective histopathological analysis. Wound Repair and Regeneration. 2009;**17**(5):649-656

[12] des Jardins-Park HE, Foster DS, Longaker MT. Fibroblasts and wound healing: An update. Regenerative Medicine. 2018;**13**(5):491-495

[13] Dalsgaard CJ, Rydh M, Haegerstrand A. Cutaneous innervation in man visualized with protein gene product 9.5 (PGP 9.5) antibodies. Histochemistry. 1989;**92**(5):385-390

[14] Caron A, Lee S, Elmquist JK, Gautron L. Leptin and brain–adipose crosstalks. Nature Reviews. Neuroscience. 2018;**19**(3):153-165

[15] Kwon O, Kim KW, Kim M-S. Leptin signalling pathways in hypothalamic neurons. Cellular and Molecular Life Sciences. 2016;**73**(7):1457-1477

[16] Maeda N, Funahashi T, Matsuzawa Y, Shimomura I. Adiponectin, a unique adipocyte-derived factor beyond hormones. Atherosclerosis. 2020;**292**:1-9

[17] Rivera-Gonzalez G, Shook B, Horsley V. Adipocytes in skin health and disease. Cold Spring Harbor Perspectives in Medicine. 2014;**4**(3):a015271-a015271

[18] Bordoni B, Zanier E. Skin, fascias, and scars: Symptoms and systemic connections. Journal of Multidisciplinary Healthcare. 2013;**7**:11-24

[19] Di Meglio P, Perera GK, Nestle FO. The multitasking organ: Recent insights into skin immune function. Immunity. 2011;**35**(6):857-869

[20] Jang SH, Seo JP, Ahn SH, Lee MY. Comparison of cortical activation patterns by somatosensory stimulation on the palm and dorsum of the hand. Somatosensory & Motor Research. 2013;**30**(3):109-113

[21] Mondelli M, Aretini A, Ballerini M, Vecchiarelli B, Rossi A. Sympathetic skin response. Glabella stimulation may be more useful than peripheral nerve stimulation in clinical practice. Autonomic Neuroscience. 2011;**164**(1-2):101-104

[22] Henderson LA, Stathis A, James C, Brown R, McDonald S, Macefield VG. Real-time imaging of cortical areas involved in the generation of increases in skin sympathetic nerve activity when viewing emotionally charged images. NeuroImage. 2012;**62**(1):30-40

[23] Bordoni B, Zanier E. Clinical and symptomatological reflections: The fascial system. Journal of Multidisciplinary Healthcare. 2014;**7**: 401-411

[24] Miranda A, Peles S, Rudolph C, Shaker R, Sengupta JN. Altered visceral sensation in response to somatic pain in the rat☆. Gastroenterology. 2004;**126**(4):1082-1089

[25] Albrecht PJ, Hou Q, Argoff CE, Storey JR, Wymer JP, Rice FL. Excessive Peptidergic sensory innervation of cutaneous arteriole-venule shunts (AVS) in the palmar glabrous skin of fibromyalgia patients: Implications for widespread deep tissue pain and fatigue. Pain Medicine. 2013;**14**(6):895-915

[26] Peppin JF, Albrecht PJ, Argoff C, Gustorff B, Pappagallo M, Rice FL, et al. Skin matters: A review of topical treatments for chronic pain. Part one: Skin physiology and delivery systems. Pain and therapy. 2015;**4**(1):17-32

[27] Driscoll M. Fascia – The unsung hero of spine biomechanics. Journal of Bodywork and Movement Therapies. 2018;**22**(1):90-91

[28] Adstrum S, Nicholson H. A history of fascia. Clinical Anatomy. 2019;**32**(7):862-870

[29] Adstrum S, Hedley G, Schleip R, Stecco C, Yucesoy CA. Defining the fascial system. Journal of Bodywork and Movement Therapies. 2017;**21**(1):173-177

[30] Stecco C, Adstrum S, Hedley G, Schleip R, Yucesoy CA. Update on fascial nomenclature. Journal of Bodywork and Movement Therapies. 2018;**22**(2):354

[31] Avila Gonzalez CA, Driscoll M, Schleip R, Wearing S, Jacobson E, Findley T, et al. Frontiers in fascia research. Journal of Bodywork and Movement Therapies. 2018;**22**(4): 873-880

[32] Stecco C, Fede C, Macchi V, Porzionato A, Petrelli L, Biz C, et al. The fasciacytes: A new cell devoted to fascial gliding regulation. Clinical Anatomy. 2018;**31**(5):667-676

[33] Hughes EJ, McDermott K, Funk MF. Evaluation of hyaluronan content in areas of densification compared to adjacent areas of fascia. Journal of

Bodywork and Movement Therapies. 2019;**23**(2):324-328

[34] Stecco C, Porzionato A, Lancerotto L, Stecco A, Macchi V, Ann Day J, et al. Histological study of the deep fasciae of the limbs. Journal of Bodywork and Movement Therapies. 2008;**12**(3):225-230

[35] Stecco C, Stern R, Porzionato A, Macchi V, Masiero S, Stecco A, et al. Hyaluronan within fascia in the etiology of myofascial pain. Surgical and Radiologic Anatomy. 2011;**33**(10):891-896

[36] Wilke J, Krause F, Vogt L, Banzer W. What is evidence-based about myofascial chains: A systematic review. Archives of Physical Medicine and Rehabilitation. 2016;**97**(3):454-461

[37] Kjaer M, Langberg H, Heinemeier K, Bayer ML, Hansen M, Holm L, et al. From mechanical loading to collagen synthesis, structural changes and function in human tendon. Scandinavian Journal of Medicine & Science in Sports. 2009;**19**(4):500-510

[38] Myers B. Wound Management: Principles and Practices. 3rd ed. Pearson: London, UK; 2012

[39] Bei Y, Wang F, Yang C, Xiao J. Telocytes in regenerative medicine. Journal of Cellular and Molecular Medicine. 2015;**19**(7):1441-1454

[40] Scarr G. Biotensegrity: The Structural Basis of Life. Pencaitland, UK: Handspring Publishing Limited; 2014

[41] Krause F, Wilke J, Vogt L, Banzer W. Intermuscular force transmission along myofascial chains: A systematic review. Journal of Anatomy. 2016;**228**(6):910-918

[42] Tidball JG. Force transmission across muscle cell membranes. Journal of Biomechanics. 1991;**24**:43-52

[43] Zügel M, Maganaris CN, Wilke J, Jurkat-Rott K, Klingler W, Wearing SC, et al. Fascial tissue research in sports medicine: From molecules to tissue adaptation, injury and diagnostics: Consensus statement. British Journal of Sports Medicine. 2018;**52**(23):1497-1497

[44] Dischiavi SL, Wright AA, Hegedus EJ, Bleakley CM. Biotensegrity and myofascial chains: A global approach to an integrated kinetic chain. Medical Hypotheses. 2018;**110**:90-96

[45] Tak I, Glasgow P, Langhout R, Weir A, Kerkhoffs G, Agricola R. Hip range of motion is lower in professional soccer players with hip and groin symptoms or previous injuries, independent of cam deformities. The American Journal of Sports Medicine. 2016;**44**(3):682-688

[46] Tozzi P. Selected fascial aspects of osteopathic practice. Journal of Bodywork and Movement Therapies. 2012;**16**(4):503-519

[47] Stecco C, Gagey O, Belloni A, Pozzuoli A, Porzionato A, Macchi V, et al. Anatomy of the deep fascia of the upper limb. Second part: Study of innervation. Morphologie. 2007;**91**(292):38-43

[48] van der Wal J. The architecture of the connective tissue in the musculoskeletal system-an often overlooked functional parameter as to proprioception in the locomotor apparatus. International Journal of Therapeutic Massage & Bodywork: Research, Education, & Practice. 2009;**2**(4):9-23

[49] Bordoni B, Myers T. A review of the theoretical Fascial models: Biotensegrity, fascintegrity, and myofascial chains. Cureus. 2020;**12**(2):e7092

[50] Varela F, Frenk S. The organ of form: Towards a theory of biological shape. Journal of Social and Biological Systems. 1987;**10**(1):73-83

[51] Susan S, editor. Gray's Anatomy: The Anatomical Basis of Clinical Practice. 41st ed. Amsterdam, The Netherlands: Elsevier; 2015

[52] Karamanos NK, Theocharis AD, Neill T, Iozzo RV. Matrix modeling and remodeling: A biological interplay regulating tissue homeostasis and diseases. Matrix Biology. 2019;**75-76**:1-11

[53] Gantwerker EA, Hom DB. Skin: Histology and physiology of wound healing. Clinics in Plastic Surgery. 2012;**39**(1):85-97

[54] Bran GM, Goessler UR, Hormann K, Riedel F, Sadick H. Keloids: Current concepts of pathogenesis (review). International Journal of Molecular Medicine. 2009;**24**(3):283-293

[55] Lichtman MK, Otero-Vinas M, Falanga V. Transforming growth factor beta (TGF-β) isoforms in wound healing and fibrosis. Wound Repair and Regeneration. 2016;**24**(2):215-222

[56] Sorg H, Tilkorn DJ, Hager S, Hauser J, Mirastschijski U. Skin wound healing: An update on the current knowledge and concepts. European Surgical Research. 2017;**58**(1-2):81-94

[57] Bijlard E, Uiterwaal L, Kouwenberg CAE, Mureau MAM, Hovius SER, Huygen FJPM. A systematic review on the prevalence, etiology, and pathophysiology of intrinsic pain in dermal scar tissue. Pain Physician. 2017;**20**(2):1-13

[58] Zhang L, Laato M. Innervation of normal and hypertrophic human scars and experimental wounds in the rat. Annales Chirurgiae et Gynaecologiae. 2001;**90**(Suppl 215):29-32

[59] Ogawa R. Keloid and hypertrophic scars are the result of chronic inflammation in the reticular dermis. International Journal of Molecular Sciences. 2017;**18**(3):606

[60] Karkampouna S, Kreulen M, Obdeijn MC, Kloen P, Dorjée AL, Rivellese F, et al. Connective tissue degeneration: Mechanisms of palmar fascia degeneration (Dupuytren's disease). Current Molecular Biology Reports. 2016;**2**(3):133-140

[61] Roseborough I, Grevious M, Lee R. Prevention and treatment of excessive dermal scarring. Journal of the National Medical Association. 2004;**96**(1):108-116

[62] Akaishi S, Ogawa R, Hyakusoku H. Keloid and hypertrophic scar: Neurogenic inflammation hypotheses. Medical Hypotheses. 2008;**71**(1):32-38

[63] Ogawa R. Mechanobiology of scarring. Wound Repair and Regeneration. 2011;**19**:s2-s9

[64] Miyamoto J, Nagasao T, Miyamoto S, Nakajima T. Biomechanical analysis of stresses occurring in vertical and transverse scars on the lower leg. Plastic and Reconstructive Surgery. 2009;**124**(6):1974-1979

[65] Wolfram D, Tzankov A, Pülzl P, Piza-Katzer H. Hypertrophic scars and keloids—A review of their pathophysiology, risk factors, and therapeutic management. Dermatologic Surgery. 2009;**35**(2):171-181

[66] Midwood KS, Williams LV, Schwarzbauer JE. Tissue repair and the dynamics of the extracellular matrix. The International Journal of Biochemistry & Cell Biology. 2004;**36**(6):1031-1037

[67] el Hayderi L, Nikkels-Tassoudji N, Nikkels AF. Incidence of and risk factors for cutaneous scarring after herpes zoster. American Journal of Clinical Dermatology. 2018;**19**(6):893-897

[68] Leung AKC, Kao CP, Sauve RS. Scarring resulting from chickenpox. Pediatric Dermatology. 2001;**18**(5):378-380

[69] Connolly D, Vu HL, Mariwalla K, Saedi N. Acne scarring-pathogenesis, evaluation, and treatment options. The Journal of Clinical and Aesthetic Dermatology. 2017;**10**(9):12-23

[70] Krakowski AC, Totri CR, Donelan MB, Shumaker PR. Scar Management in the pediatric and adolescent populations. Pediatrics. 2016;**137**(2):e20142065-e20142065

[71] Reinholz M, Schwaiger H, Poetschke J, Epple A, Ruzicka T, Von Braunmühl T, et al. Objective and subjective treatment evaluation of scars using optical coherence tomography, sonography, photography, and standardised questionnaires. European Journal of Dermatology. 2016;**26**(6):599-608

[72] Cheng W, Saing H, Zhou H, Han Y, Peh W, Tam PKH. Ultrasound assessment of scald scars in Asian children receiving pressure garment therapy. Journal of Pediatric Surgery. 2001;**36**(3):466-469

[73] Simons M, Kee EG, Kimble R, Tyack Z. Ultrasound is a reproducible and valid tool for measuring scar height in children with burn scars: A cross-sectional study of the psychometric properties and utility of the ultrasound and 3D camera. Burns. 2017;**43**(5):993-1001

[74] Ferriero G, Di Carlo S, Ferriero A, Salgovic L, Bravini E, Sartorio F, et al. Post-surgical scar assessment in rehabilitation: A systematic review. Physical Therapy Rehabilitation. 2015;**2**(1):2

[75] Klingler W, Velders M, Hoppe K, Pedro M, Schleip R. Clinical relevance of fascial tissue and dysfunctions. Current Pain and Headache Reports. 2014;**18**(8):439

[76] Martínez Rodríguez R, Galán del Río F. Mechanistic basis of manual therapy in myofascial injuries. Sonoelastographic evolution control. Journal of Bodywork and Movement Therapies. 2013;**17**(2):221-234

[77] Guo R, Xiang X, Wang L, Zhu B, Cheng S, Qiu L. Quantitative assessment of keloids using ultrasound shear wave elastography. Ultrasound in Medicine & Biology. 2020;**46**(5):1169-1178

[78] DeJong HM, Abbott S, Zelesco M, Kennedy BF, Ziman MR, Wood FM. The validity and reliability of using ultrasound elastography to measure cutaneous stiffness, a systematic review. International Journal of Burns and Trauma. 2017;7(7):124-141

[79] Perry DM, McGrouther DA, Bayat A. Current tools for noninvasive objective assessment of skin scars. Plastic and Reconstructive Surgery. 2010;**126**(3):912-923

[80] Gold M, Berman B, Clementoni M, Gauglitz G, Nahai F, Murcia C. Updated international clinical recommendations on scar management: Part 1--evaluating the evidence. Dermatologic Surgery. 2014;**40**(8):817-824

[81] Gold MH, McGuire M, Mustoe TA, Pusic A, Sachdev M, Waibel J, et al. Updated international clinical recommendations on scar management: Part 2--algorithms for scar prevention and treatment. Dermatologic Surgery. 2014;**40**(8):825-831

[82] Arno AI, Gauglitz GG, Barret JP, Jeschke MG. Up-to-date approach to manage keloids and hypertrophic scars: A useful guide. Burns. 2014;**40**(7):1255-1266

[83] Arno AI, Gauglitz GG, Barret JP, Jeschke MG. New molecular medicine-based scar management strategies. Burns. 2014;**40**(4):539-551

[84] Wasserman JB, Steele-Thornborrow JL, Yuen JS, Halkiotis M, Riggins EM.

Chronic caesarian section scar pain treated with fascial scar release techniques: A case series. Journal of Bodywork and Movement Therapies. 2016;**20**(4):906-913

[85] Nikolajsen L, Sørensen HC, Jensen TS, Kehlet H. Chronic pain following caesarean section. Acta Anaesthesiologica Scandinavica. 2004;**48**(1):111-116

[86] de Brito Cançado TO, Omais M, Ashmawi HA, Torres MLA. Chronic pain after cesarean section. Influence of anesthetic/surgical technique and postoperative analgesia. Brazilian Journal of Anesthesiology. 2012;**62**(6):762-774

[87] Scott JR, Muangman P, Gibran NS. Making sense of hypertrophic scar: A role for nerves. Wound Repair and Regeneration. 2007;**15**(Suppl 1): S27-S31

[88] Shayani V, Siegert C, Favia P. The role of laparoscopic adhesiolysis in the treatment of patients with chronic abdominal pain or recurrent bowel obstruction. JSLS. 2002;**6**(2):111-114

[89] Kindermann G, Debus-Thiede G. 18 postoperative urological complications after radical surgery for cervical cancer. Baillière's Clinical Obstetrics and Gynaecology. 1988;**2**(4):933-941

[90] Isla A, Alvarez F. Fibrosis epidural espinal postdiscectomía lumbar y barrera antiadhesiva. Neurocirugia. 2001;**12**(5):439-446

[91] Lewit K, Olsanska S. Clinical importance of active scars: Abnormal scars as a cause of myofascial pain. Journal of Manipulative and Physiological Therapeutics. 2004;**27**(6):399-402

[92] Kobesova A, Morris CE, Lewit K, Safarova M. Twenty-year-old pathogenic "active" postsurgical scar: A case study of a patient with persistent right lower quadrant pain. Journal of Manipulative and Physiological Therapeutics. 2007;**30**(3):234-238

[93] Valouchová P, Lewit K. Surface electromyography of abdominal and back muscles in patients with active scars. Journal of Bodywork and Movement Therapies. 2009;**13**(3):262-267

[94] Wasserman JB, Copeland M, Upp M, Abraham K. Effect of soft tissue mobilization techniques on adhesion-related pain and function in the abdomen: A systematic review. Journal of Bodywork and Movement Therapies. 2019;**23**(2):262-269

[95] Serra-Añó P, Inglés M, Bou-Catalá C, Iraola-Lliso A, Espí-López GV. Effectiveness of myofascial release after breast cancer surgery in women undergoing conservative surgery and radiotherapy: A randomized controlled trial. Supportive Care in Cancer. 2019;**27**(7): 2633-2641

[96] McKay RMTE. Assessing the effectiveness of massage therapy for bilateral cleft lip reconstruction scars. The International Journal of Therapeutic Massage & Bodywork: Research, Education, & Practice. 2014;**7**(2):3-9

[97] Myers TW. Anatomy Trains: Myofascial Meridians for Manual and Movement Therapists. 2nd ed. London, UK: Churchill Livingstone; 2008

[98] Alvira-Lechuz J, Espiau MR, Alvira-Lechuz E. Treatment of the scar after arthroscopic surgery on a knee. Journal of Bodywork and Movement Therapies. 2017;**21**(2):328-333

[99] Benjamin M. The fascia of the limbs and back--a review. Journal of Anatomy. 2009;**214**(1):1-18

[100] Stecco A, Stern R, Fantoni I, De Caro R, Stecco C. Fascial disorders:

Implications for treatment. PM & R: The Journal of Injury, Function, and Rehabilitation. 2016;**8**(2):161-168

[101] Bednar DA, Orr FW, Simon GT. Observations on the pathomorphology of the thoracolumbar fascia in chronic mechanical back pain. A microscopic study. Spine (Phila Pa 1976). 1995; **20**(10):1161-1164

[102] Langevin HM, Fox JR, Koptiuch C, Badger GJ, Greenan-Naumann AC, Bouffard NA, et al. Reduced thoracolumbar fascia shear strain in human chronic low back pain. BMC Musculoskeletal Disorders. 2011;**12**:203

[103] Chaitow L. Somatic dysfunction and fascia's gliding-potential. Journal of Bodywork and Movement Therapies. 2014;**18**(1):1-3

[104] Wilke J, Schleip R, Yucesoy CA, Banzer W. Not merely a protective packing organ? A review of fascia and its force transmission capacity. Journal of Applied Physiology. 2018;**124**(1):234-244

[105] Schleip R, Zorn A, Klingler W. Biomechanical properties of fascial tissues and their role as pain generators. The Journal of Musculoskeletal Pain. 2010;**18**(4):393-395

[106] Kwong EH, Findley TW. Fascia–current knowledge and future directions in physiatry: Narrative review. Journal of Rehabilitation Research and Development. 2014;**51**(6):875-884

[107] Gibson W, Arendt-Nielsen L, Taguchi T, Mizumura K, Graven-Nielsen T. Increased pain from muscle fascia following eccentric exercise: Animal and human findings. Experimental Brain Research. 2009;**194**(2):299-308

[108] Ajimsha MS, Daniel B, Chithra S. Effectiveness of myofascial release in the management of chronic low back pain in nursing professionals. Journal of Bodywork and Movement Therapies. 2014;**18**(2):273-281

[109] Day JA, Stecco C, Stecco A. Application of fascial manipulation© technique in chronic shoulder pain—Anatomical basis and clinical implications. Journal of Bodywork and Movement Therapies. 2009;**13**(2):128-135

[110] Langevin HM, Bishop J, Maple R, Badger GJ, Fox JR. Effect of stretching on thoracolumbar fascia injury and movement restriction in a porcine model. American Journal of Physical Medicine & Rehabilitation. 2018;**97**(3):187-191

[111] Henry R, Cahill CM, Wood G, Hroch J, Wilson R, Cupido T, et al. Myofascial pain in patients waitlisted for total knee arthroplasty. Pain Research & Management. 2012;**17**(5):321-327

[112] Earl J. A small scale study to establish if an abdominal scar is a factor in lower back pain [dissertation]. 2015. Available from: https://jackieearl.co.uk/images/Dissertation_Final_Copy.pdf [Accessed: 12 June 2020]

[113] Willard FH, Vleeming A, Schuenke MD, Danneels L, Schleip R. The thoracolumbar fascia: Anatomy, function and clinical considerations. Journal of Anatomy. 2012;**221**(6):507-536

[114] Ljungqvist A, Schwellnus MP, Bachl N, Collins M, Cook J, Khan KM, et al. International Olympic Committee consensus statement: Molecular basis of connective tissue and muscle injuries in sport. Clinics in Sports Medicine. 2008;**27**(1):231-239

[115] Langevin HM, Stevens-Tuttle D, Fox JR, Badger GJ, Bouffard NA, Krag MH, et al. Ultrasound evidence of altered lumbar connective tissue structure in human subjects with chronic low back pain. BMC Musculoskeletal Disorders. 2009;**10**(1):151

[116] Lauder G, West N, Siren G. myoActivation: A structured process for chronic pain resolution. In: Cascella M, editor. From Conventional to Innovative Approaches for Pain Treatment. London: IntechOpen; 2019. DOI: 10.5772/intechopen.84377

[117] Miazga S, West N, Ng M, Lauder G. myoActivation, a structured system for assessment and management of chronic pain: A retrospective review of pediatric cases. In: University of British Columbia Department of Anesthesiology, Pharmacology & Therapeutics 14th Annual Research Day. Canada: Vancouver; 2020

[118] Minasny B. Understanding the process of fascial unwinding. International Journal of Therapeutic Massage & Bodywork: Research, Education, & Practice. 2009;**2**(3):10-17

[119] Wasserman JB, Abraham K, Massery M, Chu J, Farrow A, Marcoux BC. Soft tissue mobilization techniques are effective in treating chronic pain following cesarean section. Journal of Women's Health Physical Therapy. 2018;**42**(3):111-119

[120] Chung MK, LaRiccia PJ. Successful integrative medicine assessment and treatment of chronic pain associated with breast surgery: A report of 3 cases. Holistic Nursing Practice. 2017;**31**(1):21-29

[121] Costa IMC, Costa MC. Microneedling for varicella scars in a dark-skinned teenager. Dermatologic Surgery. 2014;**40**(3):333-334

[122] Alster TS, Graham PM. Microneedling: A review and practical guide. Dermatologic Surgery. 2018;**44**(3):397-404

[123] Orentreich DS, Orentreich N. Subcutaneous incisionless (subcision) surgery for the correction of depressed scars and wrinkles. Dermatologic Surgery. 1995;**21**(6):543-549

[124] Ramaut L, Hoeksema H, Pirayesh A, Stillaert F, Monstrey S. Microneedling: Where do we stand now? A systematic review of the literature. Journal of Plastic, Reconstructive & Aesthetic Surgery. 2018;**71**(1):1-14

[125] Hou A, Cohen B, Haimovic A, Elbuluk N. Microneedling: A comprehensive review. Dermatologic Surgery. 2017;**43**(3):321-339

[126] Schwarz M, Laaff H. A prospective controlled assessment of microneedling with the dermaroller device. Plastic and Reconstructive Surgery. 2011;**127**(6):146e-148e

[127] Nair P, Arora T. Microneedling using dermaroller a means of collagen induction therapy. Gujarat Medical Journal. 2014;**69**(1):24-27

[128] Aust MC, Fernandes D, Kolokythas P, Kaplan HM, Vogt PM. Percutaneous collagen induction therapy: An alternative treatment for scars, wrinkles, and skin laxity. Plastic and Reconstructive Surgery. 2008;**121**(4):1421-1429

[129] Aust MC, Knobloch K, Reimers K, Redeker J, Ipaktchi R, Altintas MA, et al. Percutaneous collagen induction therapy: An alternative treatment for burn scars. Burns. 2010;**36**(6):836-843

[130] Aust MC, Reimers K, Kaplan HM, Stahl F, Repenning C, Scheper T, et al. Percutaneous collagen induction–regeneration in place of cicatrisation? Journal of Plastic, Reconstructive & Aesthetic Surgery. 2011;**64**(1):97-107

[131] Doddaballapur S. Microneedling with dermaroller. Journal of Cutaneous and Aesthetic Surgery. 2009;**2**(2):110

[132] Fabbrocini G, Fardella N, Monfrecola A, Proietti I, Innocenzi D. Acne scarring treatment using skin needling. Clinical and Experimental Dermatology. 2009;**34**(8):874-879

[133] Bonati LM, Epstein GK, Strugar TL. Microneedling in all skin types: A review. Journal of Drugs in Dermatology. 2017;**16**(4):308-313

[134] Cagnie B, Dewitte V, Barbe T, Timmermans F, Delrue N, Meeus M. Physiologic effects of dry needling. Current Pain and Headache Reports. 2013;**17**(8):348

[135] Liu X, Zhu B, Zhang SX. Relationship between electroacupuncture analgesia and descending pain inhibitory mechanism of nucleus raphe magnus. Pain. 1986;**24**(3):383-396

[136] Lauder GR, Huang J, West NC. Unrecognized myofascial components of pediatric complex pain: myoActivation, a structured solution for assessment and management. Current Trends in Medicine. 2019;**1**(1):1-16

[137] Tozzi P. Does fascia hold memories? Journal of Bodywork and Movement Therapies. 2014;**18**(2):259-265

[138] Rothschild B. The Body Remembers: The Psychophysiology of Trauma and Trauma Treatment. New York: W. W. Norton & Company; 2000

[139] Hakala P, Rimpelä A, Salminen JJ, Virtanen SM, Rimpelä M. Back, neck, and shoulder pain in Finnish adolescents: National cross sectional surveys. BMJ. 2002;**325**(7367):743

[140] Sperotto F, Brachi S, Vittadello F, Zulian F. Musculoskeletal pain in schoolchildren across puberty: A 3-year follow-up study. Pediatric Rheumatology Online Journal. 2015;**13**:16

[141] Huguet A, Tougas ME, Hayden J, McGrath PJ, Stinson JN, Chambers CT. Systematic review with meta-analysis of childhood and adolescent risk and prognostic factors for musculoskeletal pain. Pain. 2016;**157**(12):2640-2656

[142] Silva GRR, Pitangui ACR, Xavier MKA, Correia-Júnior MAV, De Araújo RC. Prevalence of musculoskeletal pain in adolescents and association with computer and videogame use. Jornal de Pediatria. 2016;**92**(2):188-196

[143] Queiroz LB, Lourenço B, Silva LEV, Lourenço DMR, Silva CA. Musculoskeletal pain and musculoskeletal syndromes in adolescents are related to electronic devices. Jornal de Pediatria. 2018;**94**(6): 673-679

[144] Leino-Arjas P, Rajaleid K, Mekuria G, Nummi T, Virtanen P, Hammarström A. Trajectories of musculoskeletal pain from adolescence to middle age: The role of early depressive symptoms, a 27-year follow-up of the northern Swedish cohort. Pain. 2018;**159**(1):67-74

[145] Kyu HH, Pinho C, Wagner JA, Brown JC, Bertozzi-Villa A, Charlson FJ, et al. Global and national burden of diseases and injuries among children and adolescents between 1990 and 2013. JAMA Pediatrics. 2016;**170**(3):267

[146] King S, Chambers CT, Huguet A, MacNevin RC, McGrath PJ, Parker L, et al. The epidemiology of chronic pain in children and adolescents revisited: A systematic review. Pain. 2011;**152**(12):2729-2738

[147] Jones GT, Macfarlane GJ. Epidemiology of low back pain in children and adolescents. Archives of Disease in Childhood. 2005;**90**(3):312-316

[148] Salminen JJ. The adolescent back. A field survey of 370 Finnish schoolchildren. Acta Paediatrica Scandinavica. Supplement. 1984;**315**: 1-122

[149] Oksanen AM, Laimi K, Löyttyniemi E, Kunttu K. Trends of

weekly musculoskeletal pain from 2000 to 2012: National study of Finnish university students. European Journal of Pain. 2014;**18**(9):1316-1322

[150] Mikkelsson M, El-Metwally A, Kautiainen H, Auvinen A, Macfarlane GJ, Salminen JJ. Onset, prognosis and risk factors for widespread pain in schoolchildren: A prospective 4-year follow-up study. Pain. 2008;**138**(3): 681-687

[151] Gobina I, Villberg J, Välimaa R, Tynjälä J, Whitehead R, Cosma A, et al. Prevalence of self-reported chronic pain among adolescents: Evidence from 42 countries and regions. European Journal of Pain. 2019;**23**(2):316-326

[152] van den Heuvel MM, Jansen PW, Bindels PJE, Bierma-Zeinstra SMA, van Middelkoop M. Musculoskeletal pain in 6-year-old children. Pain. 2020;**161**(6):1278-1285

[153] Friedrichsdorf SJ, Giordano J, Desai Dakoji K, Warmuth A, Daughtry C, Schulz CA. Chronic pain in children and adolescents: Diagnosis and treatment of primary pain disorders in head, abdomen, muscles and joints. Children. 2016;**3**(4):pii: E42

[154] Lee YJ, Kim S-H, Chung SW, Lee Y-K, Koo K-H. Causes of chronic hip pain undiagnosed or misdiagnosed by primary physicians in young adult patients: A retrospective descriptive study. Journal of Korean Medical Science. 2018;**33**(52):e339

[155] Feinberg BI, Feinberg RA. Persistent pain after total knee arthroplasty: Treatment with manual therapy and trigger point injections. The Journal of Musculoskeletal Pain. 1998;**6**(4):85-95

[156] Ingber RS. Iliopsoas myofascial dysfunction: A treatable cause of "failed" low back syndrome. Archives of Physical Medicine and Rehabilitation. 1989;**70**(5):382-386

[157] Tay A, Chua K, Chan K-F. Upper quarter myofascial pain syndrome in Singapore: Characteristics and treatment. The Journal of Musculoskeletal Pain. 2000;**8**(4):49-56

[158] Vadivelu N, Mitra S, Hines RL. Undergraduate medical education on pain management across the globe. Virtual Mentoring. 2013;**15**(5):421-427

[159] Canadian Medical Protective Association. What happened to the physical exam? [Internet]. 2019. Available from: https://www.cmpa-acpm.ca/en/advice-publications/browse-articles/2019/what-happened-to-the-physical-exam [Accessed: 26 July 2019]

[160] Clark BW, Derakhshan A, Desai SV. Diagnostic errors and the bedside clinical examination. The Medical Clinics of North America. 2018;**102**(3):453-464

Chapter 8

Suffering as a Diagnostic Indicator

Marek Rózycki and Robert Tobias

Abstract

Pain is the subjective sensation closely related to disease and treatment. Very often its diagnosis is more an expression of the diagnostician's experience than a description of the patient's actual condition. In particular, orthopedic and neurological patients who develop Complex Regional Pain Syndrome are misdiagnosed because the intensity of their sensations is disbelieved. Based on case studies, it seems appropriate to introduce an additional category of patient experience that will enable prompt recognition and appropriate treatment. The misdiagnoses under evaluation also exhibit frequent improper practitioner responses to patients' experience, ranging from open expressions of disbelief, through indifference, to helplessness and pessimism. This article presents case studies in which patients' expressions of suffering were not used to modify the treatment. Rather, medical professionals accepted the pain as normal under the circumstances and resulting from tissue damage. However, in these cases, the pain was a symptom of a new disease entity, in development since the original diagnosis. With improved patient communication and treatment procedures, such oversights can be avoided and new disease entities will be more readily diagnosable.

Keywords: pain, suffering, CRPS, diagnostic indicator

1. Introduction

Complex Regional Pain Syndrome or CRPS, is a chronic pain syndrome. Pain in medical treatment is frequently an expected symptom, and a normal manifestation of tissue trauma. However, when it reaches levels of intensity and duration beyond the expected, it may present as CRPS: it is no longer a symptom but a separate disease entity capable of making the affected person's life insufferable. CRPS may be triggered by a preceding condition. However, key to its diagnosis is the lack of any obvious tissue-related causes of pain. Its relative uncommonness has resulted in widely divergent reports by medical professionals over the years. Often, it was simply pain which eluded understanding. This has led to a host of labels used to describe it across time and in different countries. Currently, the following conditions are roughly equivalent to what is understood as CRPS:

1. Algoneurodystrophy

2. Sudeck's atrophy

3. Sudeck's disease

4. Sudeck's dystrophy (referring only to radiological features in osteoporosis)

5. Causalgia (also known as CRPS Type 2 when accompanied by nerve damage)
6. Peripheral trophoneurosis
7. Reflex sympathetic dystrophy - commonly abbreviated as RSD
8. Babinski-Froment sympathetic paralysis
9. Leriche's post-traumatic osteoporosis
10. Postinfarction sclerodactyly
11. Migratory osteolysis
12. Traumatic angiospasm; traumatic vasospasm
13. Hand–shoulder syndrome
14. Foot–hip syndrome
15. Complex Regional Pain Syndrome Type 1
16. Sudeck-Babinski-Leriche syndrome
17. Pourfour du Petit syndrome [1]

This multitude of labels confuses the diagnostic process and hampers appropriate reactions to the reported symptoms.

The earliest scholarly treatment of unaccountable pain dates from the 16th century. In the 1598 book "Les Oeuvres d' Ambroise Paré", the barber-surgeon to French kings describes Charles IX's suffering around the year 1570 who, after bloodletting to treat smallpox, complained of persistent burning pain coupled with muscle loss, contracture and inability to bend or straighten his arm [2]. We also have historic descriptions of chronic pain in wounded soldiers. Pain as separate from injury and treatment was described in Lessons on the Principles of Surgery, published in France in 1766 [3], where it was observed that pain may occur in areas not directly affected by earlier trauma, and affect joints and muscles without any visible skin lesion in the area affected.

In 1813, Alexander Denmark, a British surgeon who worked at the Royal Navy Hospital in Gosport, Hampshire, reported the case of a soldier who was wounded by a bullet that had passed through his upper arm. The wound itself healed quickly, however he noted in his report: "I always found him with the forearm bent and in supine position and supported by the firm grasp of the other hand. The pain was of a 'burning' nature, and so violent as to cause a continual perspiration from his face". Eventually, the arm was amputated [4], and this concluded the patient's suffering.

The American Civil War also reaped a harvest of experience in enigmatic chronic pain. Claude Bernard, Silas Weir Mitchell, George Morehouse and William Keen all described frequent intense pain in the aftermath of battle wounds in veterans and among them, reports on pain disorders from gunshot wounds and other nerve damage [5].

In the 1880s the French neurologist Jean-Martin Charcot observed dystonic movement disorders and related contractions, and hypothesized that the syndrome's genesis (described as "hysteria minor") was in unstructured changes in the nervous system which were probably biochemical or physiological in nature [6].

At the 29th Congress of the German Society of Surgeons (Deutscher Chirurgen Kongress) in 1901, Paul Sudeck delivered a paper entitled "Acute inflammatory bone atrophy", in which he discussed changes observed in patients' X-ray images. His examples included chronic atrophies causing exceptional disability. His influence can be seen in the use of his name in several of the labels given to this set of conditions.

During World War 1 René Leriche, an army surgeon in Strasbourg, hypothesized that the sympathetic nervous system was central in the rise of signs and symptoms of the conditions described by Sudeck. In 1917, he described a patient's complaints of chronic pain in the arm and numbness in the armpit where he received a gunshot wound. Leriche coined the term "sympathetic neuritis" to illustrate the role of the sympathetic nervous system in neuropathic pain.

The term "reflex sympathetic dystrophy" (RSD) was introduced by James Evans around 1947 [7]. Evans described 57 patients with a syndrome characterized by intense pain and clinical symptoms which he described as "sympathetic stimulation". The condition appeared as a consequence of fractures (21%), sprains (21%), vascular complications (19%), amputations (9%), joint or bone inflammations (5%), minor wounds (2%) and other minor injuries such as contusions (9%) and posture defects (7%). In 1973, John Bonica proposed the following three clinical stages of RSD:

- Stage 1, acute - the first three months after injury - characterized by erythema, calor, edema, significant hyperhidrosis, pain distribution unrelated to root or nerve involvement, limited range of motion and reduced muscle strength with a negative X-ray examination, but a positive scintigraphy showing hyperaccumulation;

- Stage 2, dystrophic - characterized by severe pain, skin edema, decreased hair growth, discoloration, cyanosis, persistent hyperhidrosis, muscle weakness and limited range of motion of the affected joint or joints;

- Stage 3, atrophic - characterized by lesser but nonetheless disabling pain which subsides with rest and increases with passive motion. The skin may be atrophic, thin, dry, sometimes ulcerated, cold, mottled or cyanotic in toto; possible loss of joint range of motion and muscle strength with tendon atrophy, contractures, tremors and dystonia causing a significant motor impairment of the affected limb. At this stage, the radiographic examination shows inhomogeneous regional osteoporosis (Sudeck's atrophy).

This typology is used in some countries to this day.

The name was changed to Complex Regional Pain Syndrome in 1994 and the Orlando Conference established that CRPS could be diagnosed in presence of the following conditions [8]:

1. The presence of an initiating noxious event or a cause of immobilization.

2. Continuing pain, allodynia, or hyperalgesia with which the pain is disproportionate to any inciting event.

3. Evidence at some time of edema, changes in skin blood flow, or abnormal sudomotor activity in the region of pain.

4. This diagnosis is excluded by the existence of conditions that would otherwise account for the degree of pain and dysfunction.

Bonica's typology is currently under review. Some experts suggest a fourth stage [9], in which changes become irreversible and amputation appears the only effective method of alleviating pain in the affected limb [10]. This prospect highlights the importance of diagnosing CRPS as early as possible. Only timely treatment may save the patient. It is imperative to define the process of differentiation between pain as part of the healing process, and neuropathic pain which may lead to CRPS.

Pain is considered mainly as the subjective sensation [11] of the individual patient. This definition stipulates that the sensation is unpleasant and results from the real or hypothetical possibility of body tissue damage. The definition ignores experiences which might be perceived as positive [12]. It may seem incredible, but some people perceive pain as positive and have no negative associations with it. Although we tend to ignore this, such an attitude has firm foundations in the sphere of Western European culture: consider known martyrs and ascetics who used pain for self-improvement. In some religious practices pain is an important means towards redemption, with no negative connotations at all. Whether as "punishment" or "challenge", it may come with positive implications. Aside from spiritual overtones, medical patients often report a positive attitude towards pain when their pain is lesser than expected or when they consider alternatives worse than enduring pain.

It may therefore be accepted that people respond to pain differently and this should lead us to consider pain's applicability as a diagnostic. Patients, especially those suffering from algodystonia, motor neuron dystrophy, or CRPS [13], report pain inaccurately or too late for positive prognosis. This paper summarizes information from interviews with chronic pain sufferers in order to identify actions by medical practitioners which may have led to misunderstanding the nature of the patients' conditions.

2. Experiencing painful sensations

The effect of chronic pain on the patient is, chiefly, an altered consciousness. In chronic pain, the body is in a constant state of agitation, which is an imbalance between chemical mediators responsible for conducting and attenuating pain stimuli. As a result of chemical imbalance, patients may experience symptoms such as mood disorders, anxiety or panic attacks, or even sensory processing and memory disorders [14].

For people who have not experienced such states, the nature of the suffering may be incomprehensible. Conversely, chronic sufferers may be unaware of reporting incorrectly on their experiences.

A common practice among doctors dealing with chronic pain sufferers is to use numeric rating scales, or pain scales: patients are asked to self-assess their pain on a scale from 0 (no pain) to 10. The goal of pain scales is to give the doctor an idea of pain's intensity, but their usefulness is limited by education and experience of both the doctor and the patient. The following example will illustrate the problem: a girl aged 17 with diagnosed CRPS in the leg and clubfoot, suffering pain for a year and treated symptomatically, was admitted to hospital with abdominal pain. The patient indicated that the pain was intense and assigned it the value of 5 on the pain scale. As a result, she was classified as not requiring immediate attention and asked to wait in line. Her state rapidly deteriorated. Further investigation revealed acute appendicitis and secondary peritonitis. Had she not been a chronic pain sufferer, she would have assigned her pain the value of 9 or 10.

It is important to be aware that pain scales are relative and therefore should have limited applicability. The bottom end of the scale - "zero" - signifies no pain, however there is no equally clear definition for "ten". It could signify pain leading to unconsciousness, or pain which causes the sufferer suicidal thoughts, or is greater than ever experienced. For some, the worst possible pain could be a toothache, for others a laceration. This lack of clear qualitative definition of pain on a pain scale leads to misinterpretations and "strategic assessments" both by diagnosticians and sufferers: patients often overestimate their pain in hope of receiving more urgent help; while medical professionals interpret patients' estimations as exaggerated. The only incontestable feedback from using pain scales is the existence of pain.

As shown above, applying a simple pain scale may lead to incorrect diagnoses if the patient's situation is incorrectly assessed. Orthopedic and neurologic patients suffering from CRPS as the result of medical interventions often communicate pain in the affected limb, which is interpreted by the specialists as an indicator of appropriateness of treatment and ignored. In consequence, no treatment is offered. In another example, a patient aged 16, experiencing difficulty walking, underwent a hallux valgus (bunion) operation. First her left foot was operated and after six months, in December 2018, the right foot. The post-operative wound did not heal well and in January 2019 the patient was admitted to hospital and given a course of antibiotics. Shortly afterwards she suffered an incident at school: the operated foot was struck with a door and its bones repositioned. This resulted in a further operation to reposition the bones and stabilize the foot. The patient began reporting increased pain; however, her frequent complaints became increasingly ignored by the medical staff. Both doctors and other professionals began treating the patient as hysterical and explained the pain away as natural and necessary after the operation. After several months of ineffective physiotherapy, clubfoot developed and this resulted in the CRPS diagnosis [15].

This, and other similar incidents, suggests that sufferers may not realize that when they report pain, their reports may be interpreted as imprecise and lead to inaccurate diagnoses.

Tissue damage or loss of continuity often lead to deep but reversible changes in both the peripheral and central nervous system, typically presenting as hypersensitivity and chronic pain as the body's response to inflammation of tissue surrounding affected nerve structures. These changes accompany tissue repair processes, treatments of injuries and other conditions up until full recovery of the tissue [16]. If, however, pain exceeds the normally expected healing time, the situation changes diametrically. Pain conditions lasting more than three months necessitate the modification of the treatment process to account for chronic pain conditions [17]. Chronic pain conditions render the common pain assessment methods, used with non-sufferers, useless.

The sensation of pain in general is not as good a diagnostic as its particular form which, to differentiate it from pain, may be called suffering, and be understood as the negative sensation caused by lesions or other tissue interference, felt to be unacceptable and greater than expected. Such perceptions should be a cue for medical practitioners to suspect that the pain is not "normal" for the situation and to search for alternative or expanded diagnoses and treatments. Interviews with 35 CRPS sufferers, aged 15–45, reveal the prevalent experience of insufficient reaction by medical staff to, or disregard for, reported suffering. Since CRPS develops subsequently to a pre-existing condition, the sufferers have a unique experience of pain: they are able to compare their current sensations compounded by CRPS with past, pre-syndrome experience. Their observations have been juxtaposed in the table below. CRPS-related pain experiences are categorized as "suffering"; i.e. chronic and unacceptable in intensity. Reports of such sensations should automatically trigger a reassessment of the current diagnosis and treatment plan (**Table 1**).

The genesis of CRPS development is unidentified and the condition can only be recognized when already present. Paying attention to the above-listed symptoms may help diagnose the syndrome early enough to implement prophylactic treatment.

Interpretation of	Pre-CRPS pain experiences	Pain experiences with CRPS
Genesis	Understood, justified or even desirable, e.g. as the result of operation or treatment	Outside the patient's experience range
Intensity	Changing intensity	Persistent. No pain-free periods
Control	Can be controlled (e.g. through standard doses of drugs)	Uncontrollable (standard doses of drugs bring no relief)
Duration	Usually lasts 4–6 weeks (depending on type of treatment); changes in type, intensity, or frequency over time	Constant, with occasional periods of lesser intensity (but never entirely pain-free), lasting more than 4–6 weeks. May increase in intensity or area affected
Treatment methods	Standard procedures - even if disliked by the patient - bring about the desired improvement	Certain standard treatments (such as physical medicine and rehabilitation) may lead to worsening of the patient's state, increase pain and bring no desired rehabilitation results
Outcomes if unaddressed		May lead to depression, including thoughts of suicide
		May lead to despondency and lack of cooperation with medical professionals after experiencing increased pain following treatment
		Distrust of medical and rehabilitation practitioners
		Hyperalgesia and allodynia

Table 1.
Sufferers' reported experiences before and after developing CRPS.

Countless cases justify the necessity to identify changes in suffering and to adjust treatment appropriately. The cases listed below are all from the last two years and are representative of many other such cases.

2.1 Case: symptoms non-specific to the treated condition

Girl, 17, diagnosed with CRPS after two years of symptoms. At 15, she developed intervertebral hernia as a result of a sports injury. An orthosis was fitted and the patient was prescribed physical rehabilitation. The patient reported severe pain, which did not subside after the removal of the orthosis. Further treatment included electrostimulation, acupuncture and symptomatic treatment. At 16, the patient began reporting severe stomach symptoms. Six months later, changes characteristic of CRPS began appearing on her left leg: the leg changed coloring, hair growth increased. Bone loss occurred [18–21]. CRPS spreading to organs such as the stomach is not typical. Frequently children suffer from severe musculoskeletal pain (Amplified Musculoskeletal Pain Syndrome - AMPS), which can be interpreted as Complex Regional Pain Syndrome, Reflex Sympathetic Dystrophy, Reflex Neurovascular Dystrophy, or extensive pain, such as in fibromyalgia. CRPS was eventually diagnosed and specialist treatment commenced c. 19 months after the initial appearance of CRPS symptoms. The patient's left leg and stomach remain affected by CRPS. She is fed by a gastric (nasoduodenal - ND) tube. Leg pain causes her to periodically use crutches.

2.2 Case: identification hindered by comorbidities

Girl, 12, treated for tumor. She broke her leg in an accident at school. A typical treatment followed: the bone was set and a plaster cast was used to immobilize the leg. From the very start, the patient reported increased pain which was interpreted as symptomatic of the tumor. After the removal of the plaster cast the limb was swollen and hypersensitive to touch. Symptomatic treatment and physical rehabilitation brought no results: the child continued to be in constant pain. After changes in the bone were discovered, CRPS was diagnosed. CRPS-specific treatment commenced over a year after the symptoms first appeared.

2.3 Case: incorrect fracture fixation

Man, 43, broke the scaphoid bone in his right hand in a motorcycle collision. The hand was immobilized with a plaster cast. The patient had a history of alcohol abuse. He did not report any discomfort resulting from an overtight cast: he ignored the growing pain and anesthetized himself with alcohol. After the removal of the cast, the pain did not subside and within three months symptoms characteristic of CRPS, such as swelling, color change and hypersensitivity, appeared. Because of his alcohol abuse, his reports of increasing persistent pain were ignored. Treatment began after the hand swelled and deformed.

2.4 Case: perioperative injuries

Appearance of additional pain signals during treatment for other conditions - mainly orthopedic operations - can be illustrated by five cases: two affected lower limbs, two affected upper limbs, and one affected a shoulder. The patients all reported severe pain and difficulty moving the affected limbs. In all cases their reports of abnormal pain were interpreted as normal pain. The patients were prescribed physical rehabilitation which brought no positive results. CRPS was not recognized until limb deformation was visible or bone loss was detected with radiographic imaging.

All this evidence suggests that there are major blind spots in diagnostic procedures where chronic pain is a factor, often preventing new disease entities from being discovered and treated. To rectify this situation, new procedures are required to complement existing procedures in situations which, currently, leave medical practitioners exposed to improvisation.

The following case illustrates issues caused by insufficient diagnostic procedures: girl, 15, was diagnosed with antero-inferior subluxation of the glenohumeral (shoulder) joint with muscle weakness of the shoulder girdle. The various treatments prescribed, such as Kirschner wire fixation, all followed existing procedures but, irrespective of the method used, the shoulder always slipped. In effect, the patient was discharged from several hospitals without positive prognosis. Doctors failed to act on the patient's reports of pain, treating it as natural and necessary under the circumstances. Over the next 120 days, the patient underwent various attempts to set the shoulder, leading to brachial plexus paralysis and gradual loss of functionality in the arm and the hand. The arm became hypersensitive and changed color. CRPS wasn't diagnosed until the detection of bone loss. Symptomatic treatment at a pain management clinic and arthrodesis improved the patient's comfort and returned relative independence to her.

Although medicine, as a study of humans and nature, appears to be closer to the humanities, its history shows it has more in common with the sciences. Physicians frequently see the human body as a mechanism. A rather complicated mechanism, but nevertheless one which allows us to specify procedures for pairing symptoms with treatments. The body is so complex that it could work if 99% of its components malfunction and, conversely, die with just 1% damage. Cause-and-effect medicine appears increasingly helpless when our cognitive apparatus identifies new disease entities. It seems reasonable to suggest refinements to existing medical procedures. There should be a procedure for when there are no more procedures. Let us use another example, of a girl aged 15 diagnosed with antero-inferior subluxation of the glenohumeral (shoulder) joint with muscle weakness of the shoulder girdle. The various treatments prescribed, such as Kirschner wire fixation, all followed existing procedures but, irrespective of the method used, the shoulder always slipped. In effect, the patient was discharged from several hospitals without positive prognosis. Doctors failed to act on the patient's reports of pain, treating it as normal under the circumstances, because procedures which they followed did not anticipate the particular symptoms which occurred. They failed to reach beyond standard procedures to investigate the patient's condition and offer solutions; a state of affairs unfortunately common in an underfunded national health service.

3. Pain scales modification proposal

Medical professionals must be aware that a suffering patient's experiences are impossible to imagine for non-sufferers. A correctly conducted medical interview must use methods which will ensure a correct assessment of the patient's state. Quantitative pain scales should be avoided; rather, the interviewing physician should create a space for patients to freely report on their comfort levels and also to share their own observations and insights into their symptoms. The procedure should consider the following actions:

1. Establish the time period during which the patient has experienced constant or near-constant decline in comfort. A period of four weeks or more should be flagged as potential chronic suffering.

2. Elicit description of pain in the patient's own words. Patients are usually able to identify differences in their experience. The medical professional may help by suggesting adjectives describing various experiences. The following should be offered as core descriptors:

    - burning pain
    - tingling pain
    - stabbing pain
    - painful reaction to touch (e.g. by clothing)
    - hot/cold to the touch
    - pulsation
    - numbness
    - increased or diminished pain under pressure

A longer list of adjectives, appropriate to the assessed condition, ought to be available for use during the medical interview. The list should be expanded and reviewed as the dataset of performed interviews grows.

3. Ask the patient to describe any changes to their experience prior to treatment and during the course of treatment (e.g., has a new type of pain appeared? Has pain changed type or intensity?) Any change reported should be a prompt to consider whether a new condition or another disease entity has developed.

4. Pay attention to the patient's suggestions that the painkillers used are ineffective or otherwise inadequate. For example, if dosage or strength become inadequate after surgery [22].

5. If, after surgery, pain persists in the limbs for more than 2–3 months, or otherwise more than the time expected for full tissue repair from acute trauma, sprain, fracture, or surgery, consider CRPS [23].

3.1 Changes in patient communication

Correctly conducted medical interviews are key in accurate diagnoses of pain conditions. Nevertheless, medical professionals often ignore information given by patients. Feedback from c. 50 patients diagnosed with CRPS in Poland, Germany, UK and USA reveals counterproductive language used by medical professionals in response to reports of painful conditions. It is imperative that doctors be aware of such unhelpful phrases and avoid them. Their use demonstrates that patient reports are ignored and indicates a high likelihood of an incorrect diagnosis.

1. "**You do not look ill**". Suffering, understood as unwanted, intense pain, need not be visible. Very often the professional forms a visual first impression of the patient's condition before hearing the patient's oral report. Nobody would admit disbelieving a patient, but doctors nevertheless make a "first-impressions assessment" which influences their subsequent approach and diagnosis. If the visual impression is that of a healthy individual (or healthier than the individual's own words suggest), there is a tendency to accept the more positive observation. Opposing one's own first impression may result in feelings of cognitive dissonance and incompetence.

2. "**Perhaps you should be more active**" or "**Healing must hurt**". Both of these are symptomatic of the persistent belief in the human body's ability to self-repair. Our bodies indeed have amazing capacity for regeneration, and the patient's mental attitude - belief that they can be healed - is a factor in this capacity. However, this capacity and self-belief have their limitations and ought not to be relied on in conducting treatment. If a patient experiences increased pain as a result of following the doctors' advice, they will stop cooperating. Any further reliance on self-repair will become counter-productive.

3. "**You can learn to cope**". It is impossible for a non-sufferer to confidently assert that the chronic sufferer - such as a CRPS sufferer - can ever learn to cope, and important to realize that treatment may be far from straightforward. Many conditions are untreatable and only subject to palliative care - and not everyone, and not under all circumstances, can learn to cope with that.

4. "**It is all in your head/you are making it up**". Patients often report that doctors, when confronted with reports of increasing pain or requests for more painkillers, begin suspecting mental disorders. Before doctors jump to such conclusions, they ought to consider pain-causing conditions such as CRPS.

5. "**This is the end**". As mentioned above, medical professionals may be subject to feelings of incompetence and powerlessness and this may cause unwanted reactions. Appropriate procedures are crucial to avoid situations in which a stranded professional might submit to helplessness.

6. "**You have to be more positive**". This ties in with the belief in our ability to self-repair and reveals a patronizing attitude.

7. "**Others suffer more than you**" As outlined above, it is impossible to assess the degree of pain another person is suffering. Furthermore, chronic pain sufferers and long-term users of painkillers often cannot assess their pain levels accurately.

4. Conclusions

The old joke has it that there is no such pain that your doctor cannot take it. For severe pain sufferers, faced with inattentive medical professionals, this joke loses its humor. The widespread fear of dentists and surgeons is not caused by the nature of their work, but by the pain and discomfort their work connotes. It is vital that doctors of all specialties where chronic suffering is a possibility pay special attention to how they communicate with patients. Correct identification of the cause of pain and its mutability is key to successful treatment. It is often assumed that in certain cases pain cannot be effectively removed and that it can be a desired symptom. However, this should not extend to the assumption that it is natural and can be ignored. Pain is a key diagnostic. It offers feedback on accuracy of the chosen procedures. Take, for example, dental root canal: the pain caused by touching the exposed nerve indicates that the treatment proceeds correctly. It is a specific reaction to a specific stimulus, and it allows a specific diagnosis; diagnoses based on vague understanding of unexamined and unexplained pain have no place in proper medical procedures.

Author details

Marek Rózycki[1*] and Robert Tobias[2]

1 M/D/R/K Trusted Adviser Group SP Z O.O.O, Mikolow, Poland

2 Second University of Naples, Naples, Italy

*Address all correspondence to: m.rozycki@mdrk.eu

References

[1] Kucharz, E.J. (2018). Zaburzenia nerwowo-naczyniowe. Algodystrofia. In P. Gajewski (Ed.). Interna Szczeklika (p. 2106). Kraków: Medycyna Praktyczna.

[2] Iolascon, G., et al. (2015). Complex regional pain syndrome (CRPS) type I: historical perspective and critical issues. *Clinical Cases in Mineral and Bone Metabolism 12*(Suppl 1), 4-10.

[3] Doury, P. (1981). Historical Review. In: Doury, P., Dirheimer, Y., Patton, S. *Algodystrophy*. Berlin, Heidelberg: Springer.

[4] Hooshmand, H., Phillips, E.M. (2016). Various complications of complex regional pain syndrome (CRPS). Retrieved from: www.rsdinfo.com/RSD-Articles/Various_Complications_of_Complex_Regional_Pain_Syndrome.pdf

[5] Dunglison, R. A., et al. Dictionary of Medical Science. (1874). Philadelphia: Blanchard & Lea.

[6] Cooper, M., Clark, V. (2013). Neuroinflammation, **Neuroautoimmunity**, and the Co-Morbidities of Complex Regional Pain Syndrome. *Journal of Neuroimmune Pharmacology 8*(3), 452-469

[7] Bennett, D., Brookoff, D. (2006). Complex Regional Pain Syndromes (Reflex Sympathetic Dystrophy and Causalgia) and Spinal Cord Stimulation. *Pain Medicine 7*(S1), 64-96. Retrieved from: https://academic.oup.com/painmedicine/article/7/suppl_1/S64/1818503

[8] Harden, R. N., Oaklander, A. L., Burton, A. W., Perez, R. S., Richardson, K., Swan, M., Barthel, J., Costa, B., Graciosa, J. R., Bruehl, S. (2013). Complex regional pain syndrome: practical diagnostic and treatment guidelines, 4th edition. *Pain medicine (Malden, Mass.)*, *14*(2), 180-229. https://doi.org/10.1111/pme.12033

[9] Hooshmand, H., Phillips, E.M. (no date). Spread of Complex Regional Pain Syndrome (CRPS). Vero Beach, Florida: Neurological Associates Pain Management Center. Retrieved from: https://www.rsdrx.com/RSD-Articles/rsd-articles.html

[10] Geertzen, J. H. B., Eisma, W. H. (1994). Amputation and reflex sympathetic dystrophy *Prosthetics and Orthotics International 18*, 109-1I1

[11] Cf. definitions of pain by the International Association for the Study of Pain, IASP.

[12] Ból może sprawiać przyjemność. (2013, February 27). Retrieved from: https://www.newsweek.pl/bol-moze-sprawiac-przyjemnosc/f509fg3 Norwegian neuroscientist Siri Leknes and team have shown that the touch of a hot object on the skin may be interpreted as painful or comforting; depending on context.

[13] CRPS, Complex Regional Pain Syndrome - condition in which a person experiences persistent severe and debilitating pain, usually in a single limb, often with circulatory disorders causing changes in color or temperature, extremely sensitive skin, swellings or stiffness.

[14] Muñoz, M; Esteve, R. (2005). Reports of Memory Functioning by Patients With Chronic Pain. The Clinical Journal of Pain, 21(4), 287-291. https://journals.lww.com/clinicalpain/Abstract/2005/07000/Reports_of_Memory_Functioning_by_Patients_With.1.aspx

[15] Complex Regional Pain Syndrome - CRPS, also known as Sudet's Disease,

Algodystrophy, neurodystrophy, or sympathetic dystrophy.

[16] McMahon S., & Koltzenburg, M. (2005). Wall and Melzack's Textbook of Pain (6th ed.). Edinburgh: Churchill Livingstone.

[17] Korff von M; Dunn K.M. (2008). Chronic pain reconsidered. Pain, 138(2), 267-76. https://journals.lww.com/pain/Abstract/2008/08310/Chronic_pain_reconsidered.5.aspx

[18] Costanza, C.D., Longstreth, G.F., Liu, A.L. (2004). Chronic abdominal wall pain: clinical features, health care costs, and long term outcomes. *Clinical Gastroenterology and Hepatology 2*(5), 395-399. https://pubmed.ncbi.nlm.nih.gov/15118977/

[19] Sherry, D.D., Wallace, C.A., Kelley, C., Kidder, M., Sapp, L. (1999). Short- and long-term outcomes of children with complex regional pain syndrome type I treated with exercise therapy. *Clinical Journal of Pain 15*(3), 218-223.

[20] Sherry, D.D., McGuire, T., Mellins, E., Salmonsen, K., Wallace, C.A., Nepom, B. (1991). Psychosomatic Musculoskeletal Pain in Childhood: clinical and psychological analyses of 100 children. *Pediatrics 88*(6), 1093-1099.

[21] Sherry, D.D., Wallace, C.A. Resolution of Fibromyalgia with an Intensive Exercise Program (abstract). *Clinical and Experimental Rheumatology 10*, 196.

[22] The International Association for the Study of Pain's 1994 diagnostic criteria, replaced in 2004 with the currently used Budapest Criteria, are a form of assistance; in effect a procedure for when there are no more procedures.

[23] Simanski, C.J., Althaus, A., Hoederath, S., Kreutz, K.W., Hoederath, P., Lefering, R., et al. (2014). Incidence of chronic postsurgical pain (CPSP) after general surgery. *Pain Medicine, 15*(7), 1222-9. https://pubmed.ncbi.nlm.nih.gov/24716774/

Chapter 9

Perceptions of Women toward Non-Pharmacological Methods for Pain Relief during Labor

Teketel Ermias Geltore and Abiy Tadesse Angelo

Abstract

The experience of childbirth is subjective and has multidimensional components through which every woman passes in different ways. It is one of the most beautiful episodes in mother's life, related to happiness and celebration. However, childbirth is also associated with negative emotions such as anxiety, low sense of safety, and expectation of pain. Strong and persistent pain that is associated with labor may negatively affect both mother and fetus. During labor, a woman is dealing not only with the contractions but also with the belief that the culture has made for her. Although childbirth is viewed as a normal physiological process, it can produce significant pain that requires effective pain management. The non-pharmacological approach includes a wide variety of methods to address labor pain, which prevent suffering by enhancing the psychological and spiritual components. The non-pharmacological methods of labor pain relief require patient's preparation and antenatal education. The non-pharmacological methods that used to relief labor pain are massage, acupuncture, continuous support, positioning, breathing techniques, water immersion, music therapy, and biofeedback are some of the techniques used to achieve an effective coping level for women. The aim of this chapter is to explore women's perception toward non-pharmacological methods during labor.

Keywords: attitude, non-pharmacological methods, pain relief, childbirth, pain, parturition, obstetric, perceived barriers

1. Introduction

"In pain you will bring forth children" (Gen. 3-16). Thenceforth, labor pain was considered as a punishment given by God due to Eve's sin and then asking for relief was presumably against God; for this belief in 1591, Eufane Ayane of Edinburgh was buried alive into a pit because she asked for pain relief during her difficult labor [1, 2]. Labor pain is one of the major issues women faces during childbirth; thus then, most women want to relief it. Spontaneous vaginal delivery is one of the most distressing pains that majority of women would experience during their lifetime [3–5]. A study done in United Kingdom depicted that 93.5% of the women described the pain as severe, while in Finland, 80% described intolerable [6]. Besides this, laboring mothers experienced 10.9% severe acute postpartum pain in 36 hours, 9.8% persistent pain, and 11.2% depression at 8 weeks [7]. Although strong and persistent pain during labor might not be considered as a source of complication for a healthy patient, it stimulates the sympathetic nervous system, which causes an increase in the heart rate, blood pressure, sweat production, endocrine hyperfunction, delays the patient's prognosis, and traumatic childbirth experiences. However, many of these sequelae of pain are mitigated by appropriate pain relief methods [5, 8–11]. Management of labor pain has remained a clinical issue and is as old as human kind. Labor pain perception varies in onset, timing, duration, and severity. Effective management of labor pain results in greater maternal satisfaction with the birth process [12, 13]. The study result from systematic review showed that factors that increased maternal satisfactions during labor are companionship with the caregivers, involvement in decision-making, and assuming health facility as their home [14]. Moreover, this will help women to conserve their energy to cope with the pain in a less destructive way. Non-pharmacological measures of pain relief are exploited because they are safer and tend to cause fewer interventions [15]. The aim of this chapter is to explore laboring mothers' attitude toward various non-pharmacological methods and perceived barriers to use these methods. The chapter also identified the commonly used non-pharmacological methods during childbirth.

2. Laboring mothers attitude toward non-pharmacological techniques for pain relief

Non-pharmacological methods of pain management are grouped into three: cognitive, physical, and emotional. For instance, relaxation and breathing techniques work at mind level. Massage, position change, and TENS are congregated at cutaneous level. Touch and reassurance are grouped at emotional level [9]. Even if most women report labor is painful, a good number of physicians remarkably have little awareness about it. Pain is a subjective experience involving a complex interaction of physiologic, psychosocial, cultural, and environmental influences. The study findings from narrative inquiry revealed that use of pain relief methods was missing, although women expressed need for pain relief. Moreover, the same study results showed that there was inadequate physical and emotional support for women during childbirth [16]. A literature review from India showed that some doctors perform certain interventions on women without questioning and justification. Furthermore, people who support during homebirth have no permission to enter the delivery room in health facilities [17]. On the other hand, other study findings showed that laboring mothers during childbirth were satisfied and interested in labor pain relief services. A systematic review conducted at Toronto revealed that women allocated to continuous support were more likely to have a spontaneous vaginal birth, shorter labor, and satisfaction with the care, and in contrary less likely to have intrapartum analgesia, operative deliveries, and report frustration [18]. A randomized prospective comparative study was done on 100 primigravida women in active phase of labor by dividing them into music group (n = 50) and control group (n = 50); the result showed that the music group had substantial lower serum cortisol levels than the control group. Thus, music therapy is effective in reducing stress levels and increasing satisfaction in the women during active labor [19]. The study conducted in Poland depicted that most of the women were interested in non-pharmacological methods to relieve labor pain [20]. An integrative review was employed, and the result showed that most laboring mothers were excited in each non-pharmacological method since acupuncture and acupressure worked on physiological and subjective aspects of pain. Warm bath, music therapy, aromatherapy, and breathing techniques promoted relaxation and decreased the levels of anxiety. Thermal therapies were used as local analgesia in regions affected by pain. Exercises with the Swiss ball were important for pain relief [21]. A randomized trial was conducted on 74 primigravida women, and the finding showed that the experimental group was found to have higher levels of maternal luxury during labor as well as 2 hours after delivery. Besides, they experienced less labor pain and have a shorter duration of the first stage of labor than the control groups [22]. The study conducted in Australia revealed that labor pain scoring mechanism was the same among mothers and midwives at mild-moderate pain levels, but midwives considerably undervalued the severe labor that was reported by mothers [6]. Women differ in their choices as to whether the various pain relief methods are effective in decreasing their labor pain and different pain relief approaches could enable them to relax. However, women who used medication were more likely to experience a sense of guilt, drug side effects, while non-pharmacological methods could allow women to actively work with their physiological responses and create a good team spirit with their care providers throughout in their postnatal periods [23].

3. Perceived barriers to use non-pharmacological methods

The study done in Ghana showed that some women do not obtain an ample pain management during labor because of poor antenatal education on labor pain management and insufficient support from health professionals and their families [16]. In developing countries in spite of having labor analgesic services, most women still go through sore labor due to lack of knowledge about the techniques and a negative attitude of caregivers toward the methods. Since then, the patients get little information about pain management from their relatives but not from care providers directly; in turn, this created a wide gap in communication between laboring women and obstetric care providers [1, 5, 17]. One study identified perceived barriers to use non-pharmacological techniques, for instance, lack of time, inadequate knowledge about the options, regulatory issues, and patient reluctance of analgesia [24]. Most health-care systems are often poorly developed; the provision of analgesia is seen with low importance in comparison with the treatment of other diseases, and rudimentary properties such as water and current may not be accessible [25]. Shortage of finance, unavailability of the methods, and care providers little trainings are significant barriers to improving this situation. Therefore, it is not astonishing that the provision of analgesics is problematic [26]. Many other studies' findings showed that key issues that affect the practice of labor analgesia in developing countries by caregivers are unavailability of materials, health-care delivery systems, understanding, and strong belief. From these, awareness, outlooks, and abilities of care provider are chief factors. Moreover, misunderstandings such as harm to baby and doubt on the efficacy of non-pharmacological methods [27–30] are other factors. Labor pain management in the developing world is meager. Consequently, mothers experience unmeasured grief, let alone analgesia [31].

The individual appearances of pain, as well as other the aspects that influence the perception of pain shift responsibility to the health caregiver to ensure that the laboring woman can decide about pain relief in labor meaning, midwife's activities should be influenced by the woman's preference of pain relief methods that obtainable to her. When these options are presented to them during the antenatal period, then they can easily choose the applicable methods [16]. Since pain relief in labor is an important aspect to laboring women during childbirth, efforts should be made to evaluate its improvement through confirming their satisfaction, and unalleviated, labor pains may influence negatively on the lives of parturient and her baby [3]. Some non-pharmacological techniques need professionally competent and qualified health-care providers, especially in acupuncture, TENS, and reflexology [21]. Some methods are not provided due to their cost. For instance, biofeedback and TENS units are costly and difficult to charge [9]. Evidences showed that many health-care professionals lack adequate knowledge and attitude for effective management of labor pain, leaving women and their baby to endure a reduced functional and psychological quality of life [28]. The need for women to receive complete information on the risks, the benefits, and provision of varied approaches is so that women have access to those methods that meet with their beliefs, as well as to those that they may need if their experiences differ from their expectations [23]. Regarding, service care providers' hurdles, staff's knowledge and attitudes on advancement their knowledge through incessant training programs and participating on conferences by themselves or facility regulations, that reflect on the quality and type of pain assessment and management. Therefore, inadequate knowledge remains a significant barrier to pain management. On a more positive note, health-care providers in their study said that teaching hospital environments influenced their ability to provide the techniques because more emphasis was placed on evidence-based care. As regards patient-related obstacles, in most facility settings, during labor and delivery, women were alone and often afraid by the intermittent shifting of obstetricians, midwives, and nurses [32–34]. Nurses and midwives are aware of some non-pharmacological labor pain management methods and use them in their practice. A good number of non-pharmacological techniques remain unknown to them. Some of the reasons for the usage of non-pharmacological techniques include their non-invasiveness, inexpensive nature, ease of use, safety, comfort enhancement, and bonding. Yet, barriers such as misconceptions about their efficacy, insufficient staff, and resources prevent optimal use by nurses and midwives [35]. The notion that labor pain is natural and must be endured should be changed during health education programs because it is the right of every woman to have suitable pain relief during labor. Midwives should support and encourage women during labor, and a good relationship between the midwife and the woman in labor is advocated so that women will seek professional care as well as cultural background of the woman in labor must be taken into consideration because some are socialized to be stoic. Therefore, labor pain must be assessed adequately to inform effective pain management [36]. The most commonly utilized non-pharmacological methods during childbirth include transcutaneous electrical nerve stimulation (TENS) [37–39], hypnosis [40, 41], acupuncture [42, 43], music [19], water immersion [44], continuous support [18], and biofeedback [45].

Based on the available scientific articles, the most commonly utilized non-pharmacological methods during labor and delivery are identified. Moreover, how the methods work is also reviewed.

3.1 Transcutaneous electrical nerve stimulation (TENS) for pain management in labor

A low voltage electrical impulse, which differs in frequency and intensity, will be delivered to the skin through four pads that are placed over the lower back with a boost during uterine contractions [9, 13, 46–48].

3.1.1 How does TENS work?

TENS is effective when there are large diameter nerves, with high frequency and low intensity, which results in transmission of impulses at high frequency and the release of endorphins that bind to opiate receptors, which increases pain tolerance [13, 47, 49].

3.1.2 Application of electrodes

There are various types of electrodes in terms of frequency and pulse width. Top pair of electrodes will be placed at T_{10}-L_1, and the lower pair of electrodes at S_2–S_4 (**Figure 1**) [13]. A randomized controlled trial was conducted on 1466 women from 17 trials, 13 examined TENS; 2 used acupuncture, and 2 place on the cranium. Overall, there was a slight variation in pain records between TENS and control groups. The majority of laboring mothers using TENS responded that they would be willing to use it again in their next pregnancies. There was no any evidence that TENS had any positive or negative impact on the mother and newborn [24].

3.2 Acupuncture

Acupuncture is one of Chinese traditional medicines, which became widespread and popular in some Western countries. Experts in the field assume that health is dependent on the correct flow of energy through the meridians (Qi), through the body (14 meridians). These meridians are responsible for the control the activities of the vital organs in the body. During illness, the energy flow will be imbalanced [13, 46, 49].

3.2.1 How does acupuncture work?

Acupuncture involves the insertion of fine needles into various parts of the body. The technique is aimed to treat illnesses and alleviate pain by stimulating acupuncture points. Acupuncture points used to relief labor pain are located on the hands, feet, and ears. Acupuncture stimulates nervous system, spinal cord by locking touch fibers and then block pain impulses at the pain gates, and finally help the body to release endorphins [47]. Randomized controlled trials employed found that women randomized to acupuncture had slightly reduced pain scores and decreased use of the pharmacological methods than the control groups [46]. Another randomized controlled trial was conducted on 303 nulliparous women with normal pregnancies revealed that the mean VAS scores were 66.4 in the MA

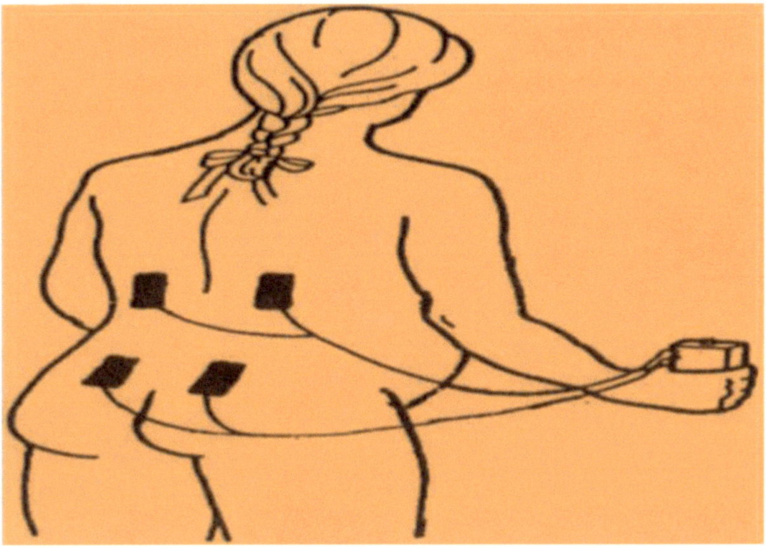

Figure 1.
A TENS unit in use [50].

group, 68.5 in the EA group, and 69.0 in the SC group. The study also showed that 2 months after birth recollection of labor pain, no significant differences were found among the groups and women's feeling in the EA group reported acupuncture as being effective for labor pain than MA, MA, spent less time in labor, and had less blood loss. Finally, the study revealed that no serious impacts of acupuncture treatment were reported [40].

3.3 Touch and massage

Massage is one of the natural pain relief methods. Touch is important in terms of positioning, decreases muscle spasms, relieves labor pain, decreases anxiety, and results in good labor outcomes [9, 13, 47, 48, 51].

3.3.1 How does touch and massage work?

In the context of physiology, touch and massage increase endorphins and oxygen supply to tissues and then stimulate nerves, which decrease pain. Studies suggest that those mothers who utilize them may have shorter labors, reduced postpartum depression, shorter hospital stays, and increased patient satisfaction. Not many potential risks were reported for mother and baby; thus, it is an excellent method to decrease labor pain [13, 48, 49, 52].

3.4 Continuous labor support

Continuous labor support refers to the nonmedical support of the woman in labor by a trained person, e.g., a doula, consistently has decreased the use of obstetric interventions [46]. Evidence indicates that continuous support during labor has a number of measurable positive impacts on key birth outcomes when compared to intermittent support like; continuous support is associated with less use of pharmacological techniques, fewer operative deliveries, and more reports of satisfaction with birth, and moreover, it has clinically meaningful benefits for women and infants [18, 46, 48, 51, 53]. **Figure 2** shows continuous labor support from the family.

3.5 Hydrotherapy

Pain alleviating mechanism of water has been known for many years. In the past decades, laboring mothers were interested in hydrotherapy due to its comfort [13].

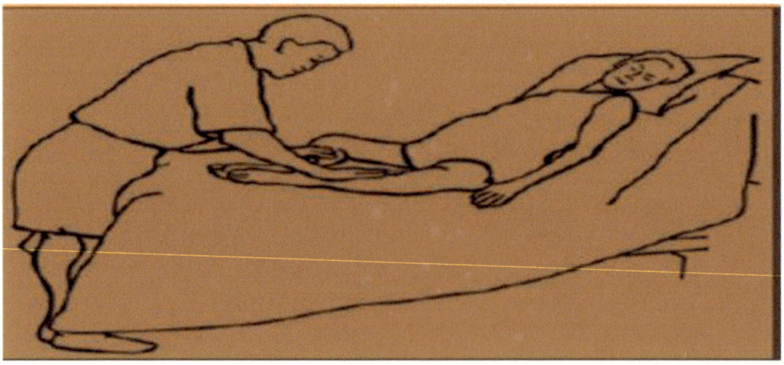

Figure 2.
Continuous support from family childbirth connection since 1918 (www.childbirthconnection.org).

3.5.1 How does hydrotherapy work?

Hydrotherapy comprises of two methods, such as an aspersion bath and sterile water injection, discussed below. The aspersion bath enhances relaxation and reduces stress levels and then decreases sense of pain. Examining the neuroendocrine parameters, this method minimizes the release of cortisol and β-endorphins, but it increases the secretion of noradrenaline [54, 55].

Intradermal injections of sterile water in the sacral area may be used to decrease back pain in labor, and it causes a burning sensation that is much more painful than saline injection and thought to relieve labor pain by counter irritation. Women who received injections of sterile water were more interested in receiving the injections in a subsequent labor than women who received saline injections [56]. Randomized control trial was conducted on 393 women using the tub during labor and a control group of 392 women receiving routine care. Women experienced less pain after water immersion than those who received routine, and more than 80% of the water immersion group said they would use the tub in subsequent labors (**Figure 3**) [57].

3.6 Music therapy

Music is a type of non-pharmacological technique, which is non-invasive, non-medical, cost-effective, and easily accessible. Music heals the soul and influences immune and endocrine function. Nowadays, many studies oriented into the therapeutic effectiveness of music in the field of obstetrics and revealed that music during childbirth promotes wellbeing of the mother and the fetus [9, 52]. Randomized control trial was done on 100 primigravida in active labor showed that there was no significant difference between both the groups in serum cortisol at pretest, whereas the group differences after the music therapy sessions indicated that the music group had significant lower serum cortisol levels compared to the control group. Thus, music therapy is effective in reducing stress levels in the women during active labor [19].

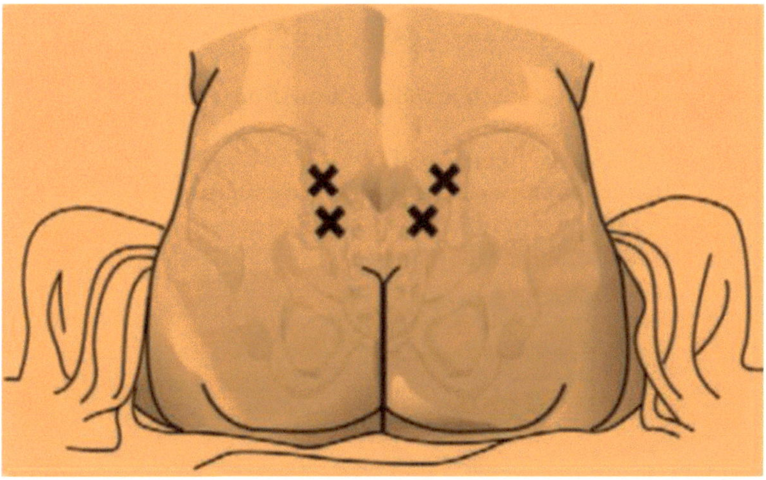

Figure 3.
Placement of intradermal water blocks: four intradermal injections of 0.05 to 0.1 mL of sterile water to form four small blebs over each posterior superior iliac spine and 3 cm below and 1 cm medial to each spine [51].

4. Conclusion

The studies revealed that transcutaneous electrical nerve stimulation, immersion bath, acupuncture and acupressure, touch, massage, continuous support, hydrotherapy, and music therapy are effective methods for pain relief during labor. Besides this, they reduce pain perception, levels of anxiety, and stress and indicated laboring mothers who used these methods did not report the need for pharmacological methods.

Although these methods are cost-effective and non-invasive, there are barriers that impediment to using the techniques as per needed. Perceived barriers can be broken up into three categories: barriers related to the patient, the clinicians, and the health-care system as a whole. To be successful in the use of non-pharmacological pain relief in labor, obstetric caregivers must have to develop positive attitude toward non-pharmacological labor analgesia and women need to be aware of different alternatives available to them.

All future randomized trials must be adequately powered in evaluation of complementary and alternative techniques for pain management in labor as they are needed for improving the quality and reporting of future trials. In particular, consideration should be given to the analysis and reporting of the person providing the intervention, for example, their training, length of experience, and relationship to the woman.

Finally, the findings of this chapter point to the need of clinical research particularly in midwifery care focusing on the use of these and other non-pharmacological strategies for pain relief during labor, aiming to humanize care for women during labor.

Conflict of interest

The authors report no conflicts of interest in this work.

Abbreviations

EA	acupuncture with a combination of both manual and electrical stimulation
MA	acupuncture with manual stimulation
SE	standard care
S_2–S_4	sacral nerve fibers 2 to 4
TENS	transcutaneous electrical nerve stimulation
T_{10}–T_{11}	thoracic nerve fibers 10 to 11
VAS	visual analog scale

Author details

Teketel Ermias Geltore[1*] and Abiy Tadesse Angelo[2]

1 Midwifery Department, School of Nursing and Midwifery, College of Health Sciences and Medicine, Wachemo University – Durame Campus, Durame, Ethiopia

2 Nursing Department, School of Nursing and Midwifery, College of Health Sciences and Medicine, Mizan Tepi University, Mizan Aman, Ethiopia

*Address all correspondence to: teketelermias@gmail.com

References

[1] Tasnim S. Perception about pain relief during normal labor among health care providers conducting delivery. MedPage Today. 2010;**22**(1):20-23. DOI: 10.3329/medtoday.v22i1.5600

[2] Pugliese PL, Cinnella G, Raimondo P, De Capraris A, Salatto P, Sforza D, et al. Implementation of epidural analgesia for labor: Is the standard of effective analgesia reachable in all women? An audit of two years. European Review for Medical and Pharmacological Sciences. 2013;**17**:1262-1268

[3] Lawani LO, Eze JN, Anozie OB, Iyoke CA, Ekem NN. Obstetric analgesia for vaginal birth in contemporary obstetrics: A survey of the practice of obstetricians in Nigeria. BMC Pregnancy and Childbirth. 2014;**14**:1. DOI: 10.1186/1471-2393-14-140

[4] El-Wahab N, Robinson N. Analgesia and anesthesia in labor. Obstetrics, Gynecology & Reproductive Medicine. 2011;**21**:137-141. DOI: 10.1016/j.ogrm.2011.02.006

[5] Karn S, Yu H, Karna S, Chen L, Qiao D. Women's awareness and attitudes towards labor analgesia influencing practice between developed and developing countries. Advances in Reproductive Sciences. 2016;**4**(2):46-52

[6] Baker A, Ferguson SA, Roach GD, Dawson D. Perceptions of labor pain by mothers and their attending midwives. Journal of Advanced Nursing. 2001;**35**:171-179

[7] Soet JE, Brack GA, Dilorio C. Prevalence and predictors of women's experience of psychological trauma during childbirth. Birth Issues in Perinatal Care. 2003;**30**:36-46

[8] Apondi C. A Survey of the knowledge attitude and practice regarding epidural labor analgesia among obstetricians at the Kenyatta National Hospital [master's thesis]. Kenya: University of Nairobi; 2012

[9] Cochrane AR. Perceptions of Labor and Delivery Clinicians on non-pharmacological Methods for Pain Relief during Labor. 2015. Available from: https://digitalcommons.brockport.edu/cgi/viewcontent.cgi?article=1093&context=honors [Accessed: March 2016]

[10] Ding T, Wang DX, Qu Y, Chen Q, Zhu SN. Epidural labor analgesia is associated with a decreased risk of postpartum depression: A prospective cohort study. Anesthesia and Analgesia. 2014;**119**(2):383-392

[11] Geltore TE et al. Perceptions of obstetric analgesia: A qualitative study among midwives attending normal vaginal deliveries in Durame Hospital, Southern Ethiopia. Journal of Pain Research. 2019;**12**:2187-2192

[12] Okojie NQ, Isah EC. Perception of epidural analgesia for labor among pregnant women in a Nigerian tertiary hospital setting. Journal of the West African College of Surgeons. 2014;**4**(4)

[13] Habanananda T. Non-pharmacological pain relief in labour. Journal of the Medical Association of Thailand. 2004;**87**(Suppl 3):S194-S202

[14] Hodnett ED. "Pain & women's satisfaction with the experience of childbirth": A systematic review. American Journal of Obstetrics and Gynecology. 2002;**186**(Suppl):S160-S172

[15] Osório SMB, Silva Júnior LG, Nicolau AIO. Evaluation of the effectiveness of non-pharmacological methods for pain relief during labor. 2014;**15**(1):174-184. DOI: 10.15253/2175-6783.2014000100022. Available from: www.revistarene.ufc.br

[16] Ampofo EA, Caine V. A narrative inquiry into women's perception and experience of labor pain: A study in the western region of Ghana. International Journal of Africa Nursing Sciences. 2015;**3**:86-93

[17] Zionts S. Ouch, that hurts: Childbirth-related pain management and the inappropriate replacement of traditional obstetrical knowledge in Kumaon, Uttarakhand, India. In: Independent Study Project (ISP) Collection Paper. Vol. 2081; 2015. Available from: http://digitalcollections.sit.edu/isp_collection/2081

[18] Hodnett ED, Gates S, Hofmeyr GJ, Sakala C. Continuous support for women during childbirth. Cochrane Database of Systematic Reviews. 2013;(7):CD003766. DOI: 10.1002/14651858.CD003766.pub5

[19] Geetha S, Anusha GK. Effect of music therapy on serum cortisol in primigravida in active labor. IOSR Journal of Dental and Medical Sciences (IOSR-JDMS). 2016;**15**(4(Ver. III)): 91-94

[20] Pilewska-Kozak AB, Klaudia P, Celina Ł-K, Beata D, Grażyna S, Magdalena B. Non-pharmacological methods of pain relief in labor in the opinion of puerperae – A preliminary report. Annals of Women's Health. 2017;**1**(1):1005

[21] Mascarenhas VH, Lima TR, Silva FM, Negreiros FS, Santos JD, Moura MA, et al. Scientifi c evidence on non-pharmacological methods for relief of labor pain. Acta Paulista de Enfermagem. 2019;**32**(3):350-357

[22] Chuntharapat S et al. Yoga during pregnancy: Effects on maternal comfort, labor pain and birth outcomes. Complementary Therapies in Clinical Practice. 2008;**14**:105-115

[23] Thomson G et al. Women's experiences of pharmacological and non-pharmacological pain relief methods for labor and childbirth: A qualitative systematic review. Reproductive Health. 2019;**16**:71. DOI: 10.1186/s12978-019-0735-4

[24] Almushait M, Ghani RA. Perception toward non-phamacological strategies in relieving labor pain: An analytic descriptive study. Journal of Natural Science Research. 2014;**4**(2):5-12

[25] Hodges SC, Mijumbi C, Okello M, McCormick BA, Walker IA, Wilson IH. Anaesthesia services in developing countries: Defining the problems. Anaesthesia. 2007;**62**:4-11

[26] Soyannwo OA. Post-operative pain control – Prescription pattern and patient experience. West African Journal of Medicine. 1999;**18**:207-210

[27] Ogboli-Nwasor E, Adaji S, Bature S, Shittu O. Pain relief in labor: A survey of awareness, attitude, and practice of health care providers in Zaria, Nigeria. Journal of Pain Research. 2011;**4**:227-232

[28] McCauley M, Stewart C, Kebede B. A survey of healthcare providers' knowledge and attitudes regarding pain relief in labor for women in Ethiopia. BMC Pregnancy and Childbirth. 2017;**17**(1):56

[29] Reena BKH, Afzal M, Mishra AK, Paul A. Labor epidural analgesia: Past, present and future. Indian Journal of Pain. 2014;**28**(2):71-81

[30] Size M, Soyannwo OA, Justins DM. Pain management in developing countries. Anaesthesia. 2007;**62** (Suppl 1):38-43

[31] Geltore TE, Taye A, Kelbore AG. Utilization of obstetric analgesia in labor pain management and associated factors among obstetric caregivers in public health facilities of Kembata Tembaro Zone, Southern Ethiopia. Journal of Pain Research. 2018;**11**:3089-3097. DOI: 10.2147/JPR.S165417

[32] Enkin M, Keirse MJ, Neilson J, Crowther C, Duley L, Hodnett E. A Guide to Effective Care in Pregnancy and Childbirth. 3rd ed. Oxford, England: Oxford University Press Journal of Midwifery and Women's Health; 2000;47(4):293-294. DOI: 10.1016/S1526-9523(02)00253-2

[33] Fielding R, Irwin MG. The knowledge and perceptions of nurses and interns regarding acute pain and postoperative pain control', HSRF project number: 822002. Hong Kong Medical Journal. 2006;**12**(Suppl 1): S31-S34

[34] Sleutel M, Schultz S, Wyble K. Nurses' views of factors that help and hinder their intrapartum care. Journal of Obstetric, Gynecologic, & Neonatal Nursing. 2007;**36**(3):203-211

[35] Boateng et al. Nurses and midwives' experiences of using non-pharmacological interventions for labor pain management: A qualitative study in Ghana. BMC Pregnancy and Childbirth. 2019;**19**:168. DOI: 10.1186/s12884-019-2311-x

[36] Aziato et al. Labour pain experiences and perceptions: A qualitative study among post-partum women in Ghana. BMC Pregnancy and Childbirth. 2017;**17**:73. DOI: 10.1186/s12884-017-1248-1

[37] Keskin EA, Onur O, Keskin HL, et al. Transcutaneous electrical nerve stimulation improves low back pain during pregnancy. Gynecologic and Obstetric Investigation. 2012;**74**(1):76-83

[38] Rodarti PAC et al. High-frequency TENS in post-episiotomy pain relief in primiparous puerpere: A randomized, controlled trial. The Journal of Obstetrics and Gynaecology Research. 2012;**38**(7):980-987

[39] Dowswell T et al. Transcutaneous electrical nerve stimulation (TENS) for pain management in labor. Cochrane Database of Systematic Reviews. 2015;2:CD007214. DOI: 10.1002/14651858.CD007214.pub2

[40] Cyna AM, McAuliffe GL, Andrew MI. Hypnosis for pain relief in labor and childbirth: A systematic review. British Journal of Anaesthesia. 2004;**93**(4):505-511

[41] Vandevusse L, Irland J, Berner MA, Fuller S, Adams D. Hypnosis for childbirth: A retrospective comparative analysis of outcomes in one obstetrician's practice. American Journal of Clinical Hypnosis. 2007;**50**(2)

[42] Lee H, Ernst E. Acupuncture for labor pain management: A systematic review. American Journal of Obstetrics and Gynecology. 2004;**191**(5):1573-1579

[43] Kvorning Ternov N et al. Acupuncture for pain relief during childbirth. Acupuncture & Electro-Therapeutics Research. 1998;**23**:19-26

[44] College of Midwives of British Columbia. Guideline for the Use of Water in Labor and Birth. British Columbia: College of Midwives; 2001

[45] Barragán Loayza IM, JC SI. Biofeedback for pain management during labor. Cochrane Database of Systematic Reviews. 2011;(6):CD006168. DOI: 10.1002/14651858.CD006168.pub2

[46] Wong C. Advances in labor analgesia. International Journal of Women's Health. 2009;**1**:139-154

[47] Jones L, Othman M, Dowswell T, et al. Pain management for women in labor: An overview of systematic reviews. Cochrane Database of Systematic Reviews. 2012;**7**(3):CD009234

[48] Ebirim LN, Buowari OY, Ghosh S. Physical and psychological aspects of

pain in obstetrics. In: Ghosh S, editor. Pain in Perspective. London, UK: InTech; 2012

[49] Gupta S, Anand Kumar GS, Singhal H. Acute pain – Labor analgesia. Indian Journal of Anaesthesia. 2006;**50**(5):363-369

[50] Simkin P, Bolding A. Update on no pharmacologic approaches to relieve labor pain and prevent suffering. Journal of Midwifery & Women's Health. 2004;**49**(6):489-504

[51] Leeman L et al. The nature and management of labor pain: Part I. Non pharmacologic pain relief. American Family Physician. 2003;**68**(6):1-8. Available from: www.aafp.org/afp

[52] Brown ST et al. Women's evaluation of intrapartum non pharmacological pain relief methods used during labor. The Journal of Perinatal Education. 2001;**10**(3)

[53] Ross-Davie M. Evidence Based Guidelines for Midwifery-Led Care in Labor. Scotland: The Royal College of Midwives; 2012

[54] Hamlac Y, Yazici S. The effect of acupressure applied to point li4 on perceived labor pains. Holistic Nursing Practice. 2017;**31**(3):167-176

[55] Henrique AJ, Gabrielloni MC, Rodney P, Barbieri M. Nonpharmacological interventions during childbirth for pain relief, anxiety, and neuroendocrine stress parameters: A randomized controlled trial. International Journal of Nursing Practice. 2018;**24**(3):12642

[56] Simkin PP, O'Hara M. No pharmacologic relief of pain during labor: Systematic reviews of five methods. American Journal of Obstetrics and Gynecology. 2002;**186**(Suppl 5):S131-S159

[57] Rush J et al. The effect of whirlpool baths in labor: A randomized controlled trial. Birth. 1996;**23**:136-143

Chapter 10

Supporting Communication Vulnerable Children to Communicate Their Pain

Ensa Johnson

Abstract

Communication vulnerable children need an alternative way to express their pain to receive appropriate pain management. In this chapter, the concept of communication vulnerability will be explained by using the social-communication model of pain as a theoretical framework. The concept of pain is difficult to describe due to its subjective nature and individuals' different experiences to pain. Clinicians and researchers find it challenging to understand the dynamic interplay between the biological, psychological and social determinants of pain. Understanding any episode of acute or chronic pain therefore necessitates considering the holistic pain picture to analyse the essentials at biological, psychological and social levels. The chapter concludes with suggestions to use augmentative and alternative strategies to support communication vulnerable children to communicate their pain.

Keywords: augmentative and alternative communication (AAC), disabilities, care, healthcare professional, paediatric patient, social-communication model of pain

1. Introduction

Pain is intrinsically private, and the concept of pain is difficult to describe and assess due to its subjective nature and individuals' unique experiences of pain [1, 2]. Up until the mid-1980s, clinicians believed that infants, toddlers and persons with disabilities, specifically those with significant communication difficulties, either do not have pain or may have very high pain thresholds [3–5]. These myths and beliefs were reinforced by McCaffery's widely accepted definition of pain at that time that stated that "pain is what the person says it is and exists whenever he or she says it does" [6, p. 95]. By default, McCaffery's definition therefore suggested that all persons with the inability to communicate their pain verbally (including the aforementioned) may not have pain.

In addition to their limited verbal ability to express pain, communication vulnerable children's neurology may also impact on their ability to show other tell-tale signs of pain that transform the parts of the brain responsible for the expression of pain [5]. For this reason, clinicians repeatedly overlooked other signs of pain [4], such as changes in the children's behaviour (withdrawal, acting clownish, having mood changes, displaying aggressive behaviour or exhibiting extreme tantrums) or changes in positioning (refusing to use the body part where pain is). This is because

IntechOpen

children with communication challenges may not display pain in the typical ways such as by crying or through facial changes [7–10]. Clinicians often mistakenly regard these kinds of "different reactions to pain" as challenging behaviour and not as children's alternative attempts of trying to express their pain [11].

Lately, clinicians have started to acknowledge that the inability to communicate pain verbally does not negate the likelihood that a person is in pain or that they require applicable pain-relieving treatment [3, 10]. The International Association for the Study of Pain (IASP) updated the definition of pain in July 2020 [2, p. 2] to: "An unpleasant sensory and emotional experience associated with, or resembling that associated with, actual or potential tissue damage". According to Raja et al. [2] the IASP also added six key notes as an expansion to the definition and to provide further context to the definition and the etymology of the word "pain." Additional notes to the latest pain definition for example highlight that a person's report of their pain should be acknowledged and respected and that verbal expressions of pain is only one of many behaviours to express pain [2]. Nevertheless, irrespective of patients' ability or inability to verbally self-report their pain, it remains the ethical obligation of all clinicians to acknowledge and relieve the most vulnerable patients' pain [12].

2. Communication vulnerability

Children with severe physical, sensory and/or cognitive disabilities affecting their receptive and expressive communication may not be able to verbally communicate their pain and other pain-related experiences [10, 13]. Children with languages or cultures different to those of the treating clinicians or with limited proficiency in the latter's language often do not have the vocabulary to express their pain [14]. Furthermore, children who are receiving treatment in intensive care units – where medical intervention such as sedation, intubation or tracheotomy can influence their ability to verbally communicate – as well as children receiving palliative end-of-life support may also not be able to communicate verbally [13]. Authors refer to these groups of children as communication vulnerable [13–15]. Communication vulnerability is defined as a reduced ability in respect of expressive and/or receptive communication and can involve permanent vulnerability (such as children with severe communication disabilities) or temporary vulnerability (such as patients in critical care units receiving medical interventions that may influence their ability to speak) [16, 17].

The inability to express pain verbally may result in communication breakdowns between the child and the clinician, which could result in risks such as non-treatment, adverse medical outcomes and increased anxiety for both patients and clinicians [18]. Clinicians often find it demanding to assess pain in communication vulnerable children [7, 19], as they have to attempt to interpret the children's bodily movements, facial expressions and physiological signs [7]. As mentioned earlier, children with communication disabilities may express their pain in atypical ways that could influence clinicians' interpretation of the children's pain [10, 11, 19]. In the latest recommendations for clinicians to follow during pain assessment of those unable to self-report, Herr et al. proposed that as a first step, clinicians should become aware of potential causes of pain [20]. The second step in pain assessment is to try to obtain self-report from all patients [20]. Therefore, it is vital that alternative means of communication should be investigated to enable children with severe communication difficulties to self-report their pain.

Hay et al. [21] promoted the use of self-reporting as the primary method for measuring the intensity and other features of pain. Thus, it was recommended that parents' proxy reports of their children's pain should only be used once the children's reports were in doubt [21, 22]. Research has confirmed that speaking children themselves can give a clear self-report of their pain experience by verbally expressing their pain or using various pain assessment tools such as the Coloured Analogue Scale or the Faces Pain Scale-Revised [23]. However, Schiavenato and Craig [24] are of the opinion that pain assessment tools do not do justice to a patient's pain experience as they oversimplify the demands for rating pain intensity without taking the type of pain into consideration. For this reason, a possible solution should be found for how communication vulnerable children can self-report their pain in ways other than by verbal accounts.

Clinicians' expertise to support communication vulnerable children in pain depends on the availability of reliable and valid information about the existence and precise nature of the child's distress [25]. Self-report and observational measures of pain can be reviewed from the perspective of a model of human communication [26]. Therefore, to gain a better understanding of this complex pain communication process, clinicians and researchers need to grasp the challenges that children with disabilities – and particularly those who are communication vulnerable – may encounter when trying to express their pain. The social communication model of pain [26, 27] offers an inclusive theoretical framework to be used in this chapter, because it explains the dynamic interaction between the biological, psychological and social determinants of pain [28]. An adapted social communication model of pain for communication vulnerable children based on the model proposed by Craig [27, 28] warrants further discussion in this chapter.

3. Social communication model of pain

Communication plays an important part in any action that aims to improve health [29]. Communication is a social, dynamic and interchanging reciprocal process that involves persons (acting as a sender or receiver) [30]. Communication comprises verbal (speech) as well as non-verbal modes (gestures, a shared glance, facial expression) [31]. Symbols (abstract or concrete) are used to convey information from the sender to the receiver in order to achieve a shared meaning in a specific context or environment [30]. In other words, communication involves sender(s) and receiver(s) conveying information through a communication channel. Effective communication occurs when the intent and meaning of one person (e.g. the sender) is understood by another person (e.g. the receiver) [31]. For communication vulnerable children, this communication process poses a serious challenge, due to their inability to communicate verbally (i.e. the communication intent is lost if the receiver does not understand the communication channel used by the sender). Although these children may have the desire to communicate their pain, research indicates that communication vulnerable children often opt not to communicate their pain because their previous communication attempts were ignored, or simply because it takes too much physical effort trying to communicate their pain [32].

The social communication model of pain was developed as a framework to explain how pain is experienced and to describe the multifaceted communication process required to adequately express and interpret pain and to have pain understood by others [26, 27]. The social communication model of pain underlines both the role of the sender who is the person in pain (e.g. the communication vulnerable child) and the ability of the receiver as the observer of the pain (e.g. clinicians) in understanding the experience of pain. Biomedical models, in contrast, focus on the sensory characteristics of pain, with no emphasis on the social factors of pain

[26, 27, 33]. Since this chapter will proceed to focus on pain communication of communication vulnerable children, **Figure 1** depicts the suggested adaptations to the social communication model of pain (based on Craig [27, 28]) as it relates to communication vulnerable children's expression of pain.

A proposed three-step pain communication process altered for communication vulnerable children highlights the different factors that may intervene in the children's pain expression, the pain assessment and the accompanying treatment [10, 27, 28]:

a. *Pain experience* – the inward personal painful pain experience that happens over time and is stimulated by both interpersonal and intrapersonal (biological and psychological) factors involves the status of the child before the event;

b. *Message* – the encoding of the pain experience (e.g. the child's understanding or making sense of the pain) and the expression of pain through expressive behaviours such as crying, exclamations or (verbal) self-report to make the pain known to observers (e.g. clinicians or parents);

c. *Observer (receiver of message)* – the process whereby observers decipher or decode pain behaviours to react and respond by providing appropriate pain management or pain-relieving treatment [34].

This model also highlights the possibility that observers' own perceptions and responses to pain as based on their own pain experiences may influence their understanding of pain as well as how they will respond to the child's pain experience. Although researchers and clinicians should be aware of their own bias towards pain, it will not be dealt with in further detail in this chapter.

In short, the adapted social communication model of pain proposes that the communication of pain begins with the communication vulnerable child who experiences pain (A); it continues to describe how this experience influences the

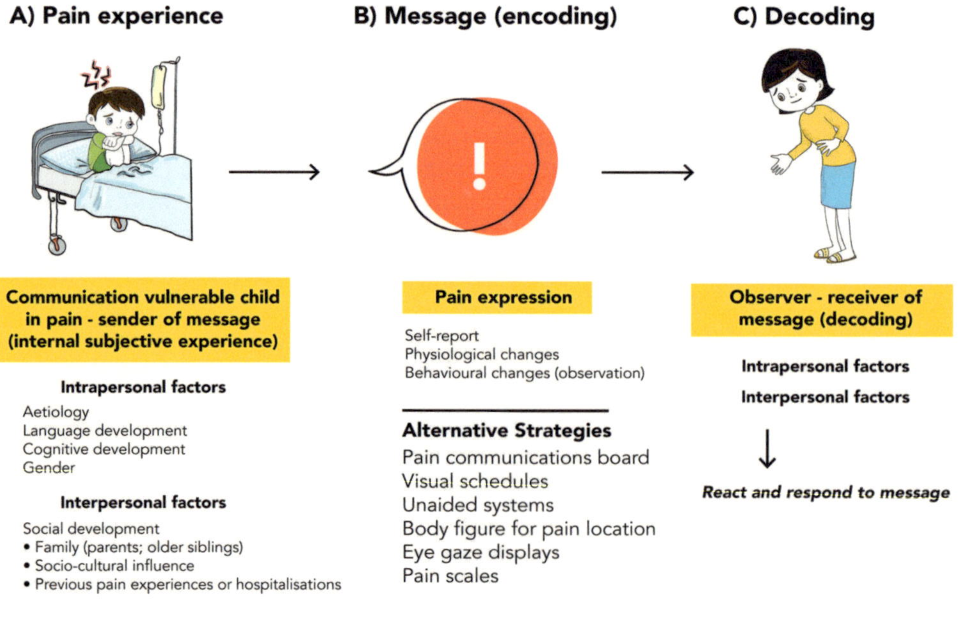

Figure 1.
Adapted social communication model of pain for communication vulnerable children (as based on Craig [27, 28]).

child to make sense of the pain (B) and to express it in atypical ways or by means of augmentative and alternative communication (AAC) modes. These pain expressions are made known to the observers (C), who decode the child's pain to take appropriate pain management actions. The adapted social communication model of pain can thus be used to help researchers and clinicians to understand the pain in communication vulnerable children. Examples are children with a variety of disabilities such as Down syndrome, intellectual disabilities, autism spectrum disorder (ASD) or cerebral palsy (CP), or children who experience temporary communication vulnerability due to medical interventions such as intubation.

The model considers that there are many ways that a child can encode (B) their pain experience (A). Thus, when decoding the child's pain, observers (C) need to be open to other modes that children may use to communicate their pain. A child's self-report of pain is influenced by the pain context as well as their emotional, sensory, cognitive, developmental and cultural composition [2, 35, 36]. The social factors and reciprocal, repeating and dynamic effects of pain communication are acknowledged during this pain account within human beings [28]. In the social communication model of pain, a clear distinction is made between historical and current biological and social factors. For example, intrapersonal factors refer to a person's temperament to react based on their biological, psychological and social histories. Craig [28] highlights that, during the pain event (A), the immediate social and physical environment has a powerful effect on both the person in pain (e.g. the communication vulnerable child) and on the observers (C). The internal subjective pain experiences of communication vulnerable children will now be discussed based on the adapted social communication model of pain for communication vulnerable children (**Figure 1**).

3.1 The internal subjective pain experiences of communication vulnerable children

The way persons express pain can give insight into their pain experiences. Pain *expressions* involve the person's observable response (such as their pain behaviours) to a noxious stimulus, whereas a person's pain *experience* is private and internal and involves severity of discomfort [27]. Based on their own experiences with pain, each individual displays different potential behavioural reactions to pain [27]. For example, children who have had negative pain experiences during needle procedures may exhibit more severe responses to pain because of their previous negative experiences. Additionally, their individual biological capabilities trigger their complicated expressions of pain [2]. Children with significant communication difficulties have different disability diagnoses with unique pain-related experiences related to these disabilities (e.g. children with CP or ASD).

3.1.1 Intrapersonal factors

Along with biological capabilities, the constructs behind pain expression are the impact of language and cognitive development as well as social interaction and experiences. The expansion of pain-related vocabulary progresses along a similar sequence as does natural language development [37, 38]. The theoretical constructs that underlie pain expression within communication vulnerable children with various aetiologies will now be discussed in more detail.

3.1.1.1 Aetiologies

All children experience pain on a regular basis. Young children with typical development may respond to everyday pain such as bumps and bruises by crying, verbalisations or spoken words to express their pain experiences. They usually start to use the word "pain" by the age of 6 years [37]. On the contrary, children with disabilities might have more pain incidents more often than their peers without disabilities. For example, children with disabilities may experience more acute pain incidents due to needle procedures (such as blood drawing or receiving blood transfusions) and recurring medical procedures and treatments (such as range-of-motion manipulation during physiotherapy for children with CP) to maintain their health [3, 39, 40].

Young children with CP experience high occurrences of chronic and acute pain [19, 41]. In an Australian study conducted by Ostojic and colleagues [19] to determine the prevalence of pain in children with CP, they found that two in three children with CP experienced acute pain and one in three children had chronic pain. Furthermore, the study revealed that children with CP, functioning on levels IV and V of the Gross Motor Function Scale (GMFCS), have a bigger risk of suffering from chronic pain [19]. This group also has communication challenges and may need alternative means to communicate their pain [19, 41]. Multi-factorial reasons for pain in children with CP could include spasticity, contractures and the incapacity to walk [19, 41, 42]. Spasticity and the inability to change their positioning to decrease pressure on certain body parts may also lead to contractures, musculoskeletal and gastrointestinal pain [43]. In a study among children with CP in South African schools, Adolfsson and colleagues [44] found that South African children with CP often experience hip dislocations– resulting from spasticity that caused hip displacements and ultimately lead to hip dislocations. As such, persons with CP have to undergo constant surgical procedures and medical interventions throughout their life span in an attempt to correct or rehabilitate orthopaedic problems associated with their condition [41, 43, 45]. All these procedures, including range-of-motion manipulation and assisted stretching, are painful experiences [44]. Communication through the use of AAC communication strategies is therefore crucial for children with CP to ensure that they can express their pain and receive appropriate pain treatment [41].

Children with intellectual disabilities are at risk of experiencing a variety of painful somatic conditions due to comorbidities such as contractures, gastro-oesophageal refluxes, and epilepsy [11, 46]. These children with intellectual disabilities often experience socio-communicative deficits typical of children with ASD, for example they may not use facial expressions or make eye contact to display pain or other emotions [11, 46, 47]. Children with intellectual disabilities also express their pain consistent with their level of cognitive and physical development and not necessarily consistent with their chronological age [46]. Some atypical expressions, such as hand flapping or hand rubbing, smiling or freezing has been observed when children with intellectual disabilities were not able to verbalise their pain [5]. Yet, according to Doody and Bailey [9], children with intellectual disability who are unable to communicate their pain in a typical manner seem to have less opportunity to receive pain treatment.

Children with Down syndrome also fall in the group of children with intellectual disability who can be expected to experience pain as a result of their disability. They are at high risk of secondary pain-related experiences such as the development of hip abnormalities and oral health issues [3, 48]. Children with Down syndrome have higher occurrences than their peers with typical development of dental problems due to frequent incidence of periodontal disease and chronic facial pain disorders [3]. They may also experience chronic pain due to congenital heart anomalies, bone fractures due to osteoporosis, or eczema – to name a few conditions [5]. Davies [48] reported that, compared to their siblings with typical development, children with Down syndrome have a decreased tendency to react to pain – but that does not mean that they are unresponsive to pain. Due to lower cognitive functioning, children with Down syndrome may not have the ability to localise the painful stimulus, because their pain-related vocabulary only tends to develop at a later stage. Their limited pain-related vocabulary may thus influence their ability to communicate pain [38].

As with children with CP, children with intellectual disabilities such as Down syndrome or ASD also experience a large number of pain incidents and they are sometimes two to three times more at risk of an injury than their peers with typical development [10, 49]. Children with ASD often display challenging and self-injurious behaviour, as well as extreme tantrums that could lead to injury and pain [10]. Some children with ASD may also have trouble expressing their pain, due to their typical delay in language development and possible cognitive impairment [10, 50]. If children with ASD do use speech, they struggle to convey their emotions and the intensity of their pain experiences due to their monotone intonation. In addition, they do not usually use the same facial expressions and gestures that their peers with typical development would do to express their feelings. The pain expressions of children with ASD are distinctively individual and may differ from those of the larger population, considering the fact that children with ASD experience socio-communicative impairments and therefore may not understand social closeness as their peers with typical development would do [3].

Besides the communication difficulties of children with disabilities, this chapter also focuses on children who experience a temporary communication vulnerability due to medical procedures (such as intubation) or life-threatening conditions (such as cancer). For example, critically ill children who have been admitted to paediatric intensive care units suffer a temporary loss of their expressive or receptive communication [13]. These communication vulnerable children show stress, frustration and anxiety, and are at a greater risk of being treated incorrectly by clinicians who wrongly decode the children's pain message [15, 51]. Even clinicians such as nurses often mention their feelings of frustration when they find it difficult to grasp what their paediatric patients are trying to communicate [7]. The vast significance of efficient alternative means of communication to ensure safe treatment of paediatric patients is therefore emphasised [15].

3.1.1.2 Language development

Spoken language is seen as the ultimate means of communicating pain [52]. Language and cognitive development influence children's use of words to describe their pain experiences in such a way that observers (clinicians) can decode the message correctly and respond appropriately with pain-relieving treatment [53]. Language learning occurs within a physical and social context determined by actual people, objects, activities and events in the child's environment [54]. Children learn about new concepts in the world while interacting with their physical environment, which forms the foundation for their lexical development [54]. For example, the words parents use to communicate with their children during painful experiences enable children to acquire new pain-related vocabulary [38]. Parents tend to talk to their children about pain on an age-appropriate level, thus enlarging their children's pain-related vocabulary. For example, when a child cries when injured, the parent might respond with exclamations or words such as "Ouch! You got hurt!" thereby enabling the child to add meaning to the painful experience and to expand their repertoire of pain-related vocabulary [55].

However, since children with severe communication difficulties do not have the same contact with their social environment as their peers with typical development, they may find the language-learning process challenging [54]. Whereas children with typical development gain new knowledge about the world they live in through their encounters with their environment, children with disabilities have reduced access to their environment. This makes it more challenging for them to acquire new concepts without having the relevant previous knowledge to build on [54]. It is consequently the adults' responsibility to guarantee that children with severe communication difficulties are exposed to a social environment that includes people, objects and possible pain experiences. This exposure to facilitate children's language development can be achieved for instance through play activities like doctor-doctor play with peers [54].

3.1.1.3 Cognitive development

Language development corresponds with cognitive development and as children mature cognitively, they can describe their pain more successfully [52]. Younger children tend to explain the bodily sensations they experience during pain in a more concrete manner (such as 'my stomach hurts') due to their limited cognitive and language skills [56]. As children's thinking develops on a symbolic level, they start to use more graphic descriptors such as "terrible" or "beating", while older children start to add intensifiers, such as "really bad" when describing their pain [53]. Since children with severe communication difficulties may not be able to verbally express their pain, Johnson et al. [57] proposed that clinicians such as speech-language therapists provide these children with preselected pain vocabulary that can be added to their AAC system to enable them to express their pain appropriately.

Apart from disability aetiology, language or cognitive development, gender is another intrapersonal factor that might have an impact on the development of children's pain-related vocabulary [37, 38, 58, 59].

3.1.1.4 Gender

Gender differences in pain expression and pain-related vocabulary – despite similar pain experiences – are often highlighted in literature [38, 60–62]. As girls typically develop expressive vocabulary sooner than boys, Frank et al. [38] found a slight advantage in girls' pain-related vocabulary, which may imply that pain-related language acquisition could be related to other factors. For example, girls tend to be more emotive and more expected to complain and also report their pain experiences more frequently than boys [52]. Contrary to girls, boys tend to be more passive or have more anger-related vocabulary in response to pain due to an injury [38]. In the event of communication vulnerable children, the differences between the reactions to pain by boys and girls are not clear [8]. However, it was found in literature that adult observers' responses to children's pain experiences tend to be influenced by gender-stereotyped attitudes, and that girls were treated in a different way than boys [62–64]. Clinicians are often biased and expect girls to experience more pain than boys [63–65].

3.1.2 Interpersonal factors

3.1.2.1 Social development

According to the adapted social communication model of pain, interpersonal factors such as family settings, children's social and cultural environment, as well as previous hospitalisations may further influence children's experience and expression of pain [27].

3.1.2.2 Family

Though some characteristics of pain-related language seem to be universal, substantial influences of family and ethnic contexts are also repeated in the specificity of pain-related language due to the nature of the social setting in which children are growing up [55, 66]. The entire family is affected by children's chronic pain experiences and these experiences are often stressful for other family members as well. The treatment prescribed to manage the child's pain can result in interferences in planned family events, thus upsetting or disrupting the overall family system [66].

From the perspective of the family systems theory, family dynamics influence the way children understand and talk about their pain [22, 62]. Parents are the role models for their children to learn words to express pain [55]. As children's cognitive and social skills develop, they learn to talk about pain by observing how their parents respond to and talk about their children's pain experiences [66]. Parents' socio-economic background, education and age may influence the way in which they respond to their children's pain. For example, in an American study by Rowe [67] – who investigated why parents from different socio-economic statuses communicate in different ways with their children – it was found that more educated parents and parents from advantaged backgrounds tended to talk more often to their children and use a bigger variety of words and longer utterances thereby expanding their children's language ability and pain-related vocabulary. Younger parents also tended to use different pain words in comparison with older parents [68].

Birth order also impacts on children's development of pain-related vocabulary [38]. Younger children observe their older siblings' use of pain words, which stimulates their own development of pain-related vocabulary [38]. It was reported that the presence of one or more older siblings has an impact on children's use of pain words compared to those children without older siblings [38]. Moreover, children with siblings who had previously been hospitalised had a larger vocabulary than those with siblings who had never been hospitalised before. This suggests that experience plays a role in the learning of pain language because these children had to deal with the illness or hospitalisations of their sibling(s) [38].

3.1.2.3 Socio-cultural influence

Apart from family practices, children develop an understanding of pain-related language within their sociolinguistic environment [66, 69]. Children's language is influenced by their cultural beliefs, social groups and communities [69]. There are differences between the beliefs of diverse cultures and their views on parents' roles in their children's language development. In some cultures, parents may not react to their children's utterances: they are of the opinion that adults must not teach children to talk, as they will eventually learn to talk on their own [67]. Some family and cultural beliefs can also result in disparities in the way children learn about pain and react to pain [36]. In some Nguni and Sotho cultures in South Africa, for example, boys are taught that they may not express their pain, because showing or expressing pain is a sign of weakness or lack of courage [70].

Clinicians should therefore acknowledge cultural differences and try to understand the culture of the communication vulnerable child. They should ask detailed questions to help understand the child's pain condition and to prevent any misunderstanding [52]. Clinicians should for instance be aware of the fact that in some cultures it is considered disgraceful to ask for pain relief, while people in other cultures believe that a godly intervention will relieve pain when necessary [62, 70].

3.1.2.4 Previous pain experiences and hospitalisations

Children's understanding (and the significance) of their first painful experience due to tissue injury will intensify with experience – either through positive or negative contextual associations [2]. Children learn the use of the word "pain" through their experiences related to injury [58]. Hospitalisations help children to develop pain vocabulary based on their personal experiences with pain. Therefore, children with previous hospitalisations who experience pain events more often and who have learnt and processed the concept of pain (and pain management) tend to have a larger pain-related vocabulary than those who have never been admitted to hospital before [38].

4. Alternative means to communicate pain

From the discussion above, it is clear that communication vulnerable children experience challenges to express their pain and need alternative means – such as AAC strategies and systems – to communicate their pain. AAC involves a variety of communication strategies that can be used to aid communication attempts of persons with communication challenges to either augment their speech or to be used as an alternative means to speech [31]. Regarding the adapted social communication model of pain, one can agree that when the communication vulnerable child is offered the use of AAC to express their pain (A), the form (or communication mode used) is less important than ensuring that the message (B) is understood by the observer (C). AAC systems are classified as either unaided or aided. Unaided AAC systems are defined as the use of only body parts to convey messages such as by pointing, making gestures, body language movements, facial expressions, and manual signing [31]. Aided AAC systems include low-technology aids that need no electronic programming (e.g. pen and paper, and symbol-based communication boards), as well as high-technology aids such as speech-generating devices [71]. Clinicians should be encouraged to incorporate AAC strategies and tools to enable communication vulnerable child patients to communicate their pain.

AAC strategies and systems have been successfully used with communication vulnerable children in various settings, including hospital settings [13, 16–18, 71–73]. Next, some potential AAC strategies are proposed to support communication vulnerable children to express their pain in order for observers (C) to understand the messages (B). The suggested AAC strategies will focus mainly on low-technology systems although all these strategies could also be incorporated in apps on digital mobile devices (smart phones or tablets) to enable communication vulnerable children as well as clinicians and researchers to gain a history of pain communication and subsequent pain treatment [74].

4.1 Pain-related communication boards

Communication boards are low-technology AAC systems used to display pictures (photographs, line drawings or graphic symbols) to enable communication vulnerable persons to communicate [31]. When designing a communication board, aspects such as the type of symbol (photograph, type of line drawing, graphic symbols or written words), the symbol size (to best accommodate the child's visual and motor skills), symbol colour (to ensure contrast and increase the ease of finding a word within a particular word class), board layout and display (e.g. using the left-to-right Fitzgerald-key outlay as a precursor to reading), as well as the child's vocabulary need should be taken into consideration [71]. For example, children with physical disabilities or limited range of movement may not be able to access symbols that are too far apart.

Johnson et al. [53] conducted a scoping review to compile a list of children's pain-related vocabulary in an attempt to provide clinicians and parents with possible pain words that children would typically use to express their pain. In this scoping review, 17 studies from diverse cultures in countries such as the United States of America, Canada, Finland, Kuwait, South Africa, Spain and Sweden were included. It was interesting to note that the meaning of children's pain-related words in the native language translated to the same English word or words [53]. The study also showed that clinicians from different countries could use this list of pain-related words to compile basic pain-related communication boards that could be further individualised for their communication vulnerable paediatric clients [53].

In a follow-up pilot study by Gerber [75], 6- to 9-year-old children were asked to choose which symbols from two symbol sets, namely Picture Communication Symbols [PCS™] and Bildstöd symbols (www.bildstod.se) that they perceived as capturing the meaning of the pain-related words identified by Johnson et al. [53] most effectively. They were also asked which symbols they prefer, and why they made this choice. The children predominantly chose the Bildstöd symbols (an open source symbol library) because they perceived these symbols as looking more "real", being colourful, and with extra features to show the intensity of the pain experienced. Hence it is recommended that clinicians familiarise themselves with the pain-related word list compiled by Johnson et al. [53] and that they use the freely available symbols from the Bildstöd platform to develop a pain-related communication board for communication vulnerable children. A further recommendation is that the pain-related words should be representative of different categories of pain-related words, namely vocabulary that can be used to (i) describe pain; (ii) direct other's actions; (iii) describe pain location; (iv) describe causes of pain; (v) describe strategies to cope with pain; (vi) reflect on strategies for pain prevention, and (vii) strategies to indicate consequences of pain or injury [57]. These categories will enable children to search quickly through the options. Adults who use AAC suggested that a body figure of a child should be included on the communication board to eliminate the use of words to describe the pain location (category (iii)) [57]. Body figures were also included in the child version of a communication board developed by Patak and colleagues [73] to be used with communication vulnerable children in intensive care settings.

4.2 Visual schedules

The discussion earlier in this chapter makes it clear that children's previous negative pain-related encounters influence how they perceive new pain experiences. Furthermore, since children with ASD and intellectual disabilities need routine to function optimally, visual schedules can be used to great benefit to prepare them for specific medical procedures. This preparation could reduce their anxiousness due to unfamiliarity with the procedure or previous negative experiences [15, 76]. A visual schedule should include a step-by-step and easily understandable format with pictures accompanied by written words (see **Figure 2** for example). These will provide children with the necessary information to help them feel that they are in control of the imminent frightening procedures [77]. Visual schedules can be offered either in paper format (low-technology) or, where applicable, in a video story-based format.

4.3 Eye gaze displays

Children with severe physical disabilities and limited movements may not be able to use their fingers to point to choices on a low-technology communication board. Therefore, the use of eye gaze displays is proposed. With eye gaze, the child

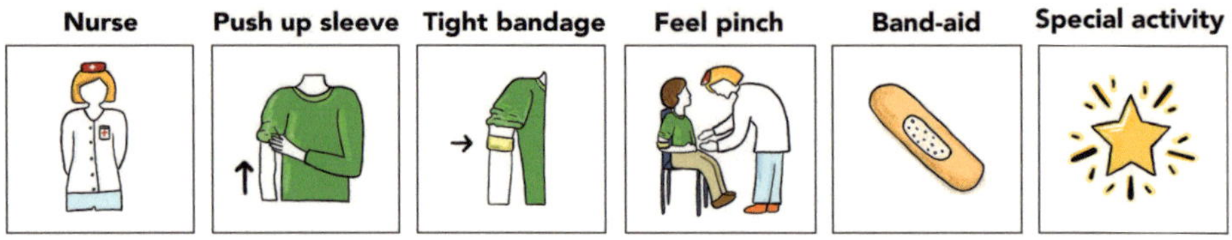

Figure 2.
Visual schedule of a needle procedure.

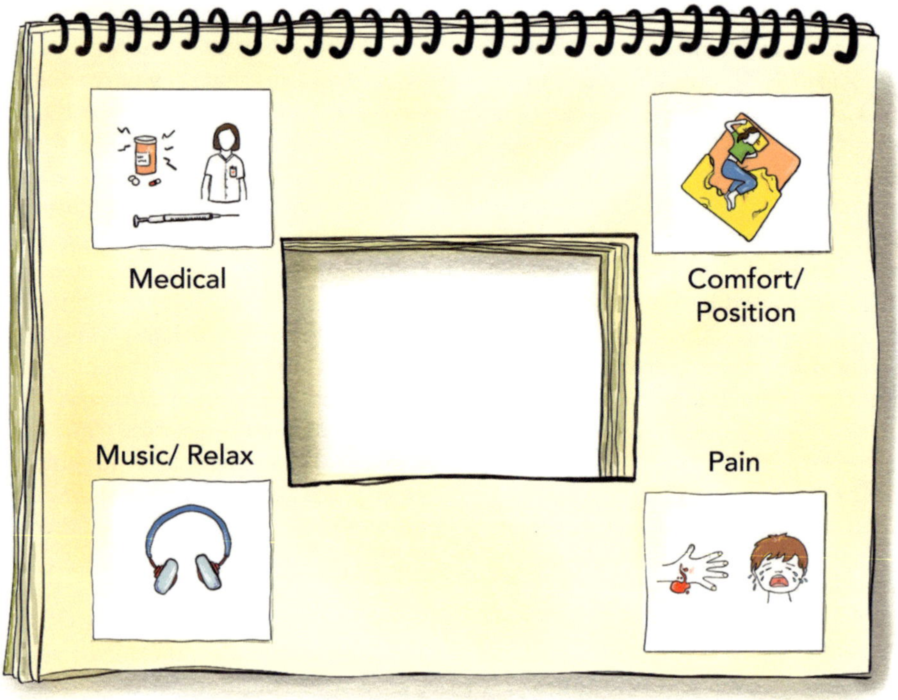

Figure 3.
Eye gaze flip chart.

is instructed to use their eyes to look at a picture or word on the display and then glance at the communication partner (observer), who will then verbally confirm the child's selection [15]. **Figure 3** is an example of an eye-gaze flipchart display.

4.4 Unaided systems

During pain assessments of communication vulnerable children, clinicians or researchers can also ask the child pain-related questions providing them three options: "Yes", "No", "Not sure". Communication vulnerable children often have clear yes/no responses (e.g. head nodding to indicate "Yes"). Should communication vulnerable children have no typical yes/no responses, the clinician can ask the child to blink their eyes ("Yes"), close their eyes ("No"), or to look away to indicate that they are not sure what to answer. In this case, the clinician should refrain from asking more than one close-ended question at a time (e.g. "Does it hurt?" and "Do you hurt in your [*body part*]?"). The clinician should rather ask only one question (e.g. "Does it hurt?") to ensure that the child can give an appropriate response.

4.5 Pain scales

Appropriate pain management relies on the ability to accurately assess pain. For children, a common method to communicate pain is the use of pain scales [13]. Pain scales that are often used in clinical and research practice typically depict faces, colours or numeric grading [13]. An example of faces pain scales that are built on how children communicate their feeling(s) in a facial expression is the Faces Pain Scale-Revised (FPS-R) [78]. Colours and numeric grading are typically used in analogue scales that are based on increments to indicate pain severity, and these allow children to show that a somewhat larger or smaller pain is experienced (examples are the Colour Analogue Scale (CAS) [79]; and the Numeric Rating Scale (NRS) [80]). In a systematic review by Birnie et al. [23] on recommendations for the selection of children's self-report rating scales for pain intensity, the FPS-R, CAS and NRS were recommended for self-report of acute pain. However, though these self-report scales are freely available, clinicians and researchers should keep in mind that they may not be effective for everyone [13]. For example, while some of these scales may not need expressive language, receptive language skills are crucial, as children are expected to comprehend and know the meaning of words such as "hurt" or "pain" when using these scales [26].

5. Conclusion

This chapter aimed to address communication vulnerable children's experiences of pain and their need for alternative ways to express their pain so as to receive appropriate pain treatment. The concept of communication vulnerability was explained framed in the context of the adapted social communication model of pain for communication vulnerable children. According to this model, there are many ways in which communication vulnerable children can encode (B) their pain experience (A). The model also emphasises the need for observers (C) to be open to other communication modes that children may use to communicate their pain. The discussion centred on the pain experiences of communication vulnerable children such as children with Down syndrome, with intellectual disabilities, autism or cerebral palsy, as well as of children in intensive care settings who experience temporary communication vulnerability. The chapter concludes with suggestions on how AAC strategies can be used to support communication vulnerable children in communicating their pain.

Acknowledgements

The author would like to thank and acknowledge Prof Stefan Nilsson from Gothenburg University and Prof Juan Bornman from the Centre for AAC, University of Pretoria for their valuable comments to improve the content of this manuscript. The author would further like to thank Ms Olivia Loots for the drawings as portrayed in the three figures in this chapter.

The funding from the National Research Foundation in South Africa to this project is also acknowledged.

Conflict of interest

The author declares no conflict of interest.

Author details

Ensa Johnson
Centre for Augmentative and Alternative Communication, University of Pretoria, Pretoria, South Africa

*Address all correspondence to: ensa.johnson@up.ac.za

References

[1] Gregory J. Use of pain scales and observational pain assessment tools in hospital settings. Nursing Standard. 2019;**34**. DOI: 10.7748/ns.2019.e11308

[2] Raja SN, Carr DB, Cohen M, Finnerup NB, Flor H, Gibson S, et al. The revised International Association for the Study of Pain definition of pain: Concepts, challenges, and compromises. Pain. 2020;**161**:1976-1982. DOI: 10.1097/j.pain.0000000000001939

[3] Bottos S, Chambers CT. The epidemiology of pain in developmental disabilities. In: Orlander TM, Symons FJ, editors. Pain in Children and Adults with Developmental Disabilities. Baltimore, Maryland: Paul Brookes Publishing Company; 2006. pp. 67-87

[4] Beacroft M, Dodd K. 'I feel pain'– audit of communication skills and understanding of pain and health needs with people with learning disabilities. British Journal of Learning Disabilities. 2011;**39**(2):139-147. DOI: 10.1111/j.1468-3156.2010.00640.x

[5] McGuire BE, Defrin R. Pain perception in people with down syndrome: A synthesis of clinical and experimental research. Frontiers in Behavioral Neuroscience. 2015;**9**:194. DOI: 10.3389/fnbeh.2015.00194

[6] McCaffery M. Nursing Practice Theories Related to Cognition, Bodily Pain, and Man-Environment Interactions. Los Angeles: University of Los Angeles; 1968

[7] Amponsah AK, Kyei EF, Agyemang JB, Boakye H, Kyei-Dompim J, Ahoto CK, et al. Nursing-related barriers to Children's pain Management at Selected Hospitals in Ghana: A descriptive qualitative study. Pain Research & Management. 2020;**2020**:1-7. DOI: 10.1155/2020/7125060

[8] Johnson E. An exploration of the common pain-related vocabulary typically-developing children use: Implications for children who use AAC [thesis]. Pretoria: University of Pretoria; 2015

[9] Doody O, Bailey E. Pain and pain assessment in people with intellectual disability: Issues and challenges in practice. British Journal of Learning Disabilities. 2017;**45**:157-165. DOI: 10.1111/bld.12189

[10] Rattaz C, Dubois A, Baghdadli A. How do people with autism spectrum disorders (ASD) experience pain? In: Battaglia A, editor. An Introduction to Pain and its Relation to Nervous System Disorders. Chichester, West Sussex, UK: John Wiley & Sons, Ltd; 2016. pp. 295-315. DOI: 10.1002/9781118455968.ch12

[11] de Knegt NC, Pieper MJC, Lobbezoo F, Schuengel C, Evenhuis HM, Passchier J, et al. Behavioral pain indicators in people with intellectual disabilities: A systematic review. The Journal of Pain. 2013;**14**(9):885-896. DOI: 10.1016/j.jpain.2013.04.016

[12] Paice JA, Coyne P. Justice in America: Ethical issues in cancer pain control. Journal of Hospice and Palliative Nursing. 2017;**19**(6):508-513. DOI: 10.1097/NJH.0000000000000384

[13] Costello J, Santiago R, Blackstone SW. Pediatric acute and intensive care in hospitals. In: Blackstone SW, Beukelman DR, Yorkson KM, editors. Patient Provider Communication: Roles for Speech-Language Pathologists and Other Health Care Professionals. San Diego, California: Plural Publishing; 2015. pp. 187-215

[14] Blackstone SW. Issues and challenges in advancing effective patient-provider communication. In: Blackstone SW, Beukelman DR, Yorkston KM, editors.

Patient-Provider Communication: Roles for Speech=Language Pathologists and Other Healthcare Professionals. San Diego: Plural Publishing; 2015. pp. 9-35

[15] Costello J. AAC intervention in the intensive care unit: The children's hospital Boston model. Augmentative and Alternative Communication. 2000;**16**(3):137-153. DOI: 10.1080/07434610012331279004

[16] Santiago R, Costello JM. AAC assessment and intervention in pediatric ICU/acute care: From referral through continuum of care. SIG 12, Augmentative and Alternative Communication. 2013;**22**(2):102-111. DOI: 10.1044/aac22.2.102

[17] Costello J, Patak L, Pritchard J. Communication vulnerable patients in the pediatric ICU: Enhancing care through augmentative and alternative communication. Journal of Pediatric Rehabilitation Medicine. 2010;**3**(4): 289-301. DOI: 10.3233/prm-2010-0140

[18] Blackstone SW, Pressman H. Patient communication in health care settings: New opportunities for augmentative and alternative communication. Augmentative and Alternative Communication. 2016;**32**(1):69-79. DOI: 10.3109/07434618.2015.1125947

[19] Ostojic K, Paget S, Kyriagis M, Morrow A. Acute and chronic pain in children and adolescents with cerebral palsy: Prevalence, interference, and management. Archives of Physical Medicine and Rehabilitation. 2020;**101**(2):213-219. DOI: 10.1016/j.apmr.2019.08.475

[20] Herr K, Coyne PJ, Ely E, Gélinas C, Manworren RCB. Pain assessment in the patient unable to self-report: Clinical practice recommendations in support of the ASPMN 2019 position statement. Pain Management Nursing. 2019;**20**(5):404-417. DOI: 10.1016/j.pmn.2019.07.007

[21] Hay I, Oates J, Giannini A, Berkowitz R, Rotenberg B. Pain perception of children undergoing nasendoscopy for investigation of voice and resonance disorders. Journal of Voice. 2009;**23**:380-388. DOI: 10.1016/j.jvoice.2007.10.008

[22] Von Baeyer CL, Marche TA, Rocha EM, Salmon K. Children's memory of pain: Overview and implications for practice. The Journal of Pain. 2004;**5**(5):241-249. DOI: 10.1016/j.jpain.2004.05.001

[23] Birnie KA, Hundert AS, Lalloo C, Nguyen C, Stinson JN. Recommendations for selection of self-report pain intensity measures in children and adolescents: A systematic review and quality assessment of measurement properties. Pain. 2019;**160**(1):5-18. DOI: 10.1097/j.pain.0000000000001377

[24] Schiavenato M, Craig KD. Pain assessment as a social transaction: Beyond the "gold standard". The Clinical Journal of Pain. 2010;**26**(8):667-676. DOI: 10.1097/AJP.0b013e3181e72507

[25] Hadjistavropoulos T, Von Baeyer CL, Craig KD. Pain assessment in persons with limited ability to communicate. In: Melzack DCTR, editor. Handbook of Pain Assessment (2nd ed). New York, NY, US: Guilford Press; 2001. p. 134-149

[26] Hadjistavropoulos T, Craig KD. A theoretical framework for understanding self-report and observational measures of pain: A communications model. Behaviour Research and Therapy. 2002;**40**(5):551-570. DOI: 10.1016/S0005-7967(01)00072-9

[27] Craig KD. The social communication model of pain. Canadian Psychology/Psychologie Canadienne. 2009;**50**(1):22-32. DOI: 10.1037/a0014772

[28] Craig KD. Social communication model of pain. Pain. 2015;**156**(7):1198-1199. DOI: 10.1097/j.pain.0000000000000185

[29] Corcoran N. Theories and models in communicating health messages. In: Communicating Health: Strategies for Health Promotion. London: Sage Publications; 2007. pp. 5-31

[30] West R, Turner LH. Introducing Communication Theory: Analysis and Application. 6th ed. New York: McGraw-Hill Education; 2018

[31] Bornman J, Tönsing KM. Augmentative and alternative communication. In: Landsberg E, Kruger D, Swart E, editors. Addressing Barriers to Learning - A South African Perspective. 4 ed. Pretoria: Van Schaik; 2019. P. 215-239

[32] Dubois A, Capdevila X, Bringuier S, Pry R. Pain expression in children with an intellectual disability. European Journal of Pain. 2010;**14**(6):654-660. DOI: 10.1016/j.ejpain.2009.10.013

[33] Craig KD. The construct and definition of pain in developmental disability. In: Oberlander TF, Symons FJ, editors. Pain in Children and Adults with Developmental Disabilities. Baltimore, Maryland: Paul Brookes Publishing Company; 2006. pp. 7-18

[34] Hadjistavropoulos T, Breau LM, Craig KD. Assessment of pain in adults and children with limited ability to communicate. In: Turck DC, Melzack R, editors. Handbook of Pain Assessment. 3rd ed. New York: The Guilford Press; 2011. pp. 260-280

[35] Finley GA, Kristjánsdóttir O, Forgeron PA. Cultural influences on the assessment of children's pain. Pain Research & Management. 2009;**14**(1):33-37. DOI: 10.1155/2009/763031

[36] Kortesluoma R, Punämaki R, Nikkonen M. Hospitalized children drawing their pain: The contents and cognitive and emotional characteristics of pain drawings. Journal of Child Health Care. 2008;**12**(4):284-300

[37] Stanford EA, Chambers CT, Craig KD. A normative analysis of the development of pain-related vocabulary in children. Pain. 2005;**114**(1-2):278-284. DOI: 10.1177%2F1367493508096204

[38] Franck L, Noble G, Liossi C. From tears to words: The development of language to express pain in young children with everyday minor illnesses and injuries. Child: Care, Health and Development. 2010;**36**(4):524-533. DOI: 10.1111/j.1365-2214.2010.01084.x

[39] Nilsson S, Finnström B, Kokinsky E. The FLACC behavioral scale for procedural pain assessment in children aged 5-16 years. Pediatric Anesthesia. 2008;**18**(8):767-774. DOI: 10.1111/j.1460-9592.2008.02655.x

[40] Breau LM, Camfield CS, McGrath PJ, Finley GA. The incidence of pain in children with severe cognitive impairments. Archives of Pediatrics & Adolescent Medicine. 2003;**157**(12):1219-1226. DOI: 10.1001/archpedi.157.12.1219

[41] McKinnon CT, Morgan PE, Antolovich GC, Clancy CH, Fahey MC, Harvey AR. Pain in children with dyskinetic and mixed dyskinetic/spastic cerebral palsy. Developmental Medicine and Child Neurology. 2020:1-8. DOI: 10.1111/dmcn.14615

[42] Novak I. Evidence-based diagnosis, health care, and rehabilitation for children with cerebral palsy. Journal of Child Neurology. 2014;**29**(8):1141-1156. DOI: 10.1177/0883073814535503

[43] Blackman JA, Svensson CI, Marchand S. Pathophysiology of chronic pain in cerebral palsy: Implications for pharmacological treatment and

research. Developmental Medicine and Child Neurology. 2018;**60**(9):861-865. DOI: 10.1111/dmcn.13930

[44] Adolfsson M, Johnson E, Nilsson S. Pain management for children with cerebral palsy in school settings in two cultures: Action and reaction approaches. Disability and Rehabilitation. 2018;**40**(18):2152-2162. DOI: 10.1080/09638288.2017.1327987

[45] Ramstad K, Jahnsen R, Skjeldal OH, Diseth TH. Characteristics of recurrent musculoskeletal pain in children with cerebral palsy aged 8 to 18 years. Developmental Medicine and Child Neurology. 2011;**53**(11):1013-1018. DOI: 10.1111/j.1469-8749.2011.04070.x

[46] Terstegen C, Koot HM, De Boer JB, Tibboel D. Measuring pain in children with cognitive impairment: Pain response to surgical procedures. Pain. 2003;**103**(1):187-198. DOI: 10.1016/s0304-3959(02)00453-0

[47] Gilbert-MacLeod CA, Craig KD, Rocha EM, Mathias MD. Everyday pain responses in children with and without developmental delays. Journal of Pediatric Psychology. 2000;**25**(5):301-308. DOI: 10.1093/jpepsy/25.5.301

[48] Davies RB. Pain in children with down syndrome: Assessment and intervention by parents. Pain Management Nursing. 2010;**11**(4):259-267. DOI: 10.1016/j.pmn.2009.09.003

[49] Yung A, Haagsma JA, Polinder S. A systematic review on the influence of pre-existing disability on sustaining injury. Accident; Analysis and Prevention. 2014;**62**:199-208. DOI: 10.1016/j.aap.2013.09.024

[50] Craig KD, Lilley CM, Gilbert CA. Social barriers to optimal pain management in infants and children. The Clinical Journal of Pain. 1996;**12**:232-242. DOI: 10.1097/00002508-199609000-00011

[51] Coyne I. Consultation with children in hospital: Children, parents' and nurses' perspectives. Journal of Clinical Nursing. 2005;**15**:61-71. DOI: 10.1111/j.1365-2702.2005.01247.x

[52] Azize PM, Humphreys A, Cattani A. The impact of language on the expression and assessment of pain in children. Intensive & Critical Care Nursing. 2011;**27**(5):235-243. DOI: 10.1016/j.iccn.2011.07.002

[53] Johnson E, Boshoff K, Bornman J. Scoping review of children's pain vocabulary. Canadian Journal of Speech-Language Pathology and Audiology. 2018;**42**(1):55-68

[54] Light J. "Let's go star fishing": Reflections on the contexts of language learning for children who use aided AAC. Augmentative and Alternative Communication. 1997;**13**(3):158-171. DOI: 10.1080/07434619712331277978

[55] Craig KD, Stanford EA, Fairbairn NS, Chambers CT. Emergent pain language communication competence in infants and children. Enfance. 2006;**1**:52-71

[56] Dubois A, Bringuier S, Capdevila X, Pry R. Vocal and verbal expression of postoperative pain in preschoolers. Pain Management Nursing. 2008;**9**(4):160-165. DOI: 10.1016/j.pmn.2007.10.003

[57] Johnson E, Bornman J, Tönsing KM. An exploration of pain-related vocabulary: Implications for AAC use with children. Augmentative and Alternative Communication. 2016;**32**(4):1-12. DOI: 10.1080/07434618.2016.1233998

[58] Jerrett M, Evans K. Children's pain vocabulary. Journal of Advanced Nursing. 1986;**11**(4):403-408. DOI: 10.1111/j.1365-2648.1986.tb01267.x

[59] Azize PM. The impact of language on the expression and assessment of

pain in children aged 4-7 years: A mixed methods study [thesis]. Plymouth: University of Plymouth; 2012

[60] Huguet A, Miró J, Nieto R. The inventory of parent/caregiver responses to the children's pain experience (IRPEDNA): Development and preliminary validation. Pain. 2008;**134**(1):128-139. DOI: 10.1016/j.pain.2007.04.004

[61] Fearon I, McGrath PJ, Achat H. 'Booboos': The study of everyday pain among young children. Pain. 1996;**68**(1):55-62. DOI: 10.1016/s0304-3959(96)03200-9

[62] Briggs E. Assessment and expression of pain. Nursing Standard. 2010;**25**(2):35-38. DOI: 10.7748/ns2010.09.25.2.35.c7986

[63] Boerner KE, Dhariwal AK. JPP student journal Club commentary: When adults evaluate a Child's pain: Considering study methodology, gender bias and parental experience. Journal of Pediatric Psychology. 2019;**44**(4): 415-417. DOI: 10.1093/jpepsy/jsz012

[64] Earp BD, Monrad JT, LaFrance M, Bargh JA, Cohen LL, Richeson JA. Featured article: Gender bias in pediatric pain assessment. Journal of Pediatric Psychology. 2019;**44**(4):403-414. DOI: 10.1093/jpepsy/jsy104

[65] Cohen LL, Cobb J, Martin SR. Gender biases in adult ratings of pediatric pain. Children's Health Care. 2014;**43**(2):87-95. DOI: 10.1080/02739615.2014.849918

[66] Palermo TM, Valrie CR, Karlson CW. Family and parent influences on pediatric chronic pain. The American Psychologist. 2014;**69**(2):142-152. DOI: 10.1037/a0035216

[67] Rowe ML. Child-directed speech: Relation to socioeconomic status, knowledge of child development and child vocabulary skill. Journal of Child Language. 2008;**35**(01):185-205. DOI: 10.1017/S0305000907008343

[68] Turck DC, Flor H, Rudy TE. Pain and families. I.: Etiology, maintenance and psychosocial impact. Pain. 1987;**30**:3-27. DOI: 10.1016/0304-3959(87)90080-7

[69] Schieffelin BB, Ochs E. Language socialization. Annual Review of Anthropology. 1986;**15**:163-191

[70] Nortjé N, Albertyn R. The cultural language of pain: A South African study. South African Family Practice. 2015;**57**(1):24-27. DOI: 10.1080/20786190.2014.977034

[71] Beukelman DR, Mirenda P. Augmentative and Alternative Communication. Supporting Shildren and Adults with Complex Communication Needs. 4th ed. Baltimore, MD: Paul. H. Brookes; 2013

[72] Blackstone SW, Ruschke K, Wilson-Stronks A, Lee C. Converging communication vulnerabilities in health care: An emerging role for speech-language pathologists and audiologists. SIG 14 Perspectives on Communication Disorders and Sciences in Culturally and Linguistically Diverse (CLD) Populations. 2011;**18**(1):3-11. DOI: 10.1044/cds18.1.3

[73] Patak L, Gawlinski A, Fung NI, Doering L, Berg J, Henneman EA. Communication boards in critical care: patients' views. Applied Nursing Research. 2006;**19**(4):182-190. DOI: 10.1016/j.apnr.2005.09.006

[74] Thurnheer SE, Gravestock I, Pichierri G, Steurer J, Burgstaller JM. Benefits of mobile apps in pain management: Systematic review. JMIR mHealth and uHealth. 2018;**6**(10):e11231. DOI: 10.2196/11231

[75] Gerber N. Exploring Graphical Representation of Pain-Related Vocabulary as Preferred by 6;0 to 9;11-Year-old Children Without Disabilities: a Stakeholder Review [unpublished Mini-dissertation]. Pretoria: University of Pretoria; 2018

[76] Vantaa Benjaminsson M, Thunberg G, Nilsson S. Using picture and text schedules to inform children: Effects on distress and pain during needle-related procedures in nitrous oxide sedation. Pain Research and Treatment. 2015;**2015**:478503. DOI: 10.1155/2015/478503

[77] Nilsson S, Holstensson J, Johansson C, Thunberg G. Children's perceptions of pictures intended to measure anxiety during hospitalization. Journal of Pediatric Nursing. 2019;**44**:63-73. DOI: 10.1016/j.pedn.2018.10.015

[78] Miró J, Huguet A. Evaluation of reliability, validity, and preference for a pediatric pain intensity scale: The Catalan version of the faces pain scale – Revised. Pain. 2004;**111**:59-64. DOI: 10.1016/j.pain.2004.05.023

[79] McGrath PA, Seifert CE, Speechley KN, Booth JC, Stitt L, Gibson MC. A new analogue scale for assessing children's pain: An initial validation study. Pain. 1996;**64**(3):435-443. DOI: 10.1016/0304-3959(95)00171-9

[80] Von Baeyer CL, Spagrud LJ, McCormick JC, Choo E, Neville K, Connelly MA. Three new datasets supporting use of the numerical rating scale (NRS-11) for children's self-reports of pain intensity. Pain. 2009;**143**(3):223-227. DOI: 10.1016/j.pain.2009.03.002

Section 3

Pharmaceuticals and Bioactives for Pain Management

Chapter 11

Nutraceutical Alternatives to Pharmaceutical Analgesics in Osteoarthritis

Shane M. Heffernan and Gillian E. Conway

Abstract

Chronic pain is a considerable health concern worldwide, effecting almost 30% of all European adults. Osteoarthritis (OA), a progressive pro-inflammatory condition, is one of the leading causes of chronic pain (effecting 13% of all those over 50 years, globally) and is the most common cause of joint pain. The prevalence of non-steroidal anti-inflammatory drug (NSAIDs) and analgesic use has been well studied and is abundant throughout the western world, with women being the greatest users and ibuprofen generally being the most reported NSAID. In the US, 65% of all OA patients are prescribed NSAIDs for pain management and form part of the current recommended strategy for OA clinical management. While some NSAIDs and analgesics are effective at improving pain and physical function, they come with significant and harmful side effects such as gastrointestinal complications, renal disturbances and severe cardiovascular events. Given these side-effects, any reduction in NSAID and analgesia use (and the resulting potentially harmful side effects) is of particular importance to OA public health. As such, a number of non-pharmaceutical alternatives (bioactive nutraceuticals) have been developed that may reduce NSAID and analgesia use while maintaining pain reduction and improvements in physical function. This chapter will discuss select nutraceuticals that are not currently in mainstream use but may have the potential to aid in the treatment of OA.

Keywords: joint pain, pain medication, non-pharmacological pain management, mechanisms of pain and action, paracetamol (acetaminophen, N-acetyl-p-aminophenol; APAP), opioids

1. Introduction

1.1 Chronic pain

Pain occurs in all demographics, with a higher prevalence in some clusters (such as the elderly) and can be either acute or chronic [1, 2]. Chronic pain is a complex interplay between biology and psychology, where the intensity/magnitude differs depending on personal, sensory, emotional experience and persists more than 3 months beyond "normal" healing time [3, 4]. This type of pain affects more than 1.5 billion people worldwide [5] and has an estimated prevalence ranging between 17-27% [6–9]. Chronic pain represents a significant financial burden that exceeds

€300 trillion (approximately 1.5%-3% of the gross domestic product across the European Union) and up to $635 billion in the United States [10, 11]. According to the International Association for the Study of Pain (IASP), the main overarching categories of chronic pain are primary (such as fibromyalgia) and secondary pain (the focus of this chapter). Secondary chronic pain is further divided into six distinct categories: cancer-related pain, postsurgical or posttraumatic pain, secondary headache/orofacial pain, secondary visceral pain, and secondary musculoskeletal pain [12, 13].

Most chronic pain begins with the occurrence of an acute injury event resulting in pain that if left untreated can develop chronically into a pathological condition and can increase the risk of future deleterious health issues such as sleep deficiency, delayed wound healing, immune dysfunction, cardiovascular problems (related to the stress response) and respiratory problems (such as pneumonia; [14, 15]). Persistent, unrelieved pain can negatively impact quality of life, daily functioning, sleep quality, work productivity and is associated with a substantial personal economic burden [16].

Pathologic pain is associated with multiple maladaptations in the nervous, endocrine, and immune systems [17–19] that often presents at multiple sites [20] and can be classified into nociceptive (somatic and visceral), neuropathic, nociplastic, or mixed [21]. Nociplastic describes pain of unknown origin that arises from altered nociception, despite no clear evidence of actual or threatened tissue damage that causes activation of peripheral nociceptors, evidence of disease or lesion of the somatosensory system causing the pain, such as early (pre structural damage) osteoarthritis [21]. Similarly, recent suggestions propose that generalised chronic pain is an expression of maladaptive plasticity within the nociceptive system [22, 23] and is relevant to the present chapter as osteoarthritic pain is generally accepted to be mainly of nociceptive origin [24].

1.2 Mechanisms of nociceptive pain

Most painful conditions initially involve the activation of dorsal root ganglion (DRG) neurons, which give rise to high threshold Aδ- and C-fibres (nociceptors) that innervate peripheral tissues (skin, bone, joints, viscera; [25]). Primary afferent neurons transduce painful stimuli action potentials through to the spinal cord (to ascending spinal neurons). Transmission of input from nociceptors, through the spinal column and to the central nerves system is mediated by monosynaptic contacts and/or through interneurons [19, 26]. In the spinal cord, neurotransmitter inhibition is mediated by the release of endogenous opioids (such as met-enkephalins and endorphins; [27]) or gamma-aminobutyric acid (GABA) which activate presynaptic opioid and/or GABA receptors on central nociceptor terminals to reduce excitatory transmitter release (**Figure 1**). The central integration of signals from excitatory and inhibitory neurotransmitters from cognitive, emotional, and environmental factors results in the perception of "pain". When the intricate balance between biological (neuronal), psychological (i.e. memory, distraction etc.) and social (i.e. attention, reward etc.) factors becomes disturbed, chronic pain develops [18].

Pain that is induced by an acute injury, initially localised, relatively proportional to the degree of tissue damage and typically increases with movement is referred to as "nociceptive pain." Specifically, as immune surveillance cells recognise the danger signals unmasked by tissue injury, the innate immune system initiates an inflammatory response to remove cellular debris and begins the healing process. Activated endothelial cells, stromal cells, and infiltrating immune cells release vasoactive and inflammatory mediators, including histamine, bradykinin, substance P, serotonin,

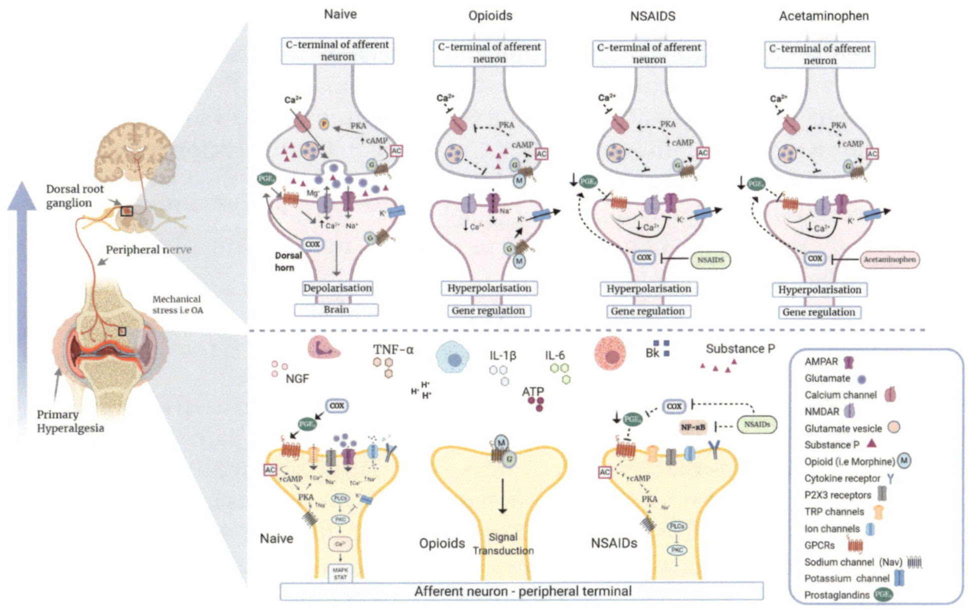

Figure 1.
Peripheral and central nociceptor pain signalling pathways following exposure to different pharmaceutical drugs. Without pharmaceutical intervention (naive state), activation of peripheral nociceptors in response to noxious stimuli, such as mechanical stress (OA) initiates the release of chemical mediators such as prostaglandins, bradykinin and cytokines at the peripheral terminal of the afferent neuron (peripheral sensitisation) which is modulated by the GPCRs, NA^+ and K^+ channels. This results in the activation of PKA, PLC releasing intracellular Ca^{2+} and the generation of action potential which transfers information to the (pre synapse) C-terminal afferent neuron (central sensitization). This triggers the release of neurotransmitters i.e. glutamate and substance P into the spinal synapse of the dorsal horn and activates AMPA or NMDA receptors on the post synaptic dorsal horn. As a result, there is an increased influx of Ca^{2+} and Na^+, inhibition of K^+ influx and depolarization of the cell membrane. These signals travel to the brain where they are transcribed into the perception of pain. Pharmaceutical invention acts by modulating various aspects of the pain signalling pathway such as opioids (opioids such as morphine bind to GPCRs preventing the presynaptic release of a number of neurotransmitters), NSAIDs (inhibit the activity of COX) and acetaminophen (inhibits the activity of COX in the central nervous system but appears to lacks peripheral anti-inflammatory properties). Figure created using Biorender.com. Abbreviations: AMPAR, α-amino-3-hydroxy-5-methyl-4-isoxazolepropionic acid receptor; ATP, adenosine triphosphate; BK, bradykinin; COX, cyclooxygenase; GPCRs, G protein-coupled receptors; IL, interleukin; NMDAR, N-methyl-D-aspartate receptor; NAV, voltage-gated sodium channels; NGF, nerve growth factor; NF-κB, nuclear factor kappa B; NSAID, nonsteroidal anti-inflammatory drug; PLC, phospholipase C; PKA, protein kinase a; PKC, protein kinase C; PGE, prostaglandin; P2X3, P2X purinoceptor 3 receptor; TNF, tumour necrosis factor; TRPV, transient receptor potential receptor.

nitric oxide, cytokines, chemokines, and prostaglandins, which amplify signal transduction in the peripheral terminals of nociceptors [26, 28]. These inflammatory mediators augment the responsiveness of nociceptors by increasing expression of pain-sensing ion channels and promoting release of pronociceptive mediators (autosensitization; [29]). This peripheral inflammation caused by local injury and continuous inputs from sensitised nociceptors promote 'central sensitization', a process that alters pain processing in the spinal dorsal horn, and in subcortical and cortical regions of the brain [30, 31]. Noxious signals associated with the injury are detected by peripheral nociceptor terminals of primary afferent neurons, transmitted via the spinal cord to the brain, processed and interpreted as highly unpleasant pain experiences [32]. Nociceptor terminals express molecules, such as transient receptor potential ion channels (TRP), voltage-gated sodium channels (Nav), voltage-gated calcium channels (VGCC), or acid-sensing ion channels (ASICs), which respond to heat, cold, acids, or mechanical stress and transduce them into action potentials [26]. The signal is then transmitted through peripheral axons to the cell bodies of the primary neurons, located in the dorsal root ganglia.

Unmyelinated C-fibres and myelinated Aδ-fibres transmit noxious stimuli, whereas thinly myelinated Aδ-fibres transmit innocuous mechanical stimuli, such as touch. The central axons of the primary neurons enter the spinal cord through the dorsal horn and synapse with secondary somatosensory neurons and, to some extent, with motor neurons to form withdrawal reflex circuits. Signal propagation to the secondary neurons is subject to modulation by descending tracts from the brainstem and by interneurons in the dorsal horn. The signal is then transmitted to the thalamus, from where tertiary afferent neurons are projected to multiple areas of the cortex involved in pain processing [33].

1.3 Mechanisms of neuropathic pain

Neuropathic pain (NP) is defined as "pain caused by a lesion or disease of the somatosensory nervous system" [34]. Chronic neuropathic pain is caused by damage to nerve fibres that respond by misappropriating sensory inputs leading to spontaneous painful sensation, through multiple mechanisms in the nervous system and its associated modulators. Peripheral nerve damage can result in chronic neuropathic pain through multiple routes [35] via peripheral pain-processing unmyelinated C-fibres and thinly-myelinated fibres because of metabolic damage, toxins, medications, cytokines, and inflammation [36]. This can result in morphological and chemical changes such as fibre density and neuronal hyperexcitability [30, 37–40]. Throughout the axon, trauma, compression, hypoxia, inflammation and chemical damage lead to fibre degeneration and alterations in gene expression [41], resulting in ectopic firing, faulty signal transmission [42], detrimental physiological alterations [43–45] and peripheral second-order targets [46–48]. This results in negative impacts on nociceptive pathways causing them to become sensitised [49], leading to maladaptive central sensitization [50] and increased responsiveness of nociceptive neurons in the central nervous system to their normal or subthreshold afferent input [51]. At the molecular level, these damaged processes disrupt second-order neuronal transduction, through alterations in receptor expression, calcium permeability, synapse location and the release of pain-promoting mediators [52–55]. The precise molecular targets of neuropathic pain stem from multiple mechanisms of peripheral nerve fibre excitation and sensitization leading to sustained electrochemical signalling and to neuropathic pain stimulus [56, 57].

1.4 Pharmaceutical treatment of chronic pain

Both acute and chronic pain are, in general, treated with a wide group of pharmaceutical medications known as "analgesics." The most frequently used are opioids, nonsteroidal anti-inflammatory drugs (NSAIDs) and paracetamol, also referred to as acetaminophen or N-acetyl-p-aminophenol [58].

1.4.1 Opioids

Opioid drugs (e.g. morphine, codeine, methadone, fentanyl and their derivatives) are the most widely used analgesic medications globally, so much so that an estimated 26.8 million people were living with 'opioid use disorder' globally in 2016, resulting in >100,000 opioid overdose deaths annually [59]. Opioids are a group of pharmaceutical formulations that interact with endogenous opioid receptors to distort neurotransmitter singling pathways through localised peripheral sensory neurons [60, 61] with the goal to reducing pain sensation. Opioid receptors are a large superfamily of seven-transmembrane G protein-coupled receptors and are classified as μ (μ1, μ2, μ3), δ (δ1, δ2), k (k1, k2, k3) and ORL1 [62, 63], of which almost all opioid drugs in use today interact with μ receptors. These receptors are inhibitory and prevent the presynaptic release of a number of neurotransmitters to inhibit the release of glutamate, calcitonin gene related protein (CGRP), and substance P. This is an important action considering the established roles of these molecules in pain signalling and nociceptive transmission (**Figure 1**; [64]). For example, morphine, extracted from opium, is by far the most commonly known opioid [59], which is thought to have been in use since the third century B.C. [22], but identified at the molecular level with high binding affinity to sites in the intestine and brain [65]. These receptors mediate an inhibitory signal of neural transmission induced by opioid drugs to produce an analgesic action (**Figure 1**). Pain stimuli are detected by nociceptors at the spinal cord dorsal horn [66] where they act on the substantia gelatinosa (inhibitory interneurons rich with opioid receptors) and are activated by the antinociceptive descending system, to control the transmission of painful stimuli from primary nerve fibres to spino-thalamic neurons [22]. Opioid receptors have an intricate relationship with inflammatory status. Early studies showed that the systemic or local application of receptor agonists elicited greater analgesic effects in inflamed compared to non-inflamed tissue (reviewed in; [67]). Furthermore, opioid receptor trafficking (movement within the neuron) is augmented, expression on DRG membranes is enhanced [68, 69] and axonal transport stimulated by cytokines and nerve growth factor that are produced within inflamed tissues [70, 71]. This enhanced/altered state resulted in increased antinociceptive function of opioid receptors on peripheral nerves [60, 72].

The major limiting factors of opioid therapy are the variety of side effects such as constipation, vomiting, myosis, cough reflex suppression, modulation of the immune system and one of the most dangerous, respiratory rhythm and respiratory depression [73, 74]. Interestingly, studies have shown that long-term use in chronic non-malignant (e.g. musculoskeletal) pain has not been proven effective [75], rather, abuse of prescription opioids have reached epidemic proportions leading to addiction, overdoses and increased death rates [76–78]. Importantly, these side effects may be drug specific and affect immune function differently [79, 80]. Nonetheless, chronic use of opioid medication can cause cellular adaptions that lead to modulation of cellular growth, inflammation, wound healing [81, 82]. For a more detailed overview of the potential side effects and opioid tolerance refer to the following references [83–86].

Regardless of the potential impact that opioid agonists could have on pain relief, meta-analyses show no improvement in clinically significant pain reduction scores, and epidemiological data suggest that quality of life and functional capacity are only minimally changed [75, 78]. Nonetheless, more data is required from larger studies (specifically in OA), however the aforementioned adverse effects and lack of analgesic efficacy has led to significant dropout rates in long-term studies [75, 78, 87–89].

1.4.2 Non-steroidal anti-inflammatory drugs (NSAIDs)

NSAIDs (particular enzyme inhibiters) are among the most widely used medications globally [90, 91] because of the lower potential for addiction (as shown by the US opioid epidemic; [92]), robust efficacy, and long history of clinical use [93].

The prevalence of 'non-aspirin' NSAID use has been well studied and is dynamic across age, body mass index and geographical ancestry, ranging between ~15-45%, women being the highest users and ibuprofen generally being the most reported [94–96]. Short-term use of NSAIDs is particularly prevalent (~50–80% per year) in athletes and soldiers (individuals that may be at risk for acute and chronic musculoskeletal injuries; [97–99]). Extended periods of NSAID treatment (e.g., more than 3 times per week for more than 3 months per year) have been reported in 10% of adults in the United States [100], a rate that can be expected to increase with age [101].

NSAIDs act primarily by mediating peripheral pain sensitization driven by inflammatory stimuli, such as acute or sport injuries, (osteo)arthritis etc. and are less effective in treating pain due to nerve damage (neuropathic pain). At the point of inflammatory pain, initiated by nociceptive stimuli, NSAIDs augment the experienced nociceptive excitability (peripheral and central sensitization; [102]). NSAIDs work differently to opioids in that they do not block central pathways of nociception, but inhibit the formation of prostanoids via competitive inhibition of arachidonic acid binding to cyclooxygenase enzyme (COX) isoform active sites [103], which sensitise nociceptive pain. There are two cyclooxygenase isoforms that are the targets of NSAIDs; COX-1 that are expressed in most tissues (including the endothelium, monocytes, gastrointestinal epithelial cells, and platelets) and controls the basal production of prostanoids (**Figure 1**) and COX-2 that are not regularly expressed in most tissues but are upregulated in response to and during the inflammatory process (in tissues such as vascular endothelium, rheumatoid synovial, endothelial cells, monocytes, and macrophages) through the actions of various inflammatory mediators such as bacterial endotoxins, tumour necrosis factor-alpha and interleukins [104]. The increase in COX-2 protein levels are the primary driving force for enhanced production of prostanoids at inflammatory sites [105, 106]. The resulting COX-2 products, particularly prostaglandin (PG) E2, potentiate this response, where PGE2 and prostacyclin (PGI2), produced during local inflammation, augment pain signalling by peripheral and central neurons [15]. PGE2 and PGI2 increase the sensitivity of pain receptors (or nociceptors) in the periphery and enhance the activity of various pain mediators [104, 107]. This mechanism propagates via brain derived PGE2 travelling through the blood–brain barrier, via venules, during systemic inflammation and lessens the inhibition of neurons in the hypothalamus [108]. Drugs that inhibit both COX isoforms with comparable potency (i.e. nonselective NSAIDs such as ibuprofen and ketoprofen) tend to preferentially activate the COX-1 pathway, while drugs with intermediate or selective target COX-2 inhibition (such as nimesulide, meloxicam, diclofenac, celecoxib, rofecoxib, etoricoxib, lumiracoxib etc.) have lesser potential for COX-1 activation [109]. This pathway selectivity is of significant importance as both COX isoform elicit different potentially harmful adverse effects.

In a recent meta-analysis (n = 220,000 patients) of placebo-controlled trials, NSAIDs (coxibs, diclofenac, ibuprofen, and naproxen, predominantly COX-1 inhibiters) significantly increased the risk of upper gastrointestinal complications [eg, ulcer perforations, bleeding, obstructions; 110]. The authors also showed an increased risk of major vascular and coronary events with high doses of coxibs and diclofenac while ibuprofen was associated with an increase in major coronary (but not vascular) events comparable with that of coxibs and oral diclofenac (predominantly COX-2 inhibiters; [110]). These data are corroborated with findings from meta-analysis of observational studies showing low risk of upper gastrointestinal complications (aceclofenac, celecoxib, and ibuprofen predominantly COX-2 inhibiters), intermediate risk (diclofenac, meloxicam, and ketoprofen etc.) and high risk (tenoxicam, naproxen, indomethacin, diflunisal, piroxicam, ketorolac, and azapropazone predominantly COX - inhibiters) depending on the NSAID, likely in a dose dependent fashion [111]. Similarly, total daily oral diclofenac had a linear dose dependent relationship cardiovascular event risk [112]. These dose dependencies are likely a product of the relative effectiveness on either COX-1 or COX-2 inhibition [113–116]. As both (non-inhabited) COX-1 and COX-2 produce cytoprotective prostanoids, inhibition of both COX isozymes (induced by NSAIDs) suppress these prostanoids and promotes damage to the gastrointestinal tract and cardiovascular tissues [109, 117]. Based on these and other safety findings, the American Heart Association recommends patients take the lowest effective dose of NSAIDs for the shortest duration of time [118].

1.4.3 Paracetamol (acetaminophen, N-acetyl-p-aminophenol; APAP)

APAP are likely to be the most commonly used pharmaceutical worldwide [119, 120], are expected to reach a global market value of USD 999.4 million in 2020 [121] and is included in the 21st World Health Organisation Model List of Essential Medicines as updated in March 2017 [122]. However, recently there have been debates from the National Institute for Health and Care Excellence, about the relevance of APAP for some conditions [123]. The efficacy of paracetamol to treat chronic pain has been questioned with systematic reviews showing limited (sometimes null) effects on chronic pain in some conditions [120, 124, 125]. Nonetheless, APAP can be beneficial for acute pain, [126–128], similar to NSAIDs and opioids [129–131]. The precise mechanism of action remains unknown, however this is most likely due to the interwoven interactions that APAP have in multiple pain pathways. Our current knowledge suggests that APAPs are metabolised by the liver into p-aminophenol, then bound with arachidonic acid, primarily in the brain, to form AM404 (N- (4-hydroxyphenyl)-5Z,8Z,11Z,14Z-eicosatetraenamide) through fatty acid amide hydrolase (FAAH) activity [132–134]. Like NSAIDs, APAP are analgesic and antipyretic, however APAP lacks peripheral anti-inflammatory properties, therefore act through the central nervous system and not peripheral tissues [135]. Current evidence suggests that there are four metabolic systems that interact to elicit the analgesic and antipyretic properties of APAP, the Eicosanoid, Opioidergic, Seretogentic and Endocannabinoid systems [136].

Briefly, like NSIADs, APAP can inhibit central cyclo-oxygenases (COX-1, COX-2) including a proposed third isoform COX-3 [137–142]. Although the results are controversial [143] it is thought that they are involved in prostaglandin (PGs) production thus the analgesic mechanism of action. Furthermore, APAP are more effective in environments with low peroxide tone and low arachidonic acid levels, such as in the central nerves system, mainly through local depletion of glutathione leading to decreased production of PGE2 [139]. Considering the antinociceptive effects of APAP, one of the main brain derived metabolites AM404 (N-arachidonoyl-phenolamine) is decrease in the presence of opioid receptor antagonist. AM404 inhibits the nociceptive activity of particular APAPs in part by modulating many neurotransmitters, including 5-HT, glutamate, and γ-aminobutyric acid [143–145]. Although the precise receptors have not been identified [146–149], serotonin antagonists block the analgesic effect of APAP through mainly indirect non-binding mechanisms [146, 150]. One possible interaction with the serotonergic pathway maybe though altering CNS monoamine neuron types in the brain that contain a major receptor for PGE2 (EP3 receptor [139]). Further to the above, AM404 can inhibit anandamide [151], with stimulation of (canobinoide 1) CB1 receptor activity (without binding) via FAAH [133], suggesting a reliance of APAP antinociceptive activity on interaction with the endocannabinoid system [134, 152]. Interestingly, AM404 is not identifiable in the blood after APAP administration [133] which might explain, to some degree, the absence of peripheral anti-inflammatory action [134]. This could help to explain why APAP may not have significant clinical effect on conditions such as osteoarthritis (further details below; [153, 154]). A recent study confirmed that APAPs act mainly on central analgesic pathways, showing that APAP modifies the activity and connectivity of analgesia via FAAH, activating a signalling cascade involving TRPV1 channels, mGlu5 receptors, PLC, DAGL and CB1 receptors, associated with the release of glutamate and GABA – through the endocannabinoid systems [155]. Though the molecular mechanisms that provide analgesia are beginning to come to light, there is also potential substantial detrimental side effects of APAPs.

APAPs are generally considered safe if administered at appropriate doses for short periods [156]. However, they remain one of the leading causes of liver disease in high-income countries [157, 158] which has led to legislative restrictions in many countries [159]. It is well accepted that APAPs cause liver injury, hepatotoxicity, mitochondrial toxicity [160, 161] and that this toxicity can be effected by interindividual variation [162]. Nonetheless, consuming APAP can increase the risks of hospitalisation for perforation, peptic ulceration and bleeding [163], relative rates of adverse cardiovascular events such as myocardial infarction, stroke, coronary heart disease and upper gastrointestinal disease such as gastroduodenal ulcers and haemorrhages [164], often in a dose response manor. However, observational studies show a favourable side effect profile for APAPs compared with NSAIDs when used in older people with chronic pain conditions [165]. Data from the most recent meta-analysis shows that APAPs are nearly four times more likely to have abnormal results on liver function tests than placebo [166].

2. Osteoarthritis

Osteoarthritis (OA) is a complex musculoskeletal condition that effects people of all ages but particularly those over 55 years [167–171]. According to the Osteoarthritis Research Society International (OARSI) OA can be defined as;

> *"...a disorder involving movable joints characterized by cell stress and extracellular matrix degradation initiated by micro- and macro-injury that activates maladaptive repair responses including pro-inflammatory pathways of innate immunity. The disease manifests first as a molecular derangement (abnormal joint tissue metabolism) followed by anatomic, and/or physiologic derangements (characterized by cartilage degradation, bone remodelling, osteophyte formation, joint inflammation and loss of normal joint function), that can culminate in illness" [172].*

OA is a pro-inflammatory branch of rheumatic disease that effects synovial joints progressively and is caused by the failure of joint tissues to repair following damage. This damage may have been caused by stresses due to an abnormality in the articular cartilage, subchondral bone, ligaments, menisci, periarticular muscles, peripheral nerves or synovium [173, 174]. While cartilage degradation is the traditionally structural trademark of OA, it is generally considered a whole joint disease with many other morphological features [175–178]. For example, an osteoarthritic joint may exhibit sclerosis in the subchondral bone, osteophytes [179], local inflammation such as synovitis [177, 178, 180, 181] and bone marrow lesions [182]. Failure of normal biological repair processes that leads to breakdown of cartilage and bone [183] is characterised by symptoms of pain, stiffness, functional disability [184] that can lead to negative impacts on fatigue, mood, sleep, overall quality of life [185, 186].

OA confers a number of modifiable and non-modifiable risk factors [174, 187]. Non-modifiable risk factors include previous joint injury [188, 189], malalignment and other mechanical factors [175, 176, 190–193], age [189], sex [194], ethnicity [195] and genetic predisposition [196–198]. Modifiable risk factors include obesity [181, 189, 199–202], metabolic syndrome [181, 203–206], in particular diabetes mellitus [207–209] and habitual diet [187, 210].

The condition is one of the most common causes of chronic pain and the most common cause of joint pain [211] with conservative estimates suggesting that there are approximately 500 million suffers worldwide [167, 212]. OA affects ~13% of all over 50's (~7% in all ages; [213]) and has no cure [214–218] while being the 11th highest contributor to years lived with disability [159].

2.1 Pain and osteoarthritis

Chronic inflammatory-associated pain can have multiple mechanisms [219–223] and can stem from mechanical stress or central sensitization either concurrently and/or vary in their influences over time [224]. Pain derived from OA can generally be characterised into two common clinical forms of pain, intermittent but severe/intense and persistent pain or aching [225]. These pain experiences can come from neuropathic and nociceptive process, as discussed above. The prevalence of neuropathic pain features at the knee in OA patients ranges from 19% to 29% [221, 226, 227]. However, recent studies of peripheral and central nerve sensitization [228], as well as nerve ending damage and regrowth [229, 230] have shown that neuropathic pain contributes substantially to the condition. This central sensitization is prominent in those that experience a high level of pain that is not proportional to radiographic evidence of structural damage [219] and contributes more to the pain experienced in women with symptomatic OA, compared to men [231]. Generally, a higher degree of central sensitization or neuropathic pain is associated with high pain intensity and a greater chance of developing chronic pain following joint replacement [232, 233]. The remaining 70-80% of knee OA pain appears to be nociceptive in nature, thus OA can be described as a chronic mild to moderate nociceptive dominant pain condition [24, 234] and should be considered as such with regards to initial treatment [24].

The diversity of pathophysiological maladaptation in OA effected joints and the low associations of these changes with pain, suggests doubt over the link between joint structural condition and the experience of pain. This is evident from the poor relationship between radiographic images and reported pain. A recent systematic review showed that the prevalence of knee pain in patients with radiographic knee OA ranged from 15% to 81% [235]. However, some studies reported associations between the structural damage of the joint (cartilage and bone) and pain [236] but at higher levels of X-ray derived pathology (Kellgren/Lawrence grade; [237]). Nonetheless, pain may still indicate a level of disease activity. In a number of studies looking more specifically at joint morphological characterises, OA pain has been associated with the rate of medial cartilage loss (also after adjustment for radiographic OA stage; [238]), osteophytes [239], more erosive OA compared to non-erosive OA [240] and changes of bone marrow lesions and synovitis [182]. These data show the complexity of the disease-pain nexus and suggests that the disease should, in the first instance (i.e. mild OA), be treated generally with lifestyle and nutritional intervention rather that pharmaceuticals that target specific pathological pathways (**Figure 1**) [241]. Regardless, pharmaceutical therapies remain the main treatment for such conditions [242].

2.2 Pharmaceutical analgesics in osteoarthritis

OA is a progressive condition with no cure where opioids, acetaminophen and non-steroidal anti-inflammatory drugs (NSAID) are the traditional, non-lifestyle, approach for early management. However, as eluded to earlier, these pharmaceutical treatments are often accompanied with significant side effects. For example, NSAIDs are the traditional approach for early clinical management of mild-to-moderate OA [241] and in the US 65% of all OA patients are prescribed NSAID for pain management - this is the current recommended strategy for OA clinical management by the leading authorities [243]. While some NSAIDs are effective at improving pain and physical function, they come with significant and potentially harmful side effects such as gastrointestinal complications, renal disturbances and severe cardiovascular events [244]. Although some of these risks may be reduced using topical administration such as Diclofenac gel/cream [245, 246]. Two recent large-scale studies have shown that, depending on the particular medication, the risk of hospital admissions (due to heart failure) can be nearly two times greater (Ketorolac; [247]) in OA/rheumatoid arthritis (n = 24,081), with ibuprofen (generally speaking, the most used NSAID) presenting with the highest rates of NSAID toxicity [248].

Approximately 34% of OA patients use Paracetamol [249], in isolation or in combination with NSAIDs. In fact, the effectiveness of Paracetamol to improve pain management has recently been called into question [124], as it has been shown to be ineffective for treating OA pain [125, 250] and may have similar side effects as ibuprofen [251], particularly when consumed at higher doses [164]. Specifically, in knee or hip OA, a recent Cochrane review concluded that Paracetamol provides no clinically important improvements in pain in the immediate and short term (up to 12 weeks; [16]). In addition, a recent network meta-analysis (56 randomised controlled trials, 22 128 participants) suggests that paracetamol was least effective for the treatment of knee and/or hip OA compared with celecoxib (NSAID) or the combination of glucosamine and chondroitin [117] – confirming other reports [252]. In contrast, some authors have concluded that paracetamol had similar efficacy to NSAIDs for the treatment of OA [253]. It is also important to remember that overuse of APAPs can cause liver injury, hepatotoxicity, mitochondrial toxicity [160, 161] which is relevant to a chronic condition with no known cure. These data led to confusion in earlier guidelines that consistently recommended the prescription of paracetamol (acetaminophen) as the first line analgesic for these conditions [90, 91, 241, 254, 255]. However, the data are now relatively clear that there is little clinically meaningful effect of Paracetamol for OA pain [153, 154].

The potential negative effects such as addiction and the physiological side effects of opioid use are well documented, as discussed above, however they remain highly prescribed for OA and are expected to triple in the coming years [256, 257]. More than half of those prescribed opioids in the first year of OA have been shown to be inappropriately dispensed [257]. The prevalence of opioid use for OA ranges from 8-26% and in Australia, with the use for knee/hip OA has being described as "alarmingly high" [257]. A number of systematic reviews and meta-analysis have been performed in recent years and have unanimously shown that the tolerability is low, efficacy for pain relief in OA is not clinically relevant and the potential harms are high [258–260]. Despite calls for guidelines to be changed on the use of opioids and the above-mentioned pharmaceuticals, their use is increasing (likely with the prevalence of the disease) and by proxy the negative consequences rising in tandem. Therefore, non-pharmaceutical food-based alternatives (termed bioactive nutraceuticals) have been developed and are beginning to be recommended as early treatment [261–263] to improve OA symptoms including pain [241, 264–266].

3. Nutraceutical alternatives and reduction in pharmacological analgesics in osteoarthritis

Given the possible side-effects of pharmaceutical treatments, any reduction in their use is of particular importance to OA public health. As such, a number of non-pharmaceutical alternatives have been developed that may reduce the use/required dose of pharmaceuticals while maintaining or improving the impacts on OA pain and physical function. The majority of these alternatives are termed "nutraceuticals" (a portmanteau of the words "nutrition" and "pharmaceutical"), coined in 1989 by Dr. Stephen DeFelice [267], founder and chairman of the Foundation for Innovation in Medicine.

While it is unlikely that Hippocrates (traditionally regarded as the father of modern medicine; died 375 BCE) actually said: "Let food be your medicine and medicine your food" [268], this is often cited in the context of nutraceuticals. A more apt and legitimate quote defines the position of nutraceuticals in health and disease as "beyond diet, before drug", coined by Ettore Novellino in 2012 [269].

There is currently no universally accepted definition of a nutraceutical [270], with the main confusion being the differences between nutraceuticals and functional foods, and the lack of regulatory definition between them (**Table 1**) [270–273]. In fact, current European regulations do not distinguish between nutraceuticals and food supplements (see the EC Regulation n. 1924/2006 of the European Parliament and Council, recently updated by the UE regulation 2015/2283), therefore neither does the European Food Safety Authority [274, 275]. However, a number of proposed definitions exist (**Table 1**) and from these definitions, for the purposes of this chapter, a nutraceutical will be defined as;

> *'a naturally derived biological substance, not synthetically created, that preserve its original active properties without chemical manipulation, can enhance health in dosages that exceed those that could be obtained from normal food digestion and has peer-reviewed scientific evidenced to base health clams'.*

Author(s)	Definition
DeFelice, [267]; coined in 1989	"A nutraceutical is any substance that is a food or part of a food and provides medical or health benefits, including the prevention and treatment of disease."
Zeisel, [271]	"......as those diet supplements that deliver a concentrated form of a presumed bioactive agent from a food, presented in a non-food matric, and used to enhance health in dosages that exceed those that could be obtained from normal food"
U.S. Nutraceutical Research and Education [276]	"a dietary supplement, food or medical food that has a benefit, which prevents or reduces the risk of a disease or health condition, including the management of a disease or health condition or the improvement of health; and is safe for human consumption in the quantity, and with the frequency required to realise such properties"
The European Nutraceutical Association [277]	"are nutritional products that provide health and medical benefits, including the prevention and treatment of disease. In contrast to pharmaceuticals however, these are not synthetic substances or chemical compounds formulated for specific indications. These are products that contain nutrients (partly in concentrated form) and mostly are assigned to the category of food. Dietary supplements are a typical example for nutraceuticals, but also dietetic and functional foods may be counted among these products."
Health Canada [278]	"A nutraceutical is a product isolated or purified from foods that is generally sold in medicinal forms not usually associated with food. A nutraceutical is demonstrated to have a physiological benefit or provide protection against chronic disease"
Corzo et al. [279]	"Nutraceuticals are biological substances extracted from natural sources by non-denaturing processes to preserve their original properties without any chemical manipulation."

Table 1.
Currently used definitions to describe nutraceuticals.

As such, the following sections will discuss those nutraceuticals that are currently not in mainstream use but may have the potential to aid in treatment of OA (i.e. the well discussed Glucosamine and Chondroitin will not feature in this chapter) but are in regular use worldwide [280]. The identified nutraceuticals that have been compared to/with NSAID/analgesics for OA can be divided into three categories, defined by their origin, and are presented in **Table 2**;

1. Terrestrial Botanicals, compounds derived from 'land' plant sources (avocado/soybean, pine bark extract and turmeric/curcumin).

2. Marine Botanicals, compounds derived from 'marine' plant sources (Lithothamnion species).

3. Marine Fauna, derived from marine animals (fish oil and green lipped mussel).

3.1 Terrestrial botanicals

Turmeric/curcumin extracts (spices used mainly in South Asian cooking) or nutraceuticals combinations where turmeric/curcumin extracts are the main active ingredient, have the greatest amount of evidence for improving OA symptoms, with some recent data on NSAID and analgesics use (**Table 2**) [300]. Two studies have directly compared raw turmeric/curcumin extracts to NSAIDs and their effectiveness for OA symptoms [287, 288]. These data show that turmeric extracts either improved or were shown to be non-inferior for knee osteoarthritis (KOA) pain, pain during stair walking and resulted in less side effects (particularly the rate of abdominal pain/distention) compared to oral ibuprofen [287–289]. Furthermore, patented/propriety formulations of turmeric/curcumin extracts have been developed around the world and show some promising effects on OA (**Table 2**). Interestingly, Chandran et al. demonstrated that curcumin formulated as BCM-95® or 'BCM-95® + diclofenac sodium' showed superior 'Disease Activity Scores', American College of Rheumatology score, pain, CRP levels and erythrocyte sedimentation rate, compared to diclofenac alone (Indian population; [289]). The same formulation showed similar improvements of KOOS variables, but BCM-95® resulted in less adverse events (including flatulence) and a lower requirements for H2 blockers (0% vs. 28%; a group of medicines that reduce the amount of acid produced by the cells in the lining of the stomach), compared to diclofenac [290]. In the longest of these studies (8 months in a European cohort), the addition of Meriva® (curcuminoids 20%, phosphatidylcholine 40%, and microcrystalline cellulose 40%) to the "best available treatment", reduced NSAID and analgesia use by 63% compared to the control group ("best available treatment" only). This reduction resulted in less side-effects between 45-67%, depending on the specific adverse advent, compared to side-effects in the control group (2-12%; [293]). Similarly, an alternative preparation (C3 complex®; Curcuminoids 500-mg capsules with 5-mg Bioperine®) reduced the use of naproxen by 84% (compared to 19% in placebo) in Iranian KOA patients and a further alternative (Theracurmin®; 10% of curcumin, 2% other curcuminoids such as demethoxycurcumin and isdemethoxycurcumin, 46% glycerin, 4% gum ghatti, and 38% of water; 180 mg of curcumin) reduced dependence on celecoxib in Japanese KOA patients (from ~70% to ~30% versus ~80 to ~60% in placebo; [294]). Recently, Heidari-Beni et al. [301] presented findings from a herbal formulation containing curcumin (300 mg), gingerols (7.5 mg) and piperine (3.75 mg), taken twice a day for 4 weeks. This formulation reduced PGE_2 (see above text and **Figure 1**) of KOA patients to the same extent as Naproxen (250 mg capsules daily). There is significant mechanistic evidence to support these

DOI: http://dx.doi.org/10.5772/intechopen.95919

Proposed main active compound	Treatment regime	Effect on OA Analgesia and NSAID	Reference
Avocado/soybean unsaponifiables	Avocado/soybean unsaponifiables 300 mg or 600 mg ASU for 3 months	↓ NSAIDs and analgesics use by 50% vs. placebo ↓ pain (~50%) in both 300 mg and 600 mg vs. placebo	[281]
Avocado/soybean unsaponifiables	Piascledine/ASU (300 mg daily) for 6 months	↓ Participants using analgesics and NSAIDs (from 58.8% to 24.9%) ↓ Median pain (by ~50%) and pain intensity, pain at rest (by 100%) and pain during walking (by ~60%) ↓ Mobility score (by ~50%)	[282]
Avocado/soybean unsaponifiables	Avocado/soybean mixture, 300 mg daily orally versus celecoxib,200 mg/day orally for 8 weeks	↓ Cartilage oligomeric matrix protein (COMP) in both groups (by ~37%, Avocado/soybean and ~ 27%, celecoxib), with no differences between groups	[283]
Fish oil/*Urtica dioica*	Phytalgic (fish-oil, vitamin E, Urtica dioica) 3 capsules daily for 12 weeks	↓ NSAIDs use vs. the placebo (by ~60%) ↓ Analgesic use vs. the placebo (BY ~40%) ↓ Pain (by ~37%), stiffness (by ~43%) and function (by ~40$) vs. placebo	[284]
Green lipped mussel	600 mg of BioLex(R)-GLM extract daily or placebo for 12 weeks	↓ Paracetamol use (by ~30% post-trial) vs. placebo ↓ Stiffness (by ~19%) vs. placebo, no difference pain	[285]
Pine bark extract	Pycnogenol (pine bark extract) 100 mg for 3 months	↓ Use of drugs (by ~57%) vs. placebo ↓ Gastrointestinal complications (by ~60%) vs. placebo ↓ WOMAC score (by ~40%) vs. placebo ↑ Walking distance (by ~34%), compared to no improvement in placebo	[286]
Turmeric	Turmeric extracts (2 g extracts/day) or ibuprofen (800 mg) for 0, 2, 4 and 6 weeks	↓ Pain on walking stairs vs. ibuprofen (however, ibuprofen was greater at baseline thus throughout) No difference in pain on level walking, 100 m walking time or stair climb	[287]
Turmeric	Turmeric extracts (1500 mg extracts/day) or ibuprofen (1200 mg/day) for 4 weeks	↓ WOMAC score, pain and function compared to baseline scores at all time points, and was non-inferior to ibuprofen. ↓ Rate of abdominal pain/distention vs. ibuprofen (by ~60%)	[288]
Curcumin	BCM-95® Curcumin: 500 mg/capsule twice daily, Curcumin 500 mg + diclofenac sodium 50 mg/capsule twice daily, diclofenac 50 mg/capsule twice daily, all for 8 weeks	↓ Disease Activity Score (by ~45%), CRP (by ~52%), American College of Rheumatology score, improved pain (by ~60%), erythrocyte sedimentation rate (by ~11%), greater in Curcumin and Curcumin+ diclofenac vs. diclofenac alone	[289]

Proposed main active compound	Treatment regime	Effect on OA Analgesia and NSAID	Reference
Curcumin	BCM-95® (curcumin, demethoxycurcumin, bisdemethoxycurcumin, and volatile oils from turmeric rhizome), 500-mg three times daily versus diclofenac 50-mg tablet two times daily for 28 days	↓ Pain similar in both groups (by ~78% for both), no difference between groups ↑ KOOS variables (n = 5) similar in both groups, no difference between groups ↑ Flatulence in diclofenac vs. curcumin (by ~79%) ↓ Requirement for H2 blockers in curcumin vs. diclofenac (by 100%, i.e. zero in curcumin) ↓ Incidence of adverse effects in curcumin vs. diclofenac (by ~76%)	[290]
Curcumin	Longvida®, 800 mg patented lipophilic matrix delivering 160 mg curcumin versus Ibuprofen (400 mg) orally and daily for 12 weeks	↓ Pain in both (by ~60%), no difference between groups	[291]
Curcumin	Herbal formulation of curcumin (300 mg), gingerols (7.5 mg), and piperine (3.75 mg; Mixodin) versus Naproxen 250 mg capsules, both twice a day for 4 weeks	↓ prostaglandin E2 (PGE2) in booth groups with no difference between the two (~27 pg./mL)	[292]
Curcumin	Meriva tablets, a curcumin-phosphatidylcholine phytosome complex, 200 mg equivalent curcumin daily with best available care (BCA) compared to BCA only as control for 8 months	↓ NSAIDs use (by ~80%) vs. control ↓ Gastrointestinal complaints (by ~40%) vs. control ↓ Pain (by ~44%), stiffness (by ~28%), physical function (by ~40%), WOMAC score (by ~41%), compared to no improvements in controls ↑ Karnofsky Performance Scale (by ~22%), compared to no improvement in controls ↑ Treadmill walking distance (345% increase from baseline) compared to 89% in controls ↓ inflammatory markers sCD40L (by ~56%), IL-1β (by ~35%), IL-6(by ~27%), sVCAM-1 (by ~30%), ESR (by ~25%), compared to no change in controls	[293]
Curcumin	Theracurmin® (10% of curcumin, 2% other curcuminoids such as demethoxycurcumin and isdemethoxycurcumin, 46% glycerin, 4% gum ghatti, and 38% of water; 180 mg of curcumin) for 8 weeks	↓ NSAID (celecoxib) dependence (p = 0.0252) ↓ Pain (by ~55%) vs. placebo	[294]
Curcumin	C3 complex, 500 mg curcuminoid capsules including 5 mg Bioperine, 3 times daily for 6 weeks	↓ Naproxen use (by ~73%) vs. controls ↓ Pain (by >38%), function (by ~41%) and WOMAC score (by ~41%) vs. placebo	[295]

Proposed main active compound	Treatment regime	Effect on OA Analgesia and NSAID	Reference
Ginger	Topical ginger extract gel (4% gel Plygersic) versus sodium diclofenac gel applied 1 mL of solution 4 times a day for 6 weeks	↓ Pain (by ~27%), symptoms (by ~27%) No difference in the above between groups	[296]
Ginger	Diclofenac 50 mg orally or Ginger 750 or Ginger 750 mg and Diclofenac 50 mg orally for 12 weeks	↓ Pain and WOMAC score in all three groups, greatest improvement with Ginger (60%; 75%) the addition of ginger to Diclofenac (67%; 79%), compared to Diclofenac alone (59%; 64%) ↓ Use of rescue medication (paracetamol) in Ginger (50%) and Ginger with Diclofenac (87%) compared to Diclofenac alone (not statistically significant)	[297]
Lithothamnion species (Red Algae)	AquaminF, 267 mg Lithothamnion, 3 capsules per day, 3 times a day for 12 weeks	↑ ROM (by 5.2°) and 6MWD (By 136 ft) following 50% forced reduction from all NSAID in AquaminF vs. placebo No difference in rescue medication (acetaminophen) consumption between groups ↑ Six meter walking distance (by~92%) following 50% forced reduction from all NSAID in AquaminF vs. placebo	[298]
Lithothamnion species combination	Aquamin+, 2668 mg Lithothamnion, 268 mg seawater-derived Mg(OH)2 and pine bark extract 120 mg versus 2000 mg Glucosamine Sulphate Daily dose for 12 weeks	↓ Pain (by ~11%), symptoms (by ~7%), no change in Glucosamine ↑ Sport and recreation (by ~9%), no change in Glucosamine ↑ Timed up and go performance (by 7%), no change in Glucosamine ↓ Rescue analgesic use (by 72%) vs. Glucosamine	[299]

Table 2.
Nutraceuticals shown to reduce analgesic and NSAID use.

in vivo therapeutic effects. Turmeric/curcumin extracts have been shown to reduce proinflammatory cytokines such as tumour necrosis factor alpha, interleukin (IL)-1 beta, IL-8, IL-6 and structural degradation protases such as matrix metalloproteinases, collagenase, induce positive cell behavioural characteristics (induces apoptosis and growth arrest) and anti-oxidative properties (through stimulation of nuclear factor-erythroid-2-related factor 2 (Nrf2) [292, 302–311]). Of particular interest to the present chapter, turmeric/curcumin extracts inhibit the NFkB pathway and other proinflammatory signalling pathways including COX-2, AP-1, Egr-1, STAT (signal transducers and activators of transcription) and mitogen-activated protein (MAP) kinases [309, 310, 312]. Considering these molecular targets, turmeric/curcumin extracts appear to enact there *in vivo* effects via similar mechanisms of action as commonly used pharmaceutical agents (**Figure 1**). These data clearly point to the positive impact that turmeric/curcumin extracts, including propriety formulations, can have on NSAID and analgesia use in the short term (best effects from study durations generally ≤12 weeks). While the long-term benefits are still being investigated, the current data suggests that turmeric/curcumin extracts could be recommended as an early stage treatment adjunct.

Alternative terrestrial botanicals have shown some advantages for OA. Three studies have investigated avocado/soybean extracts and their potential in reducing NSAID and analgesics use. One large randomised control trial (n = 260) showed that after 30 days (and continued to day 90) of supplementation, the extracts (300 or 600 mg) reduced the daily intake of NSAID and analgesics compared to placebo. Furthermore, 71% (compared to 36% in placebo) of avocado/soybean extract participants reduced their daily intake by greater than 50%, [281]. Although it must be noted that the treatment was stopped in nine participants due to adverse events from the extract, however the authors did not statistically analyse incidence of adverse events of the remaining participants, but they were generally similar to placebo. These results were somewhat supported by a smaller (n = 31; part of a large cohort receiving a number of nutraceutical compounds) observational study showing that the proportion of OA patients using analgesics and NSAIDs dropped by 34% over 6 months consuming avocado/soybean extracts [282]. Although, in this large scale "real-world" (PEGASus) study cohort where analgesic and NSAID use was assessed by phone interview bi-monthly over 2 years, avocado/soybean extracts showed no effect on reducing medication use [313]. Recently, a 2-month supplementation of avocado/soybean unsaponifiables (n = 30; 300 mg daily) was compared to celecoxib (n = 30; 200 mg/day) for changes in a biomarker of cartilage breakdown (Cartilage oligomeric matrix protein; COMP). The results showed that both interventions reduced serum COMP levels with a tendency for greater improvements with avocado/soybean unsaponifiables (33.8% vs. 30.3%; $p = 0.06$; [283]). These data in addition to other mechanistic work show that avocado/soybean unsaponifiables can impact both inflammatory and structural protein biomarkers of OA pathology. Specifically they can inhibit IL-1, reduce production of stromelysin, IL-6, IL-8 and PGE-2, increase the expression of TGF-β and activate collagen synthesis [283, 314–316]. There is some debate over the efficacy of avocado/soybean extracts to alleviate analgesics and NSAID use but there is developing molecular evidence that they may elicit similar reductions on *in vivo* cartilage breakdown which requires further investigation.

Two studies investigated Ginger root extract formulations in OA NSAID use. Compared to 1% diclofenac gel, topical ginger extract (Plygersic gel) reduce KOOS variables (pain, symptoms etc.) equally after a six week intervention in mild radiographic KOA [296]. Further, oral consumption of a Ginger root extract formulation, compared (1) 50 mg of oral Diclofenac with Ginger 750, (2) Ginger 750 mg and (3) Diclofenac 50 mg for 12 weeks [297]. All interventions decreased pain and WOMAC variables but there was a reduction in rescue medication in the ginger groups, although this was not statically significant [297]. While these results are interesting, significantly more research is needed with larger more well controlled studies but there is molecular evidence to support these reported effects. Ginger root species can block the formation of inflammatory mediators such as thromboxane, leukotrienes and prostaglandins and inhibit COX and lipoxygenase in arachidonic acid metabolism [317–325] i.e. similar mechanisms to those presented in **Figure 1**.

Finally, the trade marked Pycnogenol® (pine bark extract; 100 mg) has been shown to reduces NSAID use by 58%, compared to only 1% in the placebo group in early-KOA patients over 12 weeks [286]. This resulted in reduced hospital admissions and days spent in hospital by 50% compared to placebo (n = 156; [286]). As with the above, Pycnogenol inhibits activation of NFκB pathway mediators, particularly, COX and pain-producing prostaglandins and also activates metabolomic compounds with anti-inflammatory bio-efficacy [326–328]. Again, these data are interesting and demonstrate good potential but require further *in vivo* replication in relation to NSAID and analgesic.

3.2 Marine Fauna

New Zealand Green Lipped Mussel (Perna canaliculus) lipid extracts have recently been investigated for their potentially benefits for OA symptoms. Moderate-to-severe hip and knee OA patients received 600 mg of Biolex®-GLM for 12 weeks or a placebo and were allowed to consume paracetamol for additional pain relief [285]. Participants consuming the placebo took more paracetamol each week of the 12 weeks resulting in a statically significant change at the final week ($p = 0.001$), however did not differ in NSAID equivalence score. This suggests that there may be some potential for Green Lipped Mussel to reduce analgesic medication, although less so than others mentioned herein. Again, Green Lipped Mussel appears to inhibit COX enzymes, competitive inhibition of arachidonic acid metabolism and reduce chronic inflammation [329].

A fish oil and Urtica dioica preparation has also been shown to reduce medication use in OA. A proprietary combination of omega-3 and omega-6 fatty acids, Urtica dioica (the common nettle), zinc and vitamin E (Phytalgic®) progressively reduced NSAID and analgesia use over a tree month period (n = 81; 6.5 Paracetamol 500 mg-Equivalent per week, compared to 16.5 in the placebo group; [284]). The authors ascribed this adaptation to the anti-inflammatory potential of the mineral composition, mainly from Urtica dioica within the formulation rather than the fish oil component [284]. This was most likely the case as a previous study showed no effect of cod liver oil an OA [330] and the articles referenced to show a mechanistic potential for fish oil components (n-3 and n-6 polyunsaturated fatty acids) have recently been retracted [331, 332].

3.3 Marine botanicals

The marine red Algae species Lithothamnion corallioide, rich in sea water derived minerals including Calcium and Magnesium (AquaminF®), have recently been investigated for a potential impact on NSAID usage. In a randomised control trial of moderate-to-severe KOA patients that were regularly consuming NSAIDs, AquaminF (534 mg daily) was an effective agent for improving physical performance (six minuet walking distance), when NSAID use was intentionally reduced to 50% of previous consumption, but not when NSAID consumption was reduced to zero [298]. Furthermore, Lithothamnion (2668 mg) combined with seawater-derived Mg(OH)2 (268 mg) and pine bark extract (120 mg) reduced analgesic and

NSAID use by 72% compared to Glucosamine Sulphate (2000 mg Daily dose) [299]. Mechanistically, Lithothamnion corallioide species appear to have the ability to inhibit the NFκB pathway, reduce inflammatory cytokines such as tumour necrosis factor alpha (TNF-α), interleukin 1 beta (IL-1β) and COX2, along with reduced serum TNF-α [333–336]. This suggested there is potential for Lithothamnion species to reduce the KOA-related drug dependency *in vivo* with mechanistic rationale similar to that of pharmaceuticals (**Figure 1**). It appears as though Lithothamnion species have the ability to improve physical function and analgesia with reduced NSAID use, and induce a further reduction in drug use when combined with other nutraceuticals previously shown to reduce NSAID use. With larger scale replication and confirmation, Lithothamnion species could develop into a recommended early stage treatment adjunct.

4. Discussion and conclusions

These data are of considerable interest to those suffering from OA and medical practitioners concerned with the broader health impacts of pharmaceuticals use in OA patients. There appears to be a growing body of evidence suggesting that a variety of nutraceutical compounds, many in preparatory formulations, could provide some relief from the burden of NSAID and analgesic dependence, thus their associated side-effects. Currently the data are limited with respect to replication, sample size and duration, making conclusions about long term effectiveness difficult. The one potential exception is turmeric/curcumin extracts that in a recent meta-analysis it was shown that typically 1000 mg/day of curcumin was effective for improve OA symptoms (potentially better that NSAID) over 8-12 weeks - but the authors still call for significantly more research, specifically with increased sample size and better design quality [300].

While the precise molecular mechanisms of OA progression remain unclear, it appears to be exacerbated by the activation of NFκB signalling pathway, initiated by a host of mechanical and chemical stress stimuli, including excessive mechanical stress brought about by surplus body mass, proinflammatory cytokines and extracellular matrix degradation products [337, 338]. These actions reduce the amount of articular cartilage in the joints and degrade subchondral bone, thus induce pain and difficulty in movement. As a result, OA treatments focus on relieving pain and swelling, improving joint mobility, increasing musculoskeletal strength and minimising the disabling effects of the disease [339]. The NFκB signalling pathway and inflammatory mechanisms appear to be the molecular actions of the majority of the above nutraceuticals in combination with the inhibition of COX enzymes. These imply that their mechanism of action for pain relief (and therefore potential reduction in analgesic use) are via peripheral nociceptive action with little interaction through neuropathic mechanisms (unless through local inflammatory assault of nerve fibres).

As discussed throughout, there appears to be even further benefit through combinations of nutraceuticals that may have an additive effects to reduce NSAID/analgesic use and are recommended [263]. However, additional work needs to be carried out to understand the individual effects of these combinations in addition to the synergistic impact. This requirement is evident through the work by Jacquet et al. [284] where it appears that the proposed benefit of the combination was not attributable to the ingredient that is mentioned and discussed firstly (fish oil), rather the benefit lies with Urtica dioica and mineral composition. These combinations are often proprietary formulations where the precise combinations are not publicly available. However, where this is not the case better understanding can be achieved through *in vitro* experimentation to elucidate the mechanisms of action both individually and combined.

In conclusion, this chapter has described and discussed chronic pain, specifically osteoarthritis, and presented evidence that specific nutraceuticals and combinations may have potential to either elicit the same pain reliving effect of NSAIDs and analgesics or reduce the dependency on these drugs. Specifically, the greatest evidence exists for the inclusion of turmeric/curcumin extracts as an mild-OA treatment adjunct to reduce NSAID consumption. Any reduction in the use of harmful pharmaceutical drugs should be a welcome inclusion to any treatment plan particularly when some nutraceuticals, that appear to interact with similar molecular pathways as the discussed analgesics, may be capable of offering such benefit. However, it must be noted that significantly more experimental evidence is required for a number of these bioactives and their propitiatory formulations before specific recommendations can be made.

Acknowledgements

The authors have no acknowledgements to make.

Conflict of interests

The authors declare no conflict of interest.

Author details

Shane M. Heffernan[1*] and Gillian E. Conway[2]

1 Applied Sport Technology Exercise and Medicine Research Centre (A-STEM), Faculty of Science and Engineering, Swansea University, Swansea, Wales, UK

2 In vitro Toxicology Group, Institute of Life Science, College of Medicine, Swansea University, Swansea, Wales, UK

*Address all correspondence to: s.m.heffernan@swansea.ac.uk

References

[1] Del Giorno R, Frumento P, Varrassi G, Paladini A, Coaccioli S. Assessment of chronic pain and access to pain therapy: a cross-sectional population-based study. Journal of pain research. 2017;10:2577-2584.

[2] Rekatsina M, Paladini A, Piroli A, Zis P, Pergolizzi JV, Varrassi G. Pathophysiologic Approach to Pain Therapy for Complex Pain Entities: A Narrative Review. Pain and therapy. 2020;9(1):7-21.

[3] Treede R-D, Rief W, Barke A, Aziz Q, Bennett MI, Benoliel R, et al. Chronic pain as a symptom or a disease: the IASP Classification of Chronic Pain for the International Classification of Diseases (ICD-11). Pain. 2019;160(1):19-27.

[4] Cáceres-Matos R, Gil-García E, Cabrera-León A, Porcel-Gálvez AM, Barrientos-Trigo S. Factors that influence coping with chronic noncancer pain in European countries: a systematic review of measuring instruments. Pain Management Nursing. 2020;21(2):123-133.

[5] Analysts GI. Global pain management market to reach US $60 billion by 2015 https://www.prweb.com/releases/2011/1/prweb8052240.htm: Cision; 2011. Available from: https://www.prweb.com/releases/2011/1/prweb8052240.htm.

[6] Bushnell MC, Čeko M, Low LA. Cognitive and emotional control of pain and its disruption in chronic pain. Nature Reviews Neuroscience. 2013;14(7):502-511.

[7] Cabrera-León A, Rueda M, Cantero-Braojos M. Calibrated prevalence of disabling chronic pain according to different approaches: a face-to-face cross-sectional population-based study in Southern Spain. British Medical Journal Open. 2017;7(1).

[8] Leadley RM, Armstrong N, Lee YC, Allen A, Kleijnen J. Chronic diseases in the European Union: the prevalence and health cost implications of chronic pain. Journal of Pain and Palliative Care Pharmacotherapy. 2012;26(4):310-325.

[9] Reid KJ, Harker J, Bala MM, Truyers C, Kellen E, Bekkering GE, et al. Epidemiology of chronic non-cancer pain in Europe: narrative review of prevalence, pain treatments and pain impact. Current medical research and opinion. 2011;27(2):449-462.

[10] Torralba A, Miquel A, Darba J. Situación actual del dolor crónico en España: iniciativa" Pain Proposal". Revista de la Sociedad Española del Dolor. 2014;21(1):16-22.

[11] Gaskin DJ, Richard P. The economic costs of pain in the United States. The Journal of Pain. 2012;13(8):715-724.

[12] Nicholas M, Vlaeyen JWS, Rief W, Barke A, Aziz Q, Benoliel R, et al. The IASP classification of chronic pain for ICD-11: chronic primary pain. Pain. 2019;160(1):28-37.

[13] Treede RD, Rief W, Barke A, Aziz Q, Bennett MI, Benoliel R, et al. A classification of chronic pain for ICD-11. Pain. 2015;156(6):1003-1007.

[14] Haack M, Simpson N, Sethna N, Kaur S, Mullington J. Sleep deficiency and chronic pain: potential underlying mechanisms and clinical implications. Neuropsychopharmacology : official publication of the American College of Neuropsychopharmacology. 2020;45(1):205-216.

[15] Brune K, Patrignani P. New insights into the use of currently available non-steroidal anti-inflammatory drugs. Journal of pain research. 2015;8:105-118.

[16] McCarberg BH, Nicholson BD, Todd KH, Palmer T, Penles L. The

impact of pain on quality of life and the unmet needs of pain management: results from pain sufferers and physicians participating in an Internet survey. American journal of therapeutics. 2008;15(4):312-320.

[17] Rittner HL, Brack A, Stein C. Pain and the immune system. British journal of anaesthesia. 2008;101(1):40-44.

[18] Stein C. Opioids, sensory systems and chronic pain. European journal of pharmacology. 2013;716(1-3):179-187.

[19] Stein C. Opioid Receptors. Annual review of medicine. 2016;67:433-451.

[20] Carnes D, Parsons S, Ashby D, Breen A, Foster NE, Pincus T, et al. Chronic musculoskeletal pain rarely presents in a single body site: results from a UK population study. Rheumatology. 2007;46(7):1168-1170.

[21] Kosek E, Cohen M, Baron R, Gebhart GF, Mico JA, Rice AS, et al. Do we need a third mechanistic descriptor for chronic pain states? Pain. 2016;157(7):1382-1386.

[22] Morrone LA, Scuteri D, Rombolà L, Mizoguchi H, Bagetta G. Opioids Resistance in Chronic Pain Management. Curr Neuropharmacol. 2017;15(3):444-456.

[23] Costigan M, Scholz J, Woolf CJ. Neuropathic pain: a maladaptive response of the nervous system to damage. Annual review of neuroscience. 2009;32:1-32.

[24] McAlindon TE, Driban JB, Henrotin Y, Hunter DJ, Jiang GL, Skou ST, et al. OARSI Clinical Trials Recommendations: Design, conduct, and reporting of clinical trials for knee osteoarthritis. Osteoarthritis and cartilage. 2015;23(5):747-760.

[25] Baron R, Hans G, Dickenson AH. Peripheral input and its importance for central sensitization. Annals of neurology. 2013;74(5):630-636.

[26] Basbaum AI, Bautista DM, Scherrer G, Julius D. Cellular and molecular mechanisms of pain. Cell. 2009;139(2):267-284.

[27] Corder G, Castro DC, Bruchas MR, Scherrer G. Endogenous and Exogenous Opioids in Pain. Annual review of neuroscience. 2018;41:453-473.

[28] Ji RR, Chamessian A, Zhang YQ. Pain regulation by non-neuronal cells and inflammation. Science (New York, NY). 2016;354(6312):572-577.

[29] Chen L, Yang G, Grosser T. Prostanoids and inflammatory pain. Prostaglandins & other lipid mediators. 2013;104-105:58-66.

[30] Latremoliere A, Woolf CJ. Central sensitization: a generator of pain hypersensitivity by central neural plasticity. The Journal of Pain. 2009;10(9):895-926.

[31] Descalzi G, Kim S, Zhuo M. Presynaptic and postsynaptic cortical mechanisms of chronic pain. Molecular neurobiology. 2009;40(3):253-259.

[32] Peirs C, Seal RP. Neural circuits for pain: Recent advances and current views. Science (New York, NY). 2016;354(6312):578-584.

[33] Almeida TF, Roizenblatt S, Tufik S. Afferent pain pathways: a neuroanatomical review. Brain research. 2004;1000(1-2):40-56.

[34] Jensen TS, Baron R, Haanpää M, Kalso E, Loeser JD, Rice AS, et al. A new definition of neuropathic pain. Pain. 2011;152(10):2204-2205.

[35] Kuner R, Flor H. Structural plasticity and reorganisation in chronic pain. Nature Reviews Neuroscience. 2016;18(1):20-30.

[36] White FA, Jung H, Miller RJ. Chemokines and the pathophysiology of neuropathic pain. Proceedings of the National Academy of Sciences of the United States of America. 2007;104(51):20151-20158.

[37] Rowbotham MC, Yosipovitch G, Connolly MK, Finlay D, Forde G, Fields HL. Cutaneous innervation density in the allodynic form of postherpetic neuralgia. Neurobiology of disease. 1996;3(3):205-214.

[38] Ochoa JL, Campero M, Serra J, Bostock H. Hyperexcitable polymodal and insensitive nociceptors in painful human neuropathy. Muscle and Nerve. 2005;32(4):459-472.

[39] Reichling DB, Levine JD. Critical role of nociceptor plasticity in chronic pain. Trends in neurosciences. 2009;32(12):611-618.

[40] Ratté S, Prescott SA. Afferent hyperexcitability in neuropathic pain and the inconvenient truth about its degeneracy. Current opinion in neurobiology. 2016;36:31-37.

[41] Novakovic SD, Tzoumaka E, McGivern JG, Haraguchi M, Sangameswaran L, Gogas KR, et al. Distribution of the tetrodotoxin-resistant sodium channel PN3 in rat sensory neurons in normal and neuropathic conditions. The Journal of Neuroscience 1998;18(6):2174-2187.

[42] Bridges D, Thompson SW, Rice AS. Mechanisms of neuropathic pain. British journal of anaesthesia. 2001;87(1):12-26.

[43] Gaudet AD, Popovich PG, Ramer MS. Wallerian degeneration: gaining perspective on inflammatory events after peripheral nerve injury. Journal of neuroinflammation. 2011;8:110.

[44] Huang LY, Gu Y, Chen Y. Communication between neuronal somata and satellite glial cells in sensory ganglia. Glia. 2013;61(10):1571-1581.

[45] McLachlan EM, Jänig W, Devor M, Michaelis M. Peripheral nerve injury triggers noradrenergic sprouting within dorsal root ganglia. Nature. 1993;363(6429):543-546.

[46] Woolf CJ, Mannion RJ. Neuropathic pain: aetiology, symptoms, mechanisms, and management. Lancet (London, England). 1999;353(9168):1959-1964.

[47] Sandkühler J. Models and mechanisms of hyperalgesia and allodynia. Physiological reviews. 2009;89(2):707-758.

[48] Study RE, Kral MG. Spontaneous action potential activity in isolated dorsal root ganglion neurons from rats with a painful neuropathy. Pain. 1996;65(2-3):235-242.

[49] Gracely RH, Lynch SA, Bennett GJ. Painful neuropathy: altered central processing maintained dynamically by peripheral input. Pain. 1992;51(2):175-194.

[50] Woolf CJ. Evidence for a central component of post-injury pain hypersensitivity. Nature. 1983;306(5944):686-688.

[51] Loeser JD, Treede RD. The Kyoto protocol of IASP Basic Pain Terminology. Pain. 2008;137(3):473-477.

[52] Ji RR, Berta T, Nedergaard M. Glia and pain: is chronic pain a gliopathy? Pain. 2013;154 Suppl 1(0 1):S10-28.

[53] Woolf CJ, Shortland P, Coggeshall RE. Peripheral nerve injury triggers central sprouting of myelinated afferents. Nature. 1992;355(6355):75-78.

[54] Altman R, Alarcon G, Appelrouth D, Bloch D, Borenstein D, Brandt K, et al. The American College of Rheumatology criteria for the

classification and reporting of osteoarthritis of the hip. Arthritis and rheumatism. 1991;34.

[55] Fields HL, Rowbotham M, Baron R. Postherpetic neuralgia: irritable nociceptors and deafferentation. Neurobiology of disease. 1998;5(4):209-227.

[56] Meacham K, Shepherd A, Mohapatra DP, Haroutounian S. Neuropathic Pain: Central vs. Peripheral Mechanisms. Current Pain and Headache Reports. 2017;21(6):28.

[57] Mickle AD, Shepherd AJ, Mohapatra DP. Sensory TRP channels: the key transducers of nociception and pain. Progress in molecular biology and translational science. 2015;131:73-118.

[58] Varrassi G, Pergolizzi J, Peppin JF, Paladini A. Analgesic drugs and cardiac safety. Brain and Heart Dynamics. 2020:649-670.

[59] Strang J, Volkow ND, Degenhardt L, Hickman M, Johnson K, Koob GF, et al. Opioid Use Disorder. Nature Reviews Disease Primers. 2020;6(1):3.

[60] Stein C, Hassan AH, Przewłocki R, Gramsch C, Peter K, Herz A. Opioids from immunocytes interact with receptors on sensory nerves to inhibit nociception in inflammation. Proceedings of the National Academy of Sciences of the United States of America. 1990;87(15):5935-5939.

[61] Stein C. Peripheral mechanisms of opioid analgesia. Anesthesia and analgesia. 1993;76(1):182-91.

[62] Snyder SH. Opiate receptors and beyond: 30 years of neural signaling research. Neuropharmacology. 2004;47 Suppl 1:274-285.

[63] Waldhoer M, Bartlett SE, Whistler JL. Opioid receptors. Annual review of biochemistry. 2004;73:953-990.

[64] Yaksh TL. Pharmacology and mechanisms of opioid analgesic activity. Acta anaesthesiologica Scandinavica. 1997;41(1 Pt 2):94-111.

[65] Pert CB, Snyder SH. Opiate receptor: demonstration in nervous tissue. Science (New York, NY). 1973;179(4077):1011-1014.

[66] Hemmings HC, Hopkins PM. Foundations of anesthesia: basic sciences for clinical practice: Elsevier Health Sciences; 2006.

[67] Stein C. The control of pain in peripheral tissue by opioids. The New England journal of medicine. 1995;332(25):1685-1690.

[68] Hassan AH, Ableitner A, Stein C, Herz A. Inflammation of the rat paw enhances axonal transport of opioid receptors in the sciatic nerve and increases their density in the inflamed tissue. Neuroscience. 1993;55(1):185-195.

[69] Zollner C, Shaqura MA, Bopaiah CP, Mousa S, Stein C, Schafer M. Painful inflammation-induced increase in mu-opioid receptor binding and G-protein coupling in primary afferent neurons. Molecular pharmacology. 2003;64(2):202-210.

[70] Mousa SA, Cheppudira BP, Shaqura M, Fischer O, Hofmann J, Hellweg R, et al. Nerve growth factor governs the enhanced ability of opioids to suppress inflammatory pain. Brain : a journal of neurology. 2007;130(Pt 2):502-513.

[71] Jeanjean AP, Moussaoui SM, MaloteauxJM, LaduronPM. Interleukin-1 beta induces long-term increase of axonally transported opiate receptors and substance P. Neuroscience. 1995;68(1):151-157.

[72] Zhou L, Zhang Q, Stein C, Schäfer M. Contribution of opioid

receptors on primary afferent versus sympathetic neurons to peripheral opioid analgesia. The Journal of pharmacology and experimental therapeutics. 1998;286(2):1000-1006.

[73] Martin WR. Pharmacology of opioids. Pharmacological reviews. 1983;35(4):283-323.

[74] Sharp B, Yaksh T. Pain killers of the immune system. Nature medicine. 1997;3(8):831-832.

[75] Reinecke H, Weber C, Lange K, Simon M, Stein C, Sorgatz H. Analgesic efficacy of opioids in chronic pain: recent meta-analyses. British journal of pharmacology. 2015;172(2):324-333.

[76] Paulozzi LJ. Prescription drug overdoses: a review. Journal of safety research. 2012;43(4):283-289.

[77] Vowles KE, McEntee ML, Julnes PS, Frohe T, Ney JP, van der Goes DN. Rates of opioid misuse, abuse, and addiction in chronic pain: a systematic review and data synthesis. Pain. 2015;156(4):569-576.

[78] Chou R, Cruciani RA, Fiellin DA, Compton P, Farrar JT, Haigney MC, et al. Methadone safety: a clinical practice guideline from the American Pain Society and College on Problems of Drug Dependence, in collaboration with the Heart Rhythm Society. The Journal of Pain. 2014;15(4):321-337.

[79] Sacerdote P. Opioid-induced immunosuppression. Current opinion in supportive and palliative care. 2008;2(1):14-18.

[80] Sacerdote P, Bianchi M, Gaspani L, Manfredi B, Maucione A, Terno G, et al. The effects of tramadol and morphine on immune responses and pain after surgery in cancer patients. Anesthesia and analgesia. 2000;90(6):1411-1414.

[81] Wei LN. The RNA superhighway: axonal RNA trafficking of kappa opioid receptor mRNA for neurite growth. Integr Biol. 2011;3(1):10-16.

[82] Stein C, Küchler S. Non-analgesic effects of opioids: peripheral opioid effects on inflammation and wound healing. Current pharmaceutical design. 2012;18(37):6053-6069.

[83] Schumacher M, Basbaum A, Way W. Opioid analgesics and antagonists. 9th ed. New York: Lange Medical Books/ McGraw-Hill; 2004. 497-516 p.

[84] Mesgarpour B, Griebler U, Glechner A, Kien C, Strobelberger M, Van Noord MG, et al. Extended-release opioids in the management of cancer pain: a systematic review of efficacy and safety. European journal of pain (London, England). 2014;18(5):605-616.

[85] Drewes AM, Jensen RD, Nielsen LM, Droney J, Christrup LL, Arendt-Nielsen L, et al. Differences between opioids: pharmacological, experimental, clinical and economical perspectives. British journal of clinical pharmacology. 2013;75(1):60-78.

[86] Nestler EJ, Berhow MT, Brodkin ES. Molecular mechanisms of drug addiction: adaptations in signal transduction pathways. Molecular psychiatry. 1996;1(3):190-199.

[87] Galer BS, Lee D, Ma T, Nagle B, Schlagheck TG. MorphiDex (morphine sulfate/dextromethorphan hydrobromide combination) in the treatment of chronic pain: three multicenter, randomized, double-blind, controlled clinical trials fail to demonstrate enhanced opioid analgesia or reduction in tolerance. Pain. 2005;115(3):284-295.

[88] Noble M, Treadwell JR, Tregear SJ, Coates VH, Wiffen PJ, Akafomo C, et al. Long-term opioid management for chronic noncancer pain. The Cochrane database of systematic reviews. 2010;2010(1):Cd006605.

[89] Gustavsson A, Bjorkman J, Ljungcrantz C, Rhodin A, Rivano-Fischer M, Sjolund KF, et al. Pharmaceutical treatment patterns for patients with a diagnosis related to chronic pain initiating a slow-release strong opioid treatment in Sweden. Pain. 2012;153(12):2325-2331.

[90] Chou R, Qaseem A, Snow V, Casey D, Cross JT, Jr., Shekelle P, et al. Diagnosis and treatment of low back pain: a joint clinical practice guideline from the American College of Physicians and the American Pain Society. Annals of internal medicine. 2007;147(7):478-491.

[91] Hochberg MC, Altman RD, April KT, Benkhalti M, Guyatt G, McGowan J, et al. American College of Rheumatology 2012 recommendations for the use of nonpharmacologic and pharmacologic therapies in osteoarthritis of the hand, hip, and knee. Arthritis Care Res. 2012;64(4):465-474.

[92] Gellad WF, Good CB, Shulkin DJ. Addressing the Opioid Epidemic in the United States: Lessons From the Department of Veterans AffairsAddressing the Opioid Epidemic in the United StatesAddressing the Opioid Epidemic in the United States. Journal of the American Medical Association: Internal Medicine. 2017;177(5):611.

[93] Atchison JW, Herndon CM, Rusie E. NSAIDs for musculoskeletal pain management:current perspectives and novel strategies to improve safety. Journal of Managed Care Pharmacy. 2013;19(9 Suppl A):S3-19.

[94] Gomez-Acebo I, Dierssen-Sotos T, de Pedro M, Perez-Gomez B, Castano-Vinyals G, Fernandez-Villa T, et al. Epidemiology of non-steroidal anti-inflammatory drugs consumption in Spain. The MCC-Spain study. BMC Public Health. 2018;18(1):1134.

[95] Davis JS, Lee HY, Kim J, Advani SM, Peng HL, Banfield E, et al. Use of non-steroidal anti-inflammatory drugs in US adults: changes over time and by demographic. Open Heart. 2017;4(1):e000550.

[96] Nelson DA, Marks ES, Deuster PA, O'Connor FG, Kurina LM. Association of Nonsteroidal Anti-inflammatory Drug Prescriptions With Kidney Disease Among Active Young and Middle-aged Adults. JAMA Network Open. 2019;2(2):e187896.

[97] Walker LA, Zambraski EJ, Williams RF. Widespread Use of Prescription Nonsteroidal Anti-Inflammatory Drugs Among U.S. Army Active Duty Soldiers. Military medicine. 2017;182(3):e1709-e1e12.

[98] Gorski T, Cadore EL, Pinto SS, da Silva EM, Correa CS, Beltrami FG, et al. Use of NSAIDs in triathletes: prevalence, level of awareness and reasons for use. British journal of sports medicine. 2011;45(2):85-90.

[99] Küster M, Renner B, Oppel P, Niederweis U, Brune K. Consumption of analgesics before a marathon and the incidence of cardiovascular, gastrointestinal and renal problems: a cohort study. British Medical Journal Open. 2013;3(4).

[100] Zhou Y, Boudreau DM, Freedman AN. Trends in the use of aspirin and nonsteroidal anti-inflammatory drugs in the general U.S. population. Pharmacoepidemiology and drug safety. 2014;23(1):43-50.

[101] Grosser T, Theken KN, FitzGerald GA. Cyclooxygenase Inhibition: Pain, Inflammation, and the Cardiovascular System. Clinical pharmacology and therapeutics. 2017;102(4):611-622.

[102] Hinz B, Cheremina O, Brune K. Acetaminophen (paracetamol)

is a selective cyclooxygenase-2 inhibitor in man. FASEB Journal 2008;22(2):383-390.

[103] Ricciotti E, FitzGerald GA. Prostaglandins and inflammation. Arteriosclerosis, thrombosis, and vascular biology. 2011;31(5):986-1000.

[104] Smyth EM, Grosser T, Wang M, Yu Y, FitzGerald GA. Prostanoids in health and disease. Journal of lipid research. 2009;50 Suppl(Suppl):S423-8.

[105] Rao P, Knaus EE. Evolution of nonsteroidal anti-inflammatory drugs (NSAIDs): cyclooxygenase (COX) inhibition and beyond. Journal of Pharmacy and Pharmaceutical Sciences. 2008;11(2):81s-110s.

[106] Simmons DL, Botting RM, Hla T. Cyclooxygenase isozymes: the biology of prostaglandin synthesis and inhibition. Pharmacological reviews. 2004;56(3):387-437.

[107] Murata T, Ushikubi F, Matsuoka T, Hirata M, Yamasaki A, Sugimoto Y, et al. Altered pain perception and inflammatory response in mice lacking prostacyclin receptor. Nature. 1997;388(6643):678-682.

[108] Lazarus M, Yoshida K, Coppari R, Bass CE, Mochizuki T, Lowell BB, et al. EP3 prostaglandin receptors in the median preoptic nucleus are critical for fever responses. Nature neuroscience. 2007;10(9):1131-1133.

[109] Patrignani P, Tacconelli S, Bruno A, Sostres C, Lanas A. Managing the adverse effects of nonsteroidal anti-inflammatory drugs. Expert review of clinical pharmacology. 2011;4(5):605-621.

[110] Bhala N, Emberson J, Merhi A, Abramson S, Arber N, Baron JA, et al. Vascular and upper gastrointestinal effects of non-steroidal anti-inflammatory drugs: meta-analyses of individual participant data from randomised trials. Lancet (London, England). 2013;382(9894):769-779.

[111] Castellsague J, Riera-Guardia N, Calingaert B, Varas-Lorenzo C, Fourrier-Reglat A, Nicotra F, et al. Individual NSAIDs and upper gastrointestinal complications: a systematic review and meta-analysis of observational studies (the SOS project). Drug safety. 2012;35(12):1127-1146.

[112] Odom DM, Mladsi DM, Saag KG, Sherif BN, Miles L, Ronquest N, et al. Relationship between diclofenac dose and risk of gastrointestinal and cardiovascular events: meta-regression based on two systematic literature reviews. Clinical therapeutics. 2014;36(6):906-917.

[113] Van Hecken A, Schwartz JI, Depré M, De Lepeleire I, Dallob A, Tanaka W, et al. Comparative inhibitory activity of rofecoxib, meloxicam, diclofenac, ibuprofen, and naproxen on COX-2 versus COX-1 in healthy volunteers. Journal of clinical pharmacology. 2000;40(10):1109-1120.

[114] Hinz B, Brune K. Can drug removals involving cyclooxygenase-2 inhibitors be avoided? A plea for human pharmacology. Trends in pharmacological sciences. 2008;29(8):391-397.

[115] García Rodríguez LA, Tacconelli S, Patrignani P. Role of dose potency in the prediction of risk of myocardial infarction associated with nonsteroidal anti-inflammatory drugs in the general population. Journal of the American College of Cardiology. 2008;52(20):1628-1636.

[116] McGettigan P, Henry D. Cardiovascular risk with non-steroidal anti-inflammatory drugs: systematic review of population-based controlled observational studies. PLoS medicine. 2011;8(9):e1001098.

[117] Massó González EL, Patrignani P, Tacconelli S, García Rodríguez LA. Variability among nonsteroidal antiinflammatory drugs in risk of upper gastrointestinal bleeding. Arthritis and rheumatism. 2010;62(6):1592-1601.

[118] Antman EM, Bennett JS, Daugherty A, Furberg C, Roberts H, Taubert KA. Use of nonsteroidal antiinflammatory drugs: an update for clinicians: a scientific statement from the American Heart Association. Circulation. 2007;115(12):1634-1642.

[119] Bunchorntavakul C, Reddy KR. Acetaminophen-related hepatotoxicity. Clinics in liver disease. 2013;17(4):587-607, viii.

[120] Ennis ZN, Dideriksen D, Vaegter HB, Handberg G, Pottegård A. Acetaminophen for Chronic Pain: A Systematic Review on Efficacy. Basic and Clinical Pharmacology and Toxicology. 2016;118(3):184-189.

[121] Market Research Store. Acetaminophen (Paracetamol) Market for Pharmaceuticals, Dye Industry and Chemical Industry - Global Industry Perspective, Comprehensive Analysis, Size, Share, Growth, Segment, Trends and Forecast, 2014 – 2020 2016. Available from: https://www.marketresearchstore.com/news/global-acetaminophen-paracetamol-market-148.

[122] World Health Orgnization. WHO Model Lists of Essential Medicines 2017. Available from: https://www.who.int/groups/expert-committee-on-selection-and-use-of-essential-medicines/essential-medicines-lists.

[123] Wise J. NICE keeps paracetamol in UK guidelines on osteoarthritis. British Medical Journal. 2014;348:g1545.

[124] Machado GC, Maher CG, Ferreira PH, Pinheiro MB, Lin CW, Day RO, et al. Efficacy and safety of paracetamol for spinal pain and osteoarthritis: systematic review and meta-analysis of randomised placebo controlled trials. British Medical Journal. 2015;350:h1225.

[125] da Costa BR, Reichenbach S, Keller N, Nartey L, Wandel S, Juni P, et al. Effectiveness of non-steroidal anti-inflammatory drugs for the treatment of pain in knee and hip osteoarthritis: a network meta-analysis. Lancet (London, England). 2017;390(10090):e21-e33.

[126] Rabbie R, Derry S, Moore RA. Ibuprofen with or without an antiemetic for acute migraine headaches in adults. The Cochrane database of systematic reviews. 2013;2013(4):Cd008039.

[127] Moore RA, Derry S, Aldington D, Wiffen PJ. Single dose oral analgesics for acute postoperative pain in adults - an overview of Cochrane reviews. The Cochrane database of systematic reviews. 2015;2015(9):Cd008659.

[128] Chou D, Abalos E, Gyte GM, Gülmezoglu AM. Drugs for perineal pain in the early postpartum period: generic protocol. Cochrane Database of Systematic Reviews. 2009(3).

[129] Bailey E, Worthington HV, van Wijk A, Yates JM, Coulthard P, Afzal Z. Ibuprofen and/or paracetamol (acetaminophen) for pain relief after surgical removal of lower wisdom teeth. The Cochrane database of systematic reviews. 2013(12):Cd004624.

[130] Yoon YJ, Kim JH, Kim SY, Hwang IH, Kim MR. A Comparison of Efficacy and Safety of Non-steroidal Anti-inflammatory Drugs versus Acetaminophen in the Treatment of Episodic Tension-type Headache: A Meta-analysis of Randomized Placebo-controlled Trial Studies. Korean journal of family medicine. 2012;33(5):262-271.

[131] Pathan SA, Mitra B, Cameron PA. A Systematic Review and Meta-analysis Comparing the Efficacy of Nonsteroidal Anti-inflammatory Drugs, Opioids, and Paracetamol in the Treatment of Acute Renal Colic. European urology. 2018;73(4):583-595.

[132] Dalmann R, Daulhac L, Antri M, Eschalier A, Mallet C. Supra-spinal FAAH is required for the analgesic action of paracetamol in an inflammatory context. Neuropharmacology. 2015;91:63-70.

[133] Högestätt ED, Jönsson BA, Ermund A, Andersson DA, Björk H, Alexander JP, et al. Conversion of acetaminophen to the bioactive N-acylphenolamine AM404 via fatty acid amide hydrolase-dependent arachidonic acid conjugation in the nervous system. The Journal of biological chemistry. 2005;280(36):31405-31412.

[134] Mallet C, Daulhac L, Bonnefont J, Ledent C, Etienne M, Chapuy E, et al. Endocannabinoid and serotonergic systems are needed for acetaminophen-induced analgesia. Pain. 2008;139(1):190-200.

[135] Gerriets V, Anderson J, T.M. N. Acetaminophen Treasure Island (FL): StatPearls Publishing; 2020. Available from: https://www.ncbi.nlm.nih.gov/books/NBK482369/.

[136] Smith HS. Potential analgesic mechanisms of acetaminophen. Pain physician. 2009;12(1):269-280.

[137] Chandrasekharan NV, Dai H, Roos KL, Evanson NK, Tomsik J, Elton TS, et al. COX-3, a cyclooxygenase-1 variant inhibited by acetaminophen and other analgesic/antipyretic drugs: cloning, structure, and expression. Proceedings of the National Academy of Sciences of the United States of America. 2002;99(21):13926-13931.

[138] Flower RJ, Vane JR. Inhibition of prostaglandin synthetase in brain explains the anti-pyretic activity of paracetamol (4-acetamidophenol). Nature. 1972;240(5381):410-411.

[139] Graham GG, Scott KF. Mechanism of action of paracetamol. American journal of therapeutics. 2005;12(1):46-55.

[140] Kis B, Snipes JA, Busija DW. Acetaminophen and the cyclooxygenase-3 puzzle: sorting out facts, fictions, and uncertainties. The Journal of pharmacology and experimental therapeutics. 2005;315(1):1-7.

[141] Pickering G, Loriot MA, Libert F, Eschalier A, Beaune P, Dubray C. Analgesic effect of acetaminophen in humans: first evidence of a central serotonergic mechanism. Clinical pharmacology and therapeutics. 2006;79(4):371-378.

[142] Warner TD, Mitchell JA. Cyclooxygenase-3 (COX-3): filling in the gaps toward a COX continuum? Proceedings of the National Academy of Sciences of the United States of America. 2002;99(21):13371-13373.

[143] Sandrini M, Vitale G, Ruggieri V, Pini LA. Effect of acute and repeated administration of paracetamol on opioidergic and serotonergic systems in rats. Inflammation Research. 2007;56(4):139-142.

[144] Ruggieri V, Vitale G, Pini LA, Sandrini M. Differential involvement of opioidergic and serotonergic systems in the antinociceptive activity of N-arachidonoyl-phenolamine (AM404) in the rat: comparison with paracetamol. Naunyn-Schmiedeberg's archives of pharmacology. 2008;377(3):219-229.

[145] Schoffelmeer AN, Hogenboom F, Wardeh G, De Vries TJ. Interactions between CB1 cannabinoid and mu

opioid receptors mediating inhibition of neurotransmitter release in rat nucleus accumbens core. Neuropharmacology. 2006;51(4):773-781.

[146] Pelissier T, Alloui A, Caussade F, Dubray C, Cloarec A, Lavarenne J, et al. Paracetamol exerts a spinal antinociceptive effect involving an indirect interaction with 5-hydroxytryptamine3 receptors: in vivo and in vitro evidence. The Journal of pharmacology and experimental therapeutics. 1996;278(1):8-14.

[147] Alloui A, Chassaing C, Schmidt J, Ardid D, Dubray C, Cloarec A, et al. Paracetamol exerts a spinal, tropisetron-reversible, antinociceptive effect in an inflammatory pain model in rats. European journal of pharmacology. 2002;443(1-3):71-77.

[148] Chen C, Bazan NG. Acetaminophen modifies hippocampal synaptic plasticity via a presynaptic 5-HT2 receptor. Neuroreport. 2003;14(5):743-747.

[149] Bardin L, Lavarenne J, Eschalier A. Serotonin receptor subtypes involved in the spinal antinociceptive effect of 5-HT in rats. Pain. 2000;86(1-2):11-18.

[150] Raffa RB, Codd EE. Lack of binding of acetaminophen to 5-HT receptor or uptake sites (or eleven other binding/uptake assays). Life sciences. 1996;59(2):Pl37-Pl40.

[151] Di Marzo V, Deutsch DG. Biochemistry of the endogenous ligands of cannabinoid receptors. Neurobiology of disease. 1998;5(6 Pt B):386-404.

[152] Ottani A, Leone S, Sandrini M, Ferrari A, Bertolini A. The analgesic activity of paracetamol is prevented by the blockade of cannabinoid CB1 receptors. European journal of pharmacology. 2006;531(1-3):280-281.

[153] Negrini F, Negrini S. Is paracetamol better than placebo for knee and hip osteoarthritis? A Cochrane review summary with commentary. International journal of rheumatic diseases. 2020;23(4):595-596.

[154] Leopoldino AO, Machado GC, Ferreira PH, Pinheiro MB, Day R, McLachlan AJ, et al. Paracetamol versus placebo for knee and hip osteoarthritis. The Cochrane database of systematic reviews. 2019;2(2):Cd013273.

[155] Barrière DA, Boumezbeur F, Dalmann R, Cadeddu R, Richard D, Pinguet J, et al. Paracetamol is a centrally acting analgesic using mechanisms located in the periaqueductal grey. British journal of pharmacology. 2020;177(8):1773-1792.

[156] Jóźwiak-Bebenista M, Nowak JZ. Paracetamol: mechanism of action, applications and safety concern. Acta poloniae pharmaceutica. 2014;71(1):11-23.

[157] Wei G, Bergquist A, Broomé U, Lindgren S, Wallerstedt S, Almer S, et al. Acute liver failure in Sweden: etiology and outcome. Journal of internal medicine. 2007;262(3):393-401.

[158] Tanne J. Paracetamol causes most liver failure in UK and US. British Medical Journal. 2006;332(7542):628.

[159] Wastesson JW, Martikainen JE, Zoëga H, Schmidt M, Karlstad Ø, Pottegård A. Trends in Use of Paracetamol in the Nordic Countries. Basic and Clinical Pharmacology and Toxicology. 2018;123(3):301-307.

[160] Moore M, Thor H, Moore G, Nelson S, Moldéus P, Orrenius S. The toxicity of acetaminophen and N-acetyl-p-benzoquinone imine in isolated hepatocytes is associated with thiol depletion and increased cytosolic Ca2+. The Journal of biological chemistry. 1985;260(24):13035-13040.

[161] Xie Y, McGill MR, Du K, Dorko K, Kumer SC, Schmitt TM,

et al. Mitochondrial protein adducts formation and mitochondrial dysfunction during N-acetyl-m-aminophenol (AMAP)-induced hepatotoxicity in primary human hepatocytes. Toxicology and applied pharmacology. 2015;289(2):213-222.

[162] Athersuch TJ, Antoine DJ, Boobis AR, Coen M, Daly AK, Possamai L, et al. Paracetamol metabolism, hepatotoxicity, biomarkers and therapeutic interventions: a perspective. Toxicology research. 2018;7(3):347-357.

[163] Zhang W, Nuki G, Moskowitz RW, Abramson S, Altman RD, Arden NK, et al. OARSI recommendations for the management of hip and knee osteoarthritis: part III: Changes in evidence following systematic cumulative update of research published through January 2009. Osteoarthritis and cartilage. 2010;18(4):476-499.

[164] Roberts E, Delgado Nunes V, Buckner S, Latchem S, Constanti M, Miller P, et al. Paracetamol: not as safe as we thought? A systematic literature review of observational studies. Annals of the rheumatic diseases. 2016;75(3):552-559.

[165] Rahme E, Barkun A, Nedjar H, Gaugris S, Watson D. Hospitalizations for upper and lower GI events associated with traditional NSAIDs and acetaminophen among the elderly in Quebec, Canada. The American journal of gastroenterology. 2008;103(4):872-882.

[166] Saragiotto BT, Abdel Shaheed C, Maher CG. Paracetamol for pain in adults. British Medical Journal. 2019;367:l6693.

[167] GBD. Global, regional, and national incidence, prevalence, and years lived with disability for 310 diseases and injuries, 1990-2015: a systematic analysis for the Global Burden of Disease Study 2015. Lancet (London, England). 2016;388(10053):1545-1602.

[168] GBD. Global, regional, and national incidence, prevalence, and years lived with disability for 328 diseases and injuries for 195 countries, 1990-2016: a systematic analysis for the Global Burden of Disease Study 2016. Lancet (London, England). 2017;390(10100):1211-1259.

[169] Deshpande BR, Katz JN, Solomon DH, Yelin EH, Hunter DJ, Messier SP, et al. Number of Persons With Symptomatic Knee Osteoarthritis in the US: Impact of Race and Ethnicity, Age, Sex, and Obesity. Arthritis Care Res. 2016;68(12):1743-1750.

[170] Losina E, Weinstein AM, Reichmann WM, Burbine SA, Solomon DH, Daigle ME, et al. Lifetime risk and age at diagnosis of symptomatic knee osteoarthritis in the US. Arthritis care & research. 2013;65(5):703-711.

[171] Institute of Medicine. Relieving Pain in America: A Blueprint for Transforming Prevention, Care, Education, and Research. Washington, DC: The National Academies Press; 2011. 382 p.

[172] Kraus VB, Blanco FJ, Englund M, Karsdal MA, Lohmander LS. Call for standardized definitions of osteoarthritis and risk stratification for clinical trials and clinical use. Osteoarthritis and cartilage. 2015;23(8):1233-1241.

[173] Lane NE, Brandt K, Hawker G, Peeva E, Schreyer E, Tsuji W, et al. OARSI-FDA initiative: defining the disease state of osteoarthritis. Osteoarthritis and cartilage. 2011;19(5):478-482.

[174] Eitner A, Hofmann GO, Schaible HG. Mechanisms of Osteoarthritic Pain. Studies in Humans

and Experimental Models. Frontiers in molecular neuroscience. 2017;10:349.

[175] Felson DT. Developments in the clinical understanding of osteoarthritis. Arthritis Research and Therapy. 2009;11(1):203.

[176] Hofmann GO, Marticke J, Grossstück R, Hoffmann M, Lange M, Plettenberg HK, et al. Detection and evaluation of initial cartilage pathology in man: A comparison between MRT, arthroscopy and near-infrared spectroscopy (NIR) in their relation to initial knee pain. Pathophysiology : the official journal of the International Society for Pathophysiology. 2010;17(1):1-8.

[177] Goldring MB, Otero M. Inflammation in osteoarthritis. Current opinion in rheumatology. 2011;23(5):471-478.

[178] Yusup A, Kaneko H, Liu L, Ning L, Sadatsuki R, Hada S, et al. Bone marrow lesions, subchondral bone cysts and subchondral bone attrition are associated with histological synovitis in patients with end-stage knee osteoarthritis: a cross-sectional study. Osteoarthritis and cartilage. 2015;23(11):1858-1864.

[179] Burr DB, Gallant MA. Bone remodelling in osteoarthritis. Nature reviews Rheumatology. 2012;8(11):665-673.

[180] Attur M, Krasnokutsky S, Statnikov A, Samuels J, Li Z, Friese O, et al. Low-grade inflammation in symptomatic knee osteoarthritis: prognostic value of inflammatory plasma lipids and peripheral blood leukocyte biomarkers. Arthritis & rheumatology (Hoboken, NJ). 2015;67(11):2905-2915.

[181] Berenbaum F, van den Berg WB. Inflammation in osteoarthritis: changing views. Osteoarthritis and cartilage. 2015;23(11):1823-1824.

[182] Zhang Y, Nevitt M, Niu J, Lewis C, Torner J, Guermazi A, et al. Fluctuation of knee pain and changes in bone marrow lesions, effusions, and synovitis on magnetic resonance imaging. Arthritis and rheumatism. 2011;63(3):691-699.

[183] Eckstein F, Burstein D, Link TM. Quantitative MRI of cartilage and bone: degenerative changes in osteoarthritis. NMR in Biomedicine. 2006;19(7):822-854.

[184] Link TM, Steinbach LS, Ghosh S, Ries M, Lu Y, Lane N, et al. Osteoarthritis: MR imaging findings in different stages of disease and correlation with clinical findings. Radiology. 2003;226(2):373-381.

[185] Hawker GA, French MR, Waugh EJ, Gignac MA, Cheung C, Murray BJ. The multidimensionality of sleep quality and its relationship to fatigue in older adults with painful osteoarthritis. Osteoarthritis and cartilage. 2010;18(11):1365-1371.

[186] Hawker GA, Gignac MA, Badley E, Davis AM, French MR, Li Y, et al. A longitudinal study to explain the pain-depression link in older adults with osteoarthritis. Arthritis Care Res. 2011;63(10):1382-1390.

[187] Georgiev T, Angelov AK. Modifiable risk factors in knee osteoarthritis: treatment implications. Rheumatology international. 2019;39(7):1145-1157.

[188] Gelber AC, Hochberg MC, Mead LA, Wang NY, Wigley FM, Klag MJ. Joint injury in young adults and risk for subsequent knee and hip osteoarthritis. Annals of internal medicine. 2000;133(5):321-328.

[189] Blagojevic M, Jinks C, Jeffery A, Jordan KP. Risk factors for onset of osteoarthritis of the knee in older adults: a systematic review and meta-analysis.

Osteoarthritis and cartilage. 2010;18(1):24-33.

[190] Gelber AC, Hochberg MC, Mead LA, Wang NY, Wigley FM, Klag MJ. Body mass index in young men and the risk of subsequent knee and hip osteoarthritis. The American journal of medicine. 1999;107(6):542-548.

[191] Sharma L, Song J, Felson DT, Cahue S, Shamiyeh E, Dunlop DD. The role of knee alignment in disease progression and functional decline in knee osteoarthritis. Journal of the American Medical Association. 2001;286(2):188-195.

[192] Toivanen AT, Heliövaara M, Impivaara O, Arokoski JP, Knekt P, Lauren H, et al. Obesity, physically demanding work and traumatic knee injury are major risk factors for knee osteoarthritis--a population-based study with a follow-up of 22 years. Rheumatology. 2010;49(2):308-314.

[193] Felson DT, Niu J, Gross KD, Englund M, Sharma L, Cooke TD, et al. Valgus malalignment is a risk factor for lateral knee osteoarthritis incidence and progression: findings from the Multicenter Osteoarthritis Study and the Osteoarthritis Initiative. Arthritis and rheumatism. 2013;65(2):355-362.

[194] Srikanth VK, Fryer JL, Zhai G, Winzenberg TM, Hosmer D, Jones G. A meta-analysis of sex differences prevalence, incidence and severity of osteoarthritis. Osteoarthritis and cartilage. 2005;13(9):769-781.

[195] Vina ER, Ran D, Ashbeck EL, Kwoh CK. Natural history of pain and disability among African-Americans and Whites with or at risk for knee osteoarthritis: A longitudinal study. Osteoarthritis and cartilage. 2018;26(4):471-479.

[196] Spector TD, Cicuttini F, Baker J, Loughlin J, Hart D. Genetic influences on osteoarthritis in women: a twin study. British Medical Journal. 1996;312(7036):940-943.

[197] MacGregor AJ, Antoniades L, Matson M, Andrew T, Spector TD. The genetic contribution to radiographic hip osteoarthritis in women: results of a classic twin study. Arthritis and rheumatism. 2000;43(11):2410-2416.

[198] Loughlin J. The genetic epidemiology of human primary osteoarthritis: current status. Expert reviews in molecular medicine. 2005;7(9):1-12.

[199] Grotle M, Hagen KB, Natvig B, Dahl FA, Kvien TK. Obesity and osteoarthritis in knee, hip and/ or hand: an epidemiological study in the general population with 10 years follow-up. BMC musculoskeletal disorders. 2008;9:132.

[200] Marks R. Obesity profiles with knee osteoarthritis: correlation with pain, disability, disease progression. Obesity. 2007;15(7):1867-1874.

[201] Silverwood V, Blagojevic-Bucknall M, Jinks C, Jordan JL, Protheroe J, Jordan KP. Current evidence on risk factors for knee osteoarthritis in older adults: a systematic review and meta-analysis. Osteoarthritis and cartilage. 2015;23(4):507-515.

[202] Kulkarni K, Karssiens T, Kumar V, Pandit H. Obesity and osteoarthritis. Maturitas. 2016;89:22-28.

[203] Yoshimura N, Muraki S, Oka H, Tanaka S, Kawaguchi H, Nakamura K, et al. Accumulation of metabolic risk factors such as overweight, hypertension, dyslipidaemia, and impaired glucose tolerance raises the risk of occurrence and progression of knee osteoarthritis: a 3-year follow-up of the ROAD study. Osteoarthritis and cartilage. 2012;20(11):1217-1226.

[204] Courties A, Gualillo O, Berenbaum F, Sellam J. Metabolic stress-induced joint inflammation and osteoarthritis. Osteoarthritis and cartilage. 2015;23(11):1955-1965.

[205] Wang X, Hunter D, Xu J, Ding C. Metabolic triggered inflammation in osteoarthritis. Osteoarthritis and cartilage. 2015;23(1):22-30.

[206] Berenbaum F, Griffin TM, Liu-Bryan R. Review: Metabolic Regulation of Inflammation in Osteoarthritis. Arthritis and Rheumatology. 2017;69(1):9-21.

[207] Schett G, Kleyer A, Perricone C, Sahinbegovic E, Iagnocco A, Zwerina J, et al. Diabetes is an independent predictor for severe osteoarthritis: results from a longitudinal cohort study. Diabetes care. 2013;36(2):403-409.

[208] Eymard F, Parsons C, Edwards MH, Petit-Dop F, Reginster JY, Bruyère O, et al. Diabetes is a risk factor for knee osteoarthritis progression. Osteoarthritis and cartilage. 2015;23(6):851-859.

[209] King KB, Rosenthal AK. The adverse effects of diabetes on osteoarthritis: update on clinical evidence and molecular mechanisms. Osteoarthritis and cartilage. 2015;23(6):841-850.

[210] Dai Z, Niu J, Zhang Y, Jacques P, Felson DT. Dietary intake of fibre and risk of knee osteoarthritis in two US prospective cohorts. Annals of the rheumatic diseases. 2017;76(8):1411-1419.

[211] Breivik H, Collett B, Ventafridda V, Cohen R, Gallacher D. Survey of chronic pain in Europe: prevalence, impact on daily life, and treatment. European Journal of Pain. 2006;10(4):287-.

[212] Hunter DJ, March L, Chew M. Osteoarthritis in 2020 and beyond: a Lancet Commission. Lancet (London, England). 2020;396(10264):1711-1712.

[213] Global Burden of Disease Network Collaborative. Global Burden of Disease Study 2019 (GBD 2019) Results 2019. Available from: http://ghdx.healthdata.org/gbd-results-tool.

[214] French HP, Galvin R, Horgan NF, Kenny RA. Prevalence and burden of osteoarthritis amongst older people in Ireland: findings from The Irish LongituDinal Study on Ageing (TILDA). European Journal of Public Health. 2016;26(1):192-198.

[215] Murray CJ, Lopez AD, Organization WH. The Global burden of disease: a comprehensive assessment of mortality and disability from diseases, injuries, and risk factors in 1990 and projected to 2020. Harvard University Press. 1996;1:41.

[216] Kopec JA, Sayre EC, Schwartz TA, Renner JB, Helmick CG, Badley EM, et al. Occurrence of radiographic osteoarthritis of the knee and hip among African Americans and whites: a population-based prospective cohort study. Arthritis Care Res. 2013;65(6):928-935.

[217] Wallace IJ, Worthington S, Felson DT, Jurmain RD, Wren KT, Maijanen H, et al. Knee osteoarthritis has doubled in prevalence since the mid-20th century. Proceedings of the National Academy of Sciences of the United States of America. 2017;114(35):9332-9336.

[218] van Tunen JAC, Peat G, Bricca A, Larsen LB, Søndergaard J, Thilsing T, et al. Association of osteoarthritis risk factors with knee and hip pain in a population-based sample of 29-59 year olds in Denmark: a cross-sectional analysis. BMC musculoskeletal disorders. 2018;19(1):300.

[219] Finan PH, Buenaver LF, Bounds SC, Hussain S, Park RJ,

Haque UJ, et al. Discordance between pain and radiographic severity in knee osteoarthritis: findings from quantitative sensory testing of central sensitization. Arthritis and rheumatism. 2013;65(2):363-372.

[220] Akinci A, Al Shaker M, Chang MH, Cheung CW, Danilov A, José Dueñas H, et al. Predictive factors and clinical biomarkers for treatment in patients with chronic pain caused by osteoarthritis with a central sensitisation component. International journal of clinical practice. 2016;70(1):31-44.

[221] Lluch E, Torres R, Nijs J, Van Oosterwijck J. Evidence for central sensitization in patients with osteoarthritis pain: a systematic literature review. European Journal of Pain. 2014;18(10):1367-1375.

[222] Giesecke T, Gracely RH, Grant MA, Nachemson A, Petzke F, Williams DA, et al. Evidence of augmented central pain processing in idiopathic chronic low back pain. Arthritis and rheumatism. 2004;50(2):613-623.

[223] Lee YC, Bingham CO, 3rd, Edwards RR, Marder W, Phillips K, Bolster MB, et al. Association Between Pain Sensitization and Disease Activity in Patients With Rheumatoid Arthritis: A Cross-Sectional Study. Arthritis Care Res. 2018;70(2):197-204.

[224] Felson DT. The sources of pain in knee osteoarthritis. Current opinion in rheumatology. 2005;17(5):624-628.

[225] Hawker GA, Stewart L, French MR, Cibere J, Jordan JM, March L, et al. Understanding the pain experience in hip and knee osteoarthritis--an OARSI/OMERACT initiative. Osteoarthritis and cartilage. 2008;16(4):415-422.

[226] Oteo-Álvaro Á, Ruiz-Ibán MA, Miguens X, Stern A, Villoria J, Sánchez-Magro I. High Prevalence of Neuropathic Pain Features in Patients with Knee Osteoarthritis: A Cross-Sectional Study. Pain Practice. 2015;15(7):618-626.

[227] Hochman JR, Gagliese L, Davis AM, Hawker GA. Neuropathic pain symptoms in a community knee OA cohort. Osteoarthritis and cartilage. 2011;19(6):647-654.

[228] Suokas AK, Walsh DA, McWilliams DF, Condon L, Moreton B, Wylde V, et al. Quantitative sensory testing in painful osteoarthritis: a systematic review and meta-analysis. Osteoarthritis and cartilage. 2012;20(10):1075-1085.

[229] Mapp PI, Walsh DA. Mechanisms and targets of angiogenesis and nerve growth in osteoarthritis. Nature Reviews Rheumatology. 2012;8(7):390-398.

[230] Schaible HG. Mechanisms of chronic pain in osteoarthritis. Current Rheumatology Reports. 2012;14(6):549-556.

[231] Bartley EJ, King CD, Sibille KT, Cruz-Almeida Y, Riley JL, 3rd, Glover TL, et al. Enhanced Pain Sensitivity Among Individuals With Symptomatic Knee Osteoarthritis: Potential Sex Differences in Central Sensitization. Arthritis Care Res. 2016;68(4):472-480.

[232] Petersen KK, Arendt-Nielsen L, Simonsen O, Wilder-Smith O, Laursen MB. Presurgical assessment of temporal summation of pain predicts the development of chronic postoperative pain 12 months after total knee replacement. Pain. 2015;156(1):55-61.

[233] Wylde V, Sayers A, Lenguerrand E, Gooberman-Hill R, Pyke M, Beswick AD, et al. Preoperative widespread pain sensitization and chronic pain after hip and knee replacement: a cohort analysis. Pain. 2015;156(1):47-54.

[234] European Medicines Agency. Guideline on the Clinical Development of Medicinal Products Intended for the Treatment of Pain 2016 [Available from: https://www.ema.europa.eu/en/documents/scientific-guideline/guideline-clinical-development-medicinal-products-intended-treatment-pain-first-version_en.pdf.

[235] Bedson J, Croft PR. The discordance between clinical and radiographic knee osteoarthritis: a systematic search and summary of the literature. BMC musculoskeletal disorders. 2008;9:116.

[236] Malfait AM, Schnitzer TJ. Towards a mechanism-based approach to pain management in osteoarthritis. Nature reviews Rheumatology. 2013;9(11):654-664.

[237] Neogi T, Felson D, Niu J, Nevitt M, Lewis CE, Aliabadi P, et al. Association between radiographic features of knee osteoarthritis and pain: results from two cohort studies. British Medical Journal. 2009;339:b2844.

[238] Eckstein F, Cotofana S, Wirth W, Nevitt M, John MR, Dreher D, et al. Greater rates of cartilage loss in painful knees than in pain-free knees after adjustment for radiographic disease stage: data from the osteoarthritis initiative. Arthritis and rheumatism. 2011;63(8):2257-2267.

[239] Kaukinen P, Podlipská J, Guermazi A, Niinimäki J, Lehenkari P, Roemer FW, et al. Associations between MRI-defined structural pathology and generalized and localized knee pain - the Oulu Knee Osteoarthritis study. Osteoarthritis and cartilage. 2016;24(9):1565-1576.

[240] Wittoek R, Cruyssen BV, Verbruggen G. Predictors of functional impairment and pain in erosive osteoarthritis of the interphalangeal joints: comparison with controlled inflammatory arthritis. Arthritis and rheumatism. 2012;64(5):1430-1436.

[241] McAlindon TE, Bannuru RR, Sullivan MC, Arden NK, Berenbaum F, Bierma-Zeinstra SM, et al. OARSI guidelines for the non-surgical management of knee osteoarthritis. Osteoarthritis and cartilage. 2014;22(3):363-388.

[242] Bertin P, Becquemont L, Corruble E, Derumeaux G, Falissard B, Hanon O, et al. The therapeutic management of chronic pain in ambulatory care patients aged 65 and over in France: the S.AGES Cohort. Baseline data. The Journal of Nutrition, Health and Aging. 2013;17(8):681-686.

[243] Pelletier JP, Martel-Pelletier J, Rannou F, Cooper C. Efficacy and safety of oral NSAIDs and analgesics in the management of osteoarthritis: Evidence from real-life setting trials and surveys. Seminars in Arthritis and Rheumatism. 2016;45(4 Suppl):S22-S27.

[244] Harirforoosh S, Asghar W, Jamali F. Adverse effects of nonsteroidal antiinflammatory drugs: an update of gastrointestinal, cardiovascular and renal complications. Journal of Pharmacy & Pharmaceutical Sciences. 2013;16(5):821-847.

[245] Persson MSM, Stocks J, Walsh DA, Doherty M, Zhang W. The relative efficacy of topical non-steroidal anti-inflammatory drugs and capsaicin in osteoarthritis: a network meta-analysis of randomised controlled trials. Osteoarthritis and cartilage. 2018;26(12):1575-1582.

[246] Adili A, Bhandari M. Cochrane in CORR®: Topical NSAIDs for Chronic Musculoskeletal Pain in Adults. Clinical Orthopaedics and Related Research. 2018;476(11):2128-2134.

[247] Arfe A, Scotti L, Varas-Lorenzo C, Nicotra F, Zambon A, Kollhorst B, et al.

Non-steroidal anti-inflammatory drugs and risk of heart failure in four European countries: nested case-control study. British Medical Journal. 2016;354:i4857.

[248] Solomon DH, Husni ME, Libby PA, Yeomans ND, Lincoff AM, Lupsilonscher TF, et al. The Risk of Major NSAID Toxicity with Celecoxib, Ibuprofen, or Naproxen: A Secondary Analysis of the PRECISION Trial. The American journal of medicine. 2017;130(12):1415-1422.

[249] van den Driest JJ, Pijnenburg P, Bindels PJE, Bierma-Zeinstra SMA, Schiphof D. Analgesic Use in Dutch Patients With Osteoarthritis: Frequent But Low Doses. Journal of Clinical Rheumatology. 2019;Ahead of print.

[250] Moore N, Salvo F, Duong M, Gulmez SE. Does paracetamol still have a future in osteoarthritis? Lancet (London, England). 2016;387(10033):2065-2066.

[251] McCrae JC, Morrison EE, MacIntyre IM, Dear JW, Webb DJ. Long-term adverse effects of paracetamol - a review. British journal of clinical pharmacology. 2018;84(10):2218-2230.

[252] Doherty M, Hawkey C, Goulder M, Gibb I, Hill N, Aspley S, et al. A randomised controlled trial of ibuprofen, paracetamol or a combination tablet of ibuprofen/paracetamol in community-derived people with knee pain. Annals of the rheumatic diseases. 2011;70(9):1534-1541.

[253] Stewart M, Cibere J, Sayre EC, Kopec JA. Efficacy of commonly prescribed analgesics in the management of osteoarthritis: a systematic review and meta-analysis. Rheumatology international. 2018;38(11):1985-1997.

[254] Zhang W, Doherty M, Arden N, Bannwarth B, Bijlsma J, Gunther KP, et al. EULAR evidence based recommendations for the management of hip osteoarthritis: report of a task force of the EULAR standing Committee for International Clinical Studies Including Therapeutics (ESCISIT). Annals of the rheumatic diseases. 2005;64.

[255] Jordan KM, Arden NK, Doherty M, Bannwarth B, Bijlsma JW, Dieppe P, et al. EULAR recommendations 2003: an evidence based approach to the management of knee osteoarthritis: report of a task force of the standing Committee for International Clinical Studies Including Therapeutic Trials (ESCISIT). Annals of the rheumatic diseases. 2003;62.

[256] Ackerman IN, Zomer E, Gilmartin-Thomas JF, Liew D. Forecasting the future burden of opioids for osteoarthritis. Osteoarthritis and cartilage. 2018;26(3):350-355.

[257] Thorlund JB, Turkiewicz A, Prieto-Alhambra D, Englund M. Inappropriate opioid dispensing in patients with knee and hip osteoarthritis: a population-based cohort study. Osteoarthritis and cartilage. 2020;28(2):146-153.

[258] Welsch P, Petzke F, Klose P, Häuser W. Opioids for chronic osteoarthritis pain: An updated systematic review and meta-analysis of efficacy, tolerability and safety in randomized placebo-controlled studies of at least 4 weeks double-blind duration. European Journal of Pain. 2020;24(4):685-703.

[259] Osani MC, Lohmander LS, Bannuru RR. Is There Any Role for Opioids in the Management of Knee and Hip Osteoarthritis? A Systematic Review and Meta-Analysis. Arthritis Care Res. 2020.

[260] Fuggle N, Curtis E, Shaw S, Spooner L, Bruyère O, Ntani G, et al.

Safety of Opioids in Osteoarthritis: Outcomes of a Systematic Review and Meta-Analysis. Drugs and Aging. 2019;36(Suppl 1):129-143.

[261] Liu X, Eyles J, McLachlan AJ, Mobasheri A. Which supplements can I recommend to my osteoarthritis patients? Rheumatology. 2018;57(suppl_4):iv75-iv87.

[262] Liu X, Machado GC, Eyles JP, Ravi V, Hunter DJ. Dietary supplements for treating osteoarthritis: a systematic review and meta-analysis. British journal of sports medicine. 2018;52(3):167-175.

[263] Henrotin Y, Mobasheri A. Natural Products for Promoting Joint Health and Managing Osteoarthritis. Current Rheumatology Reports. 2018;20(11):72.

[264] Kucharz EJ, Kovalenko V, Szántó S, Bruyère O, Cooper C, Reginster J-Y. A review of glucosamine for knee osteoarthritis: why patented crystalline glucosamine sulfate should be differentiated from other glucosamines to maximize clinical outcomes. Current medical research and opinion. 2016;32(6):997-1004.

[265] Fransen M, McConnell S, Harmer AR, Van der Esch M, Simic M, Bennell KL. Exercise for osteoarthritis of the knee: a Cochrane systematic review. British journal of sports medicine. 2015;49(24):1554-1557.

[266] Altman R, Lim S, Steen RG, Dasa V. Hyaluronic Acid Injections Are Associated with Delay of Total Knee Replacement Surgery in Patients with Knee Osteoarthritis: Evidence from a Large U.S. Health Claims Database. PLoS One. 2015;10(12):e0145776.

[267] DeFelice SL. The nutraceutical revolution: its impact on food industry R&D. Trend Food Science Tech. 1995;6(2):59-61.

[268] Witkamp RF, van Norren K. Let thy food be thy medicine....when possible. European journal of pharmacology. 2018;836:102-114.

[269] Santini A, Novellino E. Nutraceuticals: Beyond the diet before the drugs. Current Bioactive Compounds. 2014;10(1):1-12.

[270] Aronson JK. Defining 'nutraceuticals': neither nutritious nor pharmaceutical. British journal of clinical pharmacology. 2017;83(1):8-19.

[271] Zeisel SH. Regulation of "nutraceuticals". Science (New York, NY). 1999;285(5435):1853-1855.

[272] Espín JC, García-Conesa MT, Tomás-Barberán FA. Nutraceuticals: facts and fiction. Phytochemistry. 2007;68(22-24):2986-3008.

[273] Santini A, Tenore GC, Novellino E. Nutraceuticals: A paradigm of proactive medicine. European Journal of Pharmaceutical Sciences. 2017;96:53-61.

[274] European Food Safety Authority PoDPNA. Scientific opinion on the substantiation of health claims related to monacolin K from red yeast rice and maintenance of normal blood LDL cholesterol concentrations (ID 1648, 1700) pursuant to Article 13 (1) of Regulation (EC) No 1924/2006. European Food Safety Authority Journal. 2011;9(7):2304.

[275] European Council. EC Regulation n. 1924/2006 2006 [Available from: https://eur-lex.europa.eu/legal-content/EN/TXT/?uri=CELEX%3A02006R1924-20141213.

[276] Act USNRaE. H.R.3001– Nutraceutical Research and Education Act. (106th Congress of 1999-2000): U.S. Congress; 1999 [Available from: https://www.congress.gov/bill/106th-congress/house-bill/3001?q=%7B%22search%22%3A%5B%22Nutraceutical+Research+and+Education+Act%22%5D%7D&r=13&s=5

[277] The European Nutraceutical Association. Nutraceutical Definition: The European Nutraceutical Association; 2018 [Available from: https://www.enaonline.eu.

[278] Health Canada. Policy Paper - Nutraceuticals/Functional Foods and Health Claims On Foods 2002 [Available from: https://www.canada.ca/en/health-canada/services/food-nutrition/food-labelling/health-claims/nutraceuticals-functional-foods-health-claims-foods-policy-paper.html.

[279] Corzo L, Fernández-Novoa L, Carrera I, Martínez O, Rodríguez S, Alejo R, et al. Nutrition, Health, and Disease: Role of Selected Marine and Vegetal Nutraceuticals. Nutrients. 2020;12(3).

[280] Vaishya R, Agarwal AK, Shah A, Vijay V, Vaish A. Current status of top 10 nutraceuticals used for Knee Osteoarthritis in India. J Clin Orthop Trauma. 2018;9(4):338-348.

[281] Appelboom T, Schuermans J, Verbruggen G, Henrotin Y, Reginster JY. Symptoms modifying effect of avocado/soybean unsaponifiables (ASU) in knee osteoarthritis. A double blind, prospective, placebo-controlled study. Scandinavian Journal of Rheumatology. 2001;30(4):242-247.

[282] Gluszko P, Stasiek M. Symptom-modifying effects of oral avocado/soybean unsaponifiables in routine treatment of knee osteoarthritis in Poland. An open, prospective observational study of patients adherent to a 6-month treatment. Reumatologia. 2016;54(5):217-226.

[283] Jokar M, Azadeh H, Mirfeizi Z, Shariati Sarabi J, Hashemzadeh K. A Comparison between Avocado-Soybean Unsaponifiables and Celecoxib on Serum Levels of Cartilage Oligomeric Matrix Protein in Patients with Knee Osteoarthritis. Rheumatology Research. 2019;4(2):71-75.

[284] Jacquet A, Girodet P-O, Pariente A, Forest K, Mallet L, Moore N. Phytalgic, a food supplement, vs placebo in patients with osteoarthritis of the knee or hip: a randomised double-blind placebo-controlled clinical trial. Arthritis Research and Therapy. 2009;11(6):R192-R.

[285] Stebbings S, Gray A, Schneiders AG, Sansom A. A randomized double-blind placebo-controlled trial to investigate the effectiveness and safety of a novel green-lipped mussel extract -BioLex® -for managing pain in moderate to severe osteoarthritis of the hip and knee. BMC Complement Altern Med. 2017;17(1):416.

[286] Belcaro G, Cesarone MR, Errichi S, Zulli C, Errichi BM, Vinciguerra G, et al. Treatment of osteoarthritis with Pycnogenol. The SVOS (San Valentino Osteo-arthrosis Study). Evaluation of signs, symptoms, physical performance and vascular aspects. Phytotherapy Research. 2008;22(4):518-523.

[287] Kuptniratsaikul V, Thanakhumtorn S, Chinswangwatanakul P, Wattanamongkonsil L, Thamlikitkul V. Efficacy and safety of Curcuma domestica extracts in patients with knee osteoarthritis. The Journal of Alternative and Complementary Medicine. 2009;15(8):891-897.

[288] Kuptniratsaikul V, Dajpratham P, Taechaarpornkul W, Buntragulpoontawee M, Lukkanapichonchut P, Chootip C, et al. Efficacy and safety of Curcuma domestica extracts compared with ibuprofen in patients with knee osteoarthritis: a multicenter study. Clinical Interventions in Aging. 2014;9:451-458.

[289] Chandran B, Goel A. A randomized, pilot study to assess the efficacy and safety of curcumin

in patients with active rheumatoid arthritis. Phytotherapy Research. 2012;26(11):1719-1725.

[290] Shep D, Khanwelkar C, Gade P, Karad S. Safety and efficacy of curcumin versus diclofenac in knee osteoarthritis: a randomized open-label parallel-arm study. Trials. 2019;20(1):214.

[291] Gupte PA, Giramkar SA, Harke SM, Kulkarni SK, Deshmukh AP, Hingorani LL, et al. Evaluation of the efficacy and safety of Capsule Longvida(®) Optimized Curcumin (solid lipid curcumin particles) in knee osteoarthritis: a pilot clinical study. Journal of inflammation research. 2019;12:145-152.

[292] Heidari-Beni M, Moravejolahkami AR, Gorgian P, Askari G, Tarrahi MJ, Bahreini-Esfahani N. Herbal formulation "turmeric extract, black pepper, and ginger" versus Naproxen for chronic knee osteoarthritis: A randomized, double-blind, controlled clinical trial. Phytotherapy Research. 2020;34(8):2067-2073.

[293] Belcaro G, Cesarone MR, Dugall M, Pellegrini L, Ledda A, Grossi MG, et al. Efficacy and safety of Meriva [R], a curcumin-phosphatidylcholine complex, during extended administration in osteoarthritis patients. Alternative Medicine Review. 2010;15(4):337-345.

[294] Nakagawa Y, Mukai S, Yamada S, Matsuoka M, Tarumi E, Hashimoto T, et al. Short-term effects of highly-bioavailable curcumin for treating knee osteoarthritis: a randomized, double-blind, placebo-controlled prospective study. Journal of Orthopaedic Science. 2014;19(6):933-939.

[295] Panahi Y, Rahimnia AR, Sharafi M, Alishiri G, Saburi A, Sahebkar A. Curcuminoid treatment for knee osteoarthritis: A randomized double-blind placebo-controlled trial. Phytotherapy Research. 2014;28(11):1625-1631.

[296] Niempoog S, Siriarchavatana P, Kajsongkram T. The efficacy of Plygersic gel for use in the treatment of osteoarthritis of the knee. Journal of the Medical Association of Thailand. 2012;95 Suppl 10:S113-S119.

[297] Paramdeep G. Efficacy and tolerability of ginger (Zingiber officinale) in patients of osteoarthritis of knee. Indian journal of physiology and pharmacology. 2013;57(2):177-183.

[298] Frestedt JL, Kuskowski MA, Zenk JL. A natural seaweed derived mineral supplement (Aquamin F) for knee osteoarthritis: a randomised, placebo controlled pilot study. Nutrition Journal. 2009;8:7.

[299] Heffernan SM, McCarthy C, Eustace S, FitzPatrick RE, Delahunt E, De Vito G. Mineral rich algae with pine bark improved pain, physical function and analgesic use in mild-knee joint osteoarthritis, compared to Glucosamine: a randomized controlled pilot trial. Complementary Therapies in Medicine. 2020:In Press.

[300] Daily JW, Yang M, Park S. Efficacy of Turmeric Extracts and Curcumin for Alleviating the Symptoms of Joint Arthritis: A Systematic Review and Meta-Analysis of Randomized Clinical Trials. Journal of Medicinal Food. 2016;19(8):717-729.

[301] Heidari-Beni M, Moravejolahkami AR, Gorgian P, Askari G, Tarrahi MJ, Bahreini-Esfahani N. Herbal formulation "turmeric extract, black pepper, and ginger" versus Naproxen for chronic knee osteoarthritis: A randomized, double-blind, controlled clinical trial. Phytotherapy Research. 2020.

[302] Bengmark S. Curcumin, an atoxic antioxidant and natural NFkappaB,

cyclooxygenase-2, lipooxygenase, and inducible nitric oxide synthase inhibitor: a shield against acute and chronic diseases. J Parenter Enteral Nutr. 2006;30(1):45-51.

[303] Oyagbemi AA, Saba AB, Ibraheem AO. Curcumin: from food spice to cancer prevention. Asian Pacific journal of cancer prevention. 2009;10(6):963-967.

[304] Khanna D, Sethi G, Ahn KS, Pandey MK, Kunnumakkara AB, Sung B, et al. Natural products as a gold mine for arthritis treatment. Current opinion in pharmacology. 2007;7(3):344-351.

[305] Saja K, Babu MS, Karunagaran D, Sudhakaran PR. Anti-inflammatory effect of curcumin involves downregulation of MMP-9 in blood mononuclear cells. International immunopharmacology. 2007;7(13):1659-1667.

[306] Kim KH, Lee EN, Park JK, Lee JR, Kim JH, Choi HJ, et al. Curcumin attenuates TNF-α-induced expression of intercellular adhesion molecule-1, vascular cell adhesion molecule-1 and proinflammatory cytokines in human endometriotic stromal cells. Phytotherapy Research. 2012;26(7):1037-1047.

[307] Yang Q, Wu S, Mao X, Wang W, Tai H. Inhibition effect of curcumin on TNF-α and MMP-13 expression induced by advanced glycation end products in chondrocytes. Pharmacology. 2013;91(1-2):77-85.

[308] Jackson JK, Higo T, Hunter WL, Burt HM. The antioxidants curcumin and quercetin inhibit inflammatory processes associated with arthritis. Inflammation Research. 2006;55(4):168-175.

[309] Goel A, Boland CR, Chauhan DP. Specific inhibition of cyclooxygenase-2 (COX-2) expression by dietary curcumin in HT-29 human colon cancer cells. Cancer Letters. 2001;172(2):111-118.

[310] Goel A, Jhurani S, Aggarwal BB. Multi-targeted therapy by curcumin: how spicy is it? Mol Nutr Food Res. 2008;52(9):1010-1030.

[311] Mathy-Hartert M, Jacquemond-Collet I, Priem F, Sanchez C, Lambert C, Henrotin Y. Curcumin inhibits pro-inflammatory mediators and metalloproteinase-3 production by chondrocytes. Inflammation Research. 2009;58(12):899.

[312] Reuter S, Gupta SC, Park B, Goel A, Aggarwal BB. Epigenetic changes induced by curcumin and other natural compounds. Genes and Nutrition. 2011;6(2):93-108.

[313] Rovati LC, Girolami F, D'Amato M, Giacovelli G. Effects of glucosamine sulfate on the use of rescue non-steroidal anti-inflammatory drugs in knee osteoarthritis: Results from the Pharmaco-Epidemiology of GonArthroSis (PEGASus) study. Seminars in Arthritis and Rheumatism. 2016;45(4 Suppl):S34-S41.

[314] Henrotin YE, Sanchez C, Deberg MA, Piccardi N, Guillou GB, Msika P, et al. Avocado/soybean unsaponifiables increase aggrecan synthesis and reduce catabolic and proinflammatory mediator production by human osteoarthritic chondrocytes. The Journal of rheumatology. 2003;30(8):1825-1834.

[315] Boumediene K, Felisaz N, Bogdanowicz P, Galera P, Guillou GB, Pujol JP. Avocado/soya unsaponifiables enhance the expression of transforming growth factor beta1 and beta2 in cultured articular chondrocytes. Arthritis and rheumatism. 1999;42(1):148-156.

[316] Henrotin YE, Labasse AH, Jaspar JM, De Groote DD, Zheng SX, Guillou GB, et al. Effects of three avocado/soybean unsaponifiable mixtures on metalloproteinases, cytokines and prostaglandin E2 production by human articular chondrocytes. Clinical rheumatology. 1998;17(1):31-39.

[317] Panthong A, Kanjanapothi D, Niwatananant W, Tuntiwachwuttikul P, Reutrakul V. Anti-inflammatory activity of compound D {(E)-4-(3',4'-dimethoxyphenyl)but-3-en-2-ol} isolated from Zingiber cassumunar Roxb. Phytomedicine : international journal of phytotherapy and phytopharmacology. 1997;4(3):207-212.

[318] Jeenapongsa R, Yoovathaworn K, Sriwatanakul KM, Pongprayoon U, Sriwatanakul K. Anti-inflammatory activity of (E)-1-(3,4-dimethoxyphenyl) butadiene from Zingiber cassumunar Roxb. Journal of ethnopharmacology. 2003;87(2-3):143-148.

[319] Minghetti P, Sosa S, Cilurzo F, Casiraghi A, Alberti E, Tubaro A, et al. Evaluation of the topical anti-inflammatory activity of ginger dry extracts from solutions and plasters. Planta medica. 2007;73(15):1525-1530.

[320] Thomson M, Al-Qattan KK, Al-Sawan SM, Alnaqeeb MA, Khan I, Ali M. The use of ginger (Zingiber officinale Rosc.) as a potential anti-inflammatory and antithrombotic agent. Prostaglandins, leukotrienes, and essential fatty acids. 2002;67(6):475-478.

[321] Nurtjahja-Tjendraputra E, Ammit AJ, Roufogalis BD, Tran VH, Duke CC. Effective anti-platelet and COX-1 enzyme inhibitors from pungent constituents of ginger. Thrombosis research. 2003;111(4-5):259-265.

[322] Lantz RC, Chen GJ, Sarihan M, Sólyom AM, Jolad SD, Timmermann BN. The effect of extracts from ginger rhizome on inflammatory mediator production. Phytomedicine : international journal of phytotherapy and phytopharmacology. 2007;14(2-3):123-128.

[323] Pongprayoon U, Soontornsaratune P, Jarikasem S, Sematong T, Wasuwat S, Claeson P. Topical antiinflammatory activity of the major lipophilic constituents of the rhizome of Zingiber cassumunar. Part I: The essential oil. Phytomedicine : international journal of phytotherapy and phytopharmacology. 1997;3(4):319-322.

[324] Pongprayoon U, Tuchinda P, Claeson P, Sematong T, Reutrakul V, Soontornsaratune P. Topical antiinflammatory activity of the major lipophilic constituents of the rhizome of Zingiber cassumunar. Part II: Hexane extractives. Phytomedicine : international journal of phytotherapy and phytopharmacology. 1997;3(4):323-326.

[325] Han AR, Kim MS, Jeong YH, Lee SK, Seo EK. Cyclooxygenase-2 inhibitory phenylbutenoids from the rhizomes of Zingiber cassumunar. Chem Pharm Bull. 2005;53(11):1466-1468.

[326] Jessberger S, Högger P, Genest F, Salter DM, Seefried L. Cellular pharmacodynamic effects of Pycnogenol® in patients with severe osteoarthritis: a randomized controlled pilot study. BMC Complement Altern Med. 2017;17(1):537-.

[327] Grimm T, Skrabala R, Chovanová Z, Muchová J, Sumegová K, Liptáková A, et al. Single and multiple dose pharmacokinetics of maritime pine bark extract (pycnogenol) after oral administration to healthy volunteers. BMC Clin Pharmacol. 2006;6:4.

[328] Schäfer A, Chovanová Z, Muchová J, Sumegová K, Liptáková A,

Duracková Z, et al. Inhibition of COX-1 and COX-2 activity by plasma of human volunteers after ingestion of French maritime pine bark extract (Pycnogenol). Biomedicine and Pharmacotherapy. 2006;60(1):5-9.

[329] Ulbricht C, Chao W, Costa D, Nguyen Y, Seamon E, Weissner W. An evidence-based systematic review of green-lipped mussel (Perna canaliculus) by the natural standard research collaboration. J Diet Suppl. 2009;6.

[330] Stammers T, Sibbald B, Freeling P. Efficacy of cod liver oil as an adjunct to non-steroidal anti-inflammatory drug treatment in the management of osteoarthritis in general practice. Annals of the rheumatic diseases. 1992;51(1):128-129.

[331] Curtis CL, Rees SG, Cramp J, Flannery CR, Hughes CE, Little CB, et al. Effects of n-3 fatty acids on cartilage metabolism. The Proceedings of the Nutrition Society. 2006;65(4):434.

[332] Curtis CL, Rees SG, Little CB, Flannery CR, Hughes CE, Wilson C, et al. Pathologic indicators of degradation and inflammation in human osteoarthritic cartilage are abrogated by exposure to n-3 fatty acids. Arthritis and rheumatism. 2002;46(6):1544-1553.

[333] Murphy CT, Martin C, Doolan AM, Molloy MG, Dinan TG, Gorman D, et al. The Marine-derived, Multi-mineral formula, AquaPT Reduces TNF-α Levels in Osteoarthritis Patients. Journal of Nutrition Health Food Science. 2014;2:1-3.

[334] Frestedt JL, Walsh M, Kuskowski MA, Zenk JL. A natural mineral supplement provides relief from knee osteoarthritis symptoms: a randomized controlled pilot trial. Nutrition Journal. 2008;7:9.

[335] Ryan S, O'Gorman DM, Nolan YM. Evidence that the marine-derived multi-mineral Aquamin has anti-inflammatory effects on cortical glial-enriched cultures. Phytotherapy Research. 2011;25(5):765-767.

[336] O'Gorman DM, O'Carroll C, Carmody RJ. Evidence that marine-derived, multi-mineral, Aquamin inhibits the NF-κB signaling pathway in vitro. Phytotherapy research: PTR. 2012;26(4):630-632.

[337] Marcu KB, Otero M, Olivotto E, Borzi RM, Goldring MB. NF-kappaB signaling: multiple angles to target OA. Current drug targets. 2010;11(5):599-613.

[338] He Y, Yue Y, Zheng X, Zhang K, Chen S, Du Z. Curcumin, inflammation, and chronic diseases: how are they linked? Molecules (Basel, Switzerland). 2015;20(5):9183-9213.

[339] Moyer RF, Ratneswaran A, Beier F, Birmingham TB. Osteoarthritis year in review 2014: mechanics--basic and clinical studies in osteoarthritis. Osteoarthritis and cartilage. 2014;22(12):1989-2002.

Chapter 12

Multimodal Pharmacological Analgesia in Pain Management

Antonella Paladini and Giustino Varrassi

Abstract

The knowledge of the pathophysiology of pain has gradually evolved in recent years, allowing the development of new management strategies, more specifically addressing single pain types and patient profiles. Despite these advancements, pain management still remains an open issue, given the limitations of single agent therapies, the potential abuse/misuse of opioids and the risk of adverse events. The advent of multimodal analgesic strategies paves the way for major improvements in pain management, combining increased efficacy with better tolerability and an opioid-sparing effect. The association of analgesics with different mechanisms of action represents a successful strategy for a wide range of pain conditions, minimizing side effects and taking advantage of the additive or synergistic actions of individual agents. Last but not least, the increasing availability of oral fixed-dose combinations of analgesics will offer further advantages over extemporaneous combinations, by increasing ease of administration and patient adherence to treatment.

Keywords: acute pain, chronic pain, analgesia, multimodal, drug combination, opioid, anti-inflammatory agents, nonsteroidal, acetaminophen

1. Introduction

Whatever its cause, pain, both acute and chronic, often emerges from multiple pathogenic pathways [1], which makes drug treatment particularly difficult [2]. In recent decades, the pharmacological arsenal against pain, in addition to traditional nonsteroidal anti-inflammatory drugs (NSAIDs) and paracetamol, has been enriched, on the one hand with molecules operating on different pain mechanisms (as anticonvulsants and antidepressants), and on the other hand with opioids [3]. However, the single-agent approach to pain remains quite challenging, since a single drug, acting on a single pain component, is generally not successful to achieve a clinically meaningful pain reduction, whereas its use at high doses may cause significant side effects [2]. On the other hand, the increasing prescription of opioids for noncancer chronic pain, besides providing limited clinical advantage compared with non-opioid alternatives [4], has opened the door to problematic opioid use and addiction problems: up to 50% of patients on long-term opioid therapy develop physical dependence or tolerance, leading to problematic opioid use in 5–10% of patients and to addiction in 1–2% [5]. As a consequence, pain management is far from being optimal and patients are exposed to the risks associated with misuse of single agents [6, 7].

Considering the complexity of pain pathogenesis, which involves multiple pathways [1], and the difficulty to reach complete symptoms control, especially for chronic pain which still affects 25–35% of adults in Europe [8], multimodal pharmacological analgesia may represent a possible solution to the still unsolved problem of pain management, thanks to a number of potential advantages: first, a decrease of the administered doses of the individual components; second, the reduction of side effects; and third, a simultaneous action on different pain components [9]. Thanks to these features, multimodal pharmacological therapy gives clinicians the opportunity to make a further step forward to a fully individualized therapy of pain in its various components and clinical manifestations [3].

In this chapter, we will present the therapeutic strategies currently available to address the specific needs in the treatment of different painful conditions and the new possibilities for pain intervention according to the multimodal approach.

2. Pain management: unmet needs and future challenges

Despite the multiple treatment options available, pain remains a mostly unresolved topic in every day clinical practice. The analgesic efficacy of single drug treatment is often not sufficient to provide an adequate pain relief, since most analgesic drugs cannot be prescribed at unlimited doses due to the ceiling effect and safety concerns. Another limitation of single-agent analgesia is that it cannot address the multiple pathways underlying pain pathogenesis. Combining drugs from different classes, with different and complementary mechanisms of action, may provide a better opportunity for effective analgesia at reduced doses of individual agents, with a potential reduction of dose-related adverse events.

Based on these considerations, clinical practice is gradually moving from a traditional one-fits-all approach to a more tailored strategy. The traditional approach to pain management refers to the three-step World Health Organization (WHO) pain ladder, which recommends the following regimen, based on the intensity of the patient's pain [10]:

Step I: a non-opioid analgesic should be used for moderate pain, with co-analgesics if necessary.

Step II: if pain persists or increases, a weak opioid may be added.

Step III: if pain still persists, then a change should be made to a strong opioid.

By contrast, newer guidelines aim at treating pain according to the mechanism or mechanisms involved, i.e., neuropathic, nociceptive, or a combination of both [11]. Clinicians should seek to identify the basic pain mechanisms and treat the patient, accordingly, choosing the drug with the most appropriate mechanism of action [6].

Pain is a complex construct with sophisticated transmission pathways in the nervous system, which can be altered physiologically or pharmacologically [2]. Modulation of the transmission of pain can be divided into three approaches:

1. Modulating the upward transmission

2. Altering perception centrally

3. Modulating descending inhibitory pathways

Intervening in all three areas with multiple drugs is more effective than single drug treatment, and it allows to reduce the total dose of any one drug, thereby limiting unwanted effects [9].

Different drugs act at different areas:

i. Peripherally acting drugs:

- Local anesthetics
- NSAIDS

ii. Drugs acting in the spinal cord:

- Opiates
- NSAIDS
- N-methyl-D-aspartate (NMDA) receptor antagonists
- Gabapentinoids

iii. Drugs acting centrally:

- Opiates
- Paracetamol

iv. Drugs acting on descending pathways:

- Tramadol
- Clonidine
- 5HT3 antagonists

The principle of multimedia analgesia is the use of a number of drugs (analgesic or adjuvant) in combination to achieve the best pain relief in acute or chronic pain. Combining analgesics that act by different mechanisms of action allows modulating multiple transmission pathways and enables individual agents to act with potentially additive or synergistic effects [12].

Multimodal analgesia is widely acknowledged to be superior to a single drug approach, having demonstrated improved pain relief, with the fewest side effects [2]. This concept was pharmacologically studied in the 1960s by Houde et al. [13], then clinically suggested (especially in postoperative pain) in the 1980s [14], and a few years later diffused by Kehlet and Dahl [9], who first introduced the term "multimodal" or "blended" analgesia. Since then, multimodal analgesia has been deeply studied, demonstrating a broader spectrum of action, greater efficacy, better patient compliance, and an improved efficacy/safety ratio compared with monotherapy [12]. As a result, analgesic combinations are recommended by the WHO, American Pain Society (APS), and American College of Rheumatology (ACR) [15–17] and are commonly used in clinical practice. As regards the ease of use, fixed-dose combinations (FDCs) may offer additional advantages, including ease of administration, reduction of pill burden, and improved adherence [18].

3. Analgesic drug combinations

The pharmacological therapeutic approach of multimodal analgesia includes all the frontline drugs available, used alone or in combination according to the specific needs of the patient [19].

Drugs for pain control fall into four main categories [20]:

1. weak analgesics (paracetamol and metamizole)

2. NSAIDs (ibuprofen, diclofenac, ketoprofen, and dexketoprofen)

3. opioids (morphine, hydromorphone, and oxycodone)

4. adjuvant drugs (antidepressant, antiepileptic medications, corticosteroids, colchicine, neurotrophine, and biologic drugs)

The choice of the most appropriate drug combination should consider the pathogenic mechanisms of pain and satisfy the following criteria:

- The drugs to be combined should have different mechanisms of action and preferably act at different sites;

- The drugs to be combined should not interfere with the preexisting comorbidities of the patient; and

- FDCs should be preferred, if available, aiming at improving patient adherence to therapy.

Drug	Mechanism of action
Paracetamol	Inhibits prostaglandin synthesis in the central nervous system.
NSAIDs	Inhibit prostaglandin production by blocking cyclooxygenase both peripherally and centrally.
Opioids	Have multiple sites of action: ○ In the brain, they activate descending pain inhibitors. ○ In the periphery, they work by reducing inflammation. ○ In the spine, they decrease presynaptic calcium and sodium influx, production and release of excitatory amino acids, such as substance P, and postsynaptic excitability.
Anticonvulsants	Inhibit high-frequency neuronal firing by blocking sodium channels and reducing neuron hyperexcitability.
NMDA-receptor antagonists (ketamine)	Bind to the NMDA receptor, thereby inhibiting glutamate activation. Glutamate is an excitatory amino acid found in laminae I, II, and III of the dorsal horn of the spinal cord, where it activates primary afferent neurons.
Alpha-2 adrenergic agonists	Act on the descending pain pathways supra-spinally, activating receptors to stimulate acetylcholine release, and on the ascending pain pathways, by inhibiting substance P release from the primary afferent neurons, thus reducing transmission of pain.
Antidepressants	Alter neurotransmitters that affect pain pathways by inhibiting presynaptic neuronal reuptake of serotonin and norepinephrine at the descending pain pathway, resulting in improved inhibition of pain.

Table 1.
Mechanism of action of different analgesics (elaborated from text in Ref. [3]).

Different drugs with different mechanism(s) of action may be combined for enhanced efficacy [20]. Analgesics relieve pain through a variety of mechanisms of action along multiple sites of the nociceptive pathway (**Table 1**) [3].

Analgesic combinations are currently recommended by several guidelines and are used in clinical practice [21]. In patients with moderate-to-severe pain, the general recommendation is the combination of opioid and non-opioid analgesics [22]:

1. Among the possible combinations, paracetamol has been associated with weak (e.g., codeine or tramadol) or strong (e.g., morphine or oxycodone) opioids. Besides being less effective than NSAIDs [23, 24], paracetamol may cause gastrointestinal (GI), cardiovascular (CV), and hepatic adverse effects [25, 26].

2. NSAID/opioid combinations have the advantage of anti-inflammatory and additive analgesic effect, along with a well-demonstrated opioid-sparing activity [27]. Currently available NSAID/opioid FDCs include:

    - Hydrocodone/ibuprofen (7.5/400 mg) and oxycodone/ibuprofen (5/400 mg) are two oral, fixed-dose combination formulations, approved for the short-term management of acute, moderate-to-severe pain. A single tablet provided better analgesia than low-dose hydrocodone/oxycodone or ibuprofen administered alone, in most trials, and appeared to be more effective than a single dose of some other fixed-dose combination analgesics [28–31].

    - An FDC of the fast-acting NSAID, dexketoprofen trometamol, and the long-acting opioid, tramadol hydrochloride, have been recently developed to generate multimodal analgesia at lower and better tolerated doses than those of the single agents used alone. The different modes and sites of action of the two components, together with their complementary pharmacokinetic profiles, and the lower incidence of the typical side effects of each class [32–35] provides physicians with an effective and safe analgesic for the treatment of moderate-to-severe acute pain [36]. This FDC provides a comprehensive multimodal approach for moderate-to-severe acute pain, thanks to the central analgesic effect, peripheral analgesic action, and anti-inflammatory activity [21].

4. Multimodal analgesia: different combinations for different types of pain

Thanks to the possibility to minimize drug dosages optimizing efficacy, multimodal therapy is useful in various medical field, from acute pain management to post-trauma or postsurgical pain treatment, besides control of chronic pain and its exacerbations or reduction of pain associated with post-immobilization rehabilitation [19]. Each type of pain requires a specific analgesic therapy, which should also be personalized according to the patient's profile. The main applications of multimodal therapy to different pain conditions are the following.

4.1 Musculoskeletal pain (MP)

Given the multiplicity of mechanisms responsible for MP, the combination of analgesics with different mechanisms of action for the relief of acute and chronic skeletal muscle pain is often recommended, with the possible advantage of pharmacokinetic synergy and improved patient adherence.

The main pharmacological associations currently available for the treatment of MP are [19]:

- codeine 30 mg + paracetamol 500 mg,
- ibuprofen 150 mg + paracetamol 500 mg,
- codeine 30 mg + ibuprofen 400 mg,
- tramadol 37.5 mg + paracetamol 325 mg,
- tramadol 75 mg + dexketoprofen 25 mg, and
- oxycodone 5 mg (10 and 20 mg) + paracetamol 325 mg.

For all these combinations, careful monitoring must be performed in order to assess whether continuation of therapy, suspension, or transition to a strong opioid is necessary [19].

4.2 Osteoarthritis (OA) pain

Pain associated with rheumatologic conditions has a strong peripheral nociceptive component, although recent data also suggest a central sensitization [37]. Ideal treatment of rheumatic pain should be through a multimodal approach, integrating non-pharmacologic and pharmacologic treatments [38]. In the context of rheumatological painful conditions, the association of dexketoprofen and tramadol may represent an attractive medication for acute exacerbations of OA pain, due to its pharmacological profile: the combination of dexketoprofen and tramadol, targeting different sites of action, is suitable for OA type of pain, arising from different body structures (joints, muscles, ligaments, etc.) [21]. The rapid onset of analgesic effect of dexketoprofen, with its anti-inflammatory activity, associated to the sustained action of tramadol, makes their combination a valuable tool to achieve multimodal analgesia in OA patients [21].

4.3 Back pain

Back problems are the third reason for seeking medical help, with about 90% of people suffering from them at some point in their lives [39, 40]. Most episodes of back pain are short lasting with little or no consequence, but recurrent episodes are common and back pain is increasingly understood as a long-lasting condition with a variable course rather than episodes of unrelated occurrences [41]. The complexity of chronic back pain management highlights the need for early intervention in patients with acute back pain in order to prevent progression to chronic back pain [42]. Chronic low back pain has been shown to be secondary to both neuropathic and nociceptive pain mechanisms [43]: a multimodal approach is therefore appropriate. The pain treatment armamentarium for both acute and chronic back pain includes NSAIDs, opioids, steroids, topical medicines, and adjuvants: the choice of medication depends on a number of factors, including the duration of symptoms, severity of symptoms, expected benefits, prior response to medications, adverse effect profile, presence of comorbidities, costs, and degree of supporting evidence [44]. Most guidelines endorse (NSAIDs) and weak opioids for short periods when there is contraindication or lack of improvement with NSAIDs [45].

4.4 Fibromyalgia

Fibromyalgia is mainly a centralized pain disorder, accompanied by fatigue, sleep disturbance, and memory and mood difficulties [43]. Effective drugs combinations for this condition include tramadol + paracetamol [46], cyclobenzaprine + fluoxetine [47], pregabalin added to either quetiapine or trazodone [48], and fluoxetine + amitriptyline [49].

4.5 Postsurgical pain

Surgical pain may be nociceptive, neuropathic, mixed, psychogenic, or idiopathic, depending on the surgical procedure. The value of balanced analgesia in treating postoperative pain was recognized by Kehlet and Dahl [9] over two decades ago. Non-opioid analgesics are the cornerstone of postsurgical pain multimodal management: in addition to their opioid-sparing effects, many of these agents are highly effective in reducing postoperative pain and allowing for faster mobilization [50].

- Many current multimodal protocols include paracetamol [51–53], based on its opioid-sparing effects, despite the risk of GI, CV, and hepatic adverse events [25, 26].

- NSAIDs represent another class of medication that is highly effective for perioperative pain management: despite concerns about the increased risk of postoperative bleeding with NSAIDs, a meta-analysis revealed that ketorolac does not increase the risk of perioperative bleeding [54]. Nevertheless, this drug has shown several other side effects. Preoperative COX inhibitors (primarily selective COX-2 inhibitors) [55] and postoperative nonselective and selective NSAIDs [56] have been associated with reduced postoperative opioid consumption [57]. The combination of NSAIDs with opioids represents another tool to limit opioid use: in particular, the combination dexketoprofen/tramadol was shown to be superior vs. single components in terms of control of moderate-to-severe acute pain after abdominal hysterectomy [58] and total hip arthroplasty [59], with a safety profile fully in line with that previously known for the single agents in monotherapy. Recently, the analgesic efficacy of dexketoprofen/tramadol was compared in a head-to-head study (DAVID study) to that of tramadol/paracetamol combination in moderate-to-severe pain following surgical removal of impacted lower third molar, showing the greatest sustained analgesia during the 6-hour post dose period [60].

- Another class of analgesics commonly used in multimodal analgesic protocols is the gabapentinoids, which include gabapentin and pregabalin. Meta-analyses have demonstrated that gabapentin [61] and pregabalin [62] improve postoperative pain when part of a multimodal regimen but are associated with sedation, particularly in elderly patients.

- Other agents to consider in multimodal protocols include NMDA antagonists, such as ketamine. Ketamine has a clear opioid-sparing effect in the perioperative period [63] and may reduce long-term opioid consumption in opioid-tolerant patients [64] as well as persistent postsurgical pain when used intravenously [65].

- Multimodal and preemptive analgesia as part of an ERAS (Enhanced Recovery after Surgery) protocol facilitates early mobility and early return of bowel function and decreases postoperative morbidity [66].

4.6 Neuropathic pain

The International Association for the Study of Pain defines neuropathic pain as "Pain caused by a lesion or disease of the somatosensory system." This includes central disorders (e.g., spinal cord injury pain, multiple sclerosis pain, and post-stroke thalamic pain) as well as peripheral disorders (e.g., diabetic neuropathy and postherpetic neuralgia) [43].

Both tricyclic antidepressants and gabapentinoids are proposed as firstline agents for neuropathic pain [67]. These medications have completely different mechanisms of actions:

- gabapentinoids are alpha-2-delta calcium channel modulators;
- tricyclic antidepressants have multiple mechanisms of action, including norepinephrine and serotonin reuptake inhibition, and so are logical candidates for combination therapy.

Opioids and gabapentinoids were also studied for neuropathic pain and the combination was found to be positive [68–70]. However, given the limited trial size and the short duration of the studies conducted so far, it is not possible to make recommendations for any specific combination for neuropathic pain [43].

5. Conclusions

As illustrated above, in recent years, the WHO ladder approach has gradually been replaced with the multimodal approach, customized from patient to patient taking into account the characteristics of pain (based on pain generator, its cause, type, and intensity) and patient comorbidity. This allows to control not only chronic pain but also its exacerbations, through the association to long-term analgesic therapy of additional drugs for acute pain as needed. In this respect, multimodal therapy represents a useful tool, not only for specialists but for general practitioners as well to personalize analgesic treatment according to the patient's characteristics and needs [71].

The availability of FDCs of most recommended combinations may help in the implementation of multimodal analgesia in clinical practice, improving patient adherence to treatment and contributing to the optimization of pain management.

Acknowledgements

The authors are particularly grateful to ContentEdNet for the editorial support. Editing has also been supported by Paolo Procacci Foundation (Via Tacito 7, 00193 Roma, Italy).

Conflict of interest

The authors do not have any potential conflict of interest related to this chapter.

Author details

Antonella Paladini[1] and Giustino Varrassi[2,3]*

1 Department of MESVA, University of L'Aquila, L'Aquila, Italy

2 Paolo Procacci Foundation, Rome, Italy

3 World Institute of Pain, Winston-Salem, NC, USA

*Address all correspondence to: giuvarr@gmail.com

References

[1] Argoff CE, Albrecht P, Irving G, Rice F. Multimodal analgesia for chronic pain: Rationale and future directions. Pain Medicine. 2009;**10**(Suppl 2):S53-S66. DOI: 10.1111/j.1526-4637.2009.00669.x

[2] Raffa RB, Pergolizzi JV Jr, Tallarida RJ. The determination and application of fixed-dose analgesic combinations for treating multimodal pain. The Journal of Pain. 2010;**11**:701-709

[3] Manworren RC. Multimodal pain management and the future of a personalized medicine approach to pain. AORN Journal. 2015;**101**(3):308-318. DOI: 10.1016/j.aorn.2014.12.009

[4] Busse JW, Wang L, Kamaleldin M, et al. Opioids for chronic noncancer pain: A systematic review and meta-analysis. Journal of the American Medical Association. 2018;**320**(23):2448-2460. DOI: 10.1001/jama.2018.18472

[5] Breivik H, Gordh T, Butler S. Keeping an open mind: Achieving balance between too liberal and too restrictive prescription of opioids for chronic non-cancer pain: Using a two-edged sword. Scandinavian Journal of Pain. 2012;**3**(1):1-4. DOI: 10.1016/j.sjpain.2011.11.012

[6] Varrassi G, Müller-Schwefe G, Pergolizzi J, et al. Pharmacological treatment of chronic pain - The need for CHANGE. Current Medical Research and Opinion. 2010;**26**(5):1231-1245. DOI: 10.1185/03007991003689175

[7] O'Brien T, Christrup LL, Drewes AM, et al. European Pain Federation position paper on appropriate opioid use in chronic pain management. European Journal of Pain. 2017;**21**(1):3-19. DOI: 10.1002/ejp.970

[8] Breivik H, Eisenberg E, O'Brien T. The individual and societal burden of chronic pain in Europe: The case for strategic prioritisation and action to improve knowledge and availability of appropriate care. BMC Public Health. 2013;**13**:1229

[9] Kehlet H, Dahl JB. The value of "multimodal" or "balanced analgesia" in postoperative pain treatment. Anesthesia and Analgesia. 1993;**77**:1048-1056

[10] World Health Organization. Cancer Pain Relief with a Guide to Opioid Availability. 2nd ed. Geneva: World Health Organization; 1996

[11] Dworkin R, O'Connor AB, Backonja M, et al. Pharmacologic management of neuropathic pain: Evidence based recommendations. Pain. 2007;**132**:237-251

[12] Raffa RB, Tallarida RJ, Taylor R Jr, Pergolizzi JV Jr. Fixed-dose combinations for emerging treatment of pain. Expert Opinion on Pharmacotherapy. 2012;**13**(9):1261-1270

[13] Houde R, Wallenstein S, Beaven W. Clinical measurement of pain. In: De Stevens G, editor. Analgesics. New York, NY: Academic Press; 1965. pp. 75-122

[14] Varrassi G. Non-opioid drugs in the potentiation of postoperative analgesia [Farmaci non oppioidi nel potenziamento dell'analgesia postoperatoria]. In: Varrassi G, editor. Atti 11° Congresso Nazionale AISD. Napoli, Italy: Casa Editrice L'Antologia; 1988. pp. 53-70. Available from: https://www.researchgate.net/publication/313439665_Atti__XI_Congresso_Nazionale_AISD

[15] Schug SA, Zech D, Dorr U. Cancer pain management according to WHO

analgesic guidelines. Journal of Pain and Symptom Management. 1990;**5**:27-32

[16] Chou R, Gordon DB, de Leon-Casasola OA, et al. Management of postoperative pain: A clinical practice guideline from the American Pain Society, the American Society of Regional Anesthesia and Pain Medicine, and the American Society of Anesthesiologists' Committee on Regional Anesthesia, Executive Committee, and Administrative Council. The Journal of Pain. 2016;**17**:131-157

[17] Altman RD, Hochberg MC, Moskowitz RW, Schnitzer TJ. Recommendations for the medical management of osteoarthritis of the hip and knee: 2000 update. Arthritis and Rheumatism. 2000;**43**:1905-1915

[18] O'Brien J, Pergolizzi J, van de Laar M, et al. Fixed-dose combinations at the front line of multimodal pain management: Perspective of the nurse-prescriber. Nursing: Research and Review. 2013;**3**:9-22

[19] Gigliotti S et al. Management of musculoskeletal pain in the setting of territorial orthopedics. Minerva Ortopedica e Traumatologica. 2020;**71**(1):23-31

[20] Varrassi G, Alon E, Bagnasco M, et al. Towards an effective and safe treatment of inflammatory pain: A Delphi-guided expert consensus. Advances in Therapy. 2019;**36**(10):2618-2637. DOI: 10.1007/s12325-019-01053

[21] Varrassi G, Hanna M, Macheras G, et al. Multimodal analgesia in moderate-to-severe pain: A role for a new fixed combination of dexketoprofen and tramadol. Current Medical Research and Opinion. 2017;**33**(6):1165-1173. DOI: 10.1080/03007995.2017.1310092

[22] Chandanwale AS, Sundar S, Latchoumibady K, et al. Efficacy and safety profile of combination of tramadol-diclofenac versus tramadol- paracetamol in patients with acute musculoskeletal conditions, postoperative pain, and acute flare of osteoarthritis and rheumatoid arthritis: A phase III, 5-day open-label study. Journal of Pain Research. 2014;**7**:455-463

[23] da Costa BR, Reichenbach S, Keller N, et al. Effectiveness of nonsteroidal anti-inflammatory drugs for the treatment of pain in knee and hip osteoarthritis: A network meta-analysis. Lancet. 2016;**387**:2093-2105

[24] Machado GC, Maher CG, Ferreira PH, et al. Efficacy and safety of paracetamol for spinal pain and osteoarthritis: Systematic review and meta-analysis of randomised placebo controlled trials. BMJ (Clinical Research Edition). 2015;**350**:h1225

[25] Roberts E, Delgado Nunes V, Buckner S, et al. Paracetamol: Not as safe as we thought? A systematic literature review of observational studies. Annals of the Rheumatic Diseases. 2016;**75**:552-559

[26] Scarpignato C, Lanas A, Blandizzi C, et al. Safe prescribing of non-steroidal anti-inflammatory drugs in patients with osteoarthritis – An expert consensus addressing benefits as well as gastrointestinal and cardiovascular risks. BMC Medicine. 2015;**13**:55

[27] Varrassi G, Marinangeli F, Agro F, et al. A double-blinded evaluation of propacetamol versus ketorolac in combination with patient-controlled analgesia morphine: Analgesic efficacy and tolerability after gynecologic surgery. Anesthesia and Analgesia. 1999;**88**:611-616

[28] Kolesnikov YA, Wilson RS, Pasternak GW. The synergistic analgesic interactions between hydrocodone and

ibuprofen. Anesthesia and Analgesia. 2003;**97**:1721-1723

[29] Oldfield V, Perry CM. Oxycodone/ibuprofen combination tablet: A review of its use in the management of acute pain. Drugs. 2005;**65**:2337-2354

[30] Betancourt JW, Kupp LI, Jasper SJ, et al. Efficacy of ibuprofen hydrocodone for the treatment of postoperative pain after periodontal surgery. Journal of Periodontology. 2004;**75**:872-876

[31] Van Dyke T, Litkowski LJ, Kiersch TA, et al. Combination oxycodone 5 mg/ibuprofen 400mg for the treatment of postoperative+ pain: A double-blind, placebo- and active-controlled parallelgroup study. Clinical Therapeutics. 2004;**26**:2003-2014

[32] Rodriguez MJ, Arbos RM, Amaro SR. Dexketoprofen trometamol: Clinical evidence supporting its role as a painkiller. Expert Review of Neurotherapeutics. 2008;**8**:1625-1640

[33] Scott LJ, Perry CM. Tramadol: A review of its use in perioperative pain. Drugs. 2000;**60**:139-176

[34] Vazzana M, Andreani T, Fangueiro J, et al. Tramadol hydrochloride: Pharmacokinetics, pharmacodynamics, adverse side effects, co-administration of drugs and new drug delivery systems. Biomedicine & Pharmacotherapy. 2015;**70**:234-238

[35] Walczak JS. Analgesic properties of dexketoprofen trometamol. Pain Management. 2011;**1**:409-416

[36] Moore RA, Gay-Escoda C, Figueiredo R, et al. Dexketoprofen/tramadol: Randomised double-blind trial and confirmation of empirical theory of combination analgesics in acute pain. The Journal of Headache and Pain. 2015;**16**:541

[37] Meeus M, Vervisch S, De Clerck LS, et al. Central sensitization in patients with rheumatoid arthritis: A systematic literature review. Seminars in Arthritis and Rheumatism. 2012;**41**(4):556-567

[38] Fitzcharles MA et al. Management of chronic pain in the rheumatic diseases with insights for the clinician. Therapeutic Advances in Musculoskeletal Disease. 2011;**3**:179-190

[39] Sauver St JL et al. Why do patients visit their doctors? Assessing the most prevalent conditions in a define US population. Mayo Clinic Proceedings. 2013;**88**:56-67

[40] Nasser MJ. How to approach the problem of low back pain: An overview. Journal of Family and Community Medicine. 2005;**12**:3-9

[41] Hartvigsen J et al. What low back pain is and why we need to pay attention. Lancet. 2018;**391**:2356-2367

[42] Morlion B. Pharmacotherapy of low back pain: Targeting nociceptive and neuropathic pain components. Current Medical Research and Opinion. 2011;**27**:11-33

[43] Dale R, Stacey B. Multimodal treatment of chronic pain. The Medical Clinics of North America. 2016;**100**(1):55-64. DOI: 10.1016/j.mcna.2015.08.012

[44] Chou R. Pharmacological management of low back pain. Drugs. 2010;**70**:387-402

[45] Oliveira CB et al. Clinical practice guidelines for the management of non specific low back pain in primary care: An updated overview. European Spine Journal. 2018;**27**:2791-2803

[46] Bennett RM, Kamin M, Karim R, et al. Tramadol and acetaminophen combination tablets in the treatment of fibromyalgia pain: A double-blind,

randomized, placebo-controlled study. The American Journal of Medicine. 2003;**114**(7):537-545

[47] Cantini F, Bellandi F, Niccoli L, et al. Fluoxetine combined with cyclobenzaprine in the treatment of fibromyalgia. Minerva Medica. 1994;**85**(3):97-100. [in Italian]

[48] Calandre EP, Morillas-Arques P, Molina-Barea R, et al. Trazodone plus pregabalin combination in the treatment of fibromyalgia: A two-phase, 24-week, open-label uncontrolled study. BMC Musculoskeletal Disorders. 2011;**12**:95

[49] Goldenberg D, Mayskiy M, Mossey C, et al. A randomized, double-blind crossover trial of fluoxetine and amitriptyline in the treatment of fibromyalgia. Arthritis and Rheumatism. 1996;**39**(11):1852-1859

[50] Schwenk ES, Mariano ER. Designing the ideal perioperative pain management plan starts with multimodal analgesia. Korean Journal of Anesthesiology. 2018;**71**(5):345-352. DOI: 10.4097/kja.d.18.00217

[51] Wick CE, Grant MC, Wu CL. Postoperative multimodal analgesia pain management with nonopioid analgesics and techniques a review. JAMA Surgery. 2017;**152**(7):691-697. DOI: 10.1001/jamasurg.2017.0898

[52] Elia N, Lysakowski C, Tramèr MR. Does multimodal analgesia with acetaminophen, nonsteroidal antiinflammatory drugs, or selective cyclooxygenase-2 inhibitors and patient-controlled analgesia morphine offer advantages over morphine alone? Meta-analyses of randomized trials. Anesthesiology. 2005;**103**:1296-1304

[53] Hebl JR, Dilger JA, Byer DE, Kopp SL, Stevens SR, Pagnano MW, et al. A pre-emptive multimodal pathway featuring peripheral nerve block improves perioperative outcomes after major orthopedic surgery. Regional Anesthesia and Pain Medicine. 2008;**33**:510-517

[54] Gobble RM, Hoang HL, Kachniarz B, Orgill DP. Ketorolac does not increase perioperative bleeding: A meta-analysis of randomized controlled trials. Plastic and Reconstructive Surgery. 2014;**133**:741-755

[55] Nir RR et al. Preoperative preemptive drug administration for acute postoperative pain: A systematic review and metaanalysis. European Journal of Pain. 2016;**20**(7):1025-1043

[56] Maund E et al. Paracetamol and selective and non-selective non-steroidal anti-inflammatory drugs for the reduction in morphine-related side-effects after major surgery: A systematic review. British Journal of Anaesthesia. 2011;**106**(3):292-297

[57] Polomano RC, Fillman M, Giordano NA, Vallerand AH, Nicely KL, Jungquist CR. Multimodal analgesia for acute postoperative and trauma-related pain. The American Journal of Nursing. 2017;**117**(3 Suppl 1):S12-S26. DOI: 10.1097/01.NAJ.0000513527.71934.73

[58] Moore RA et al. Dexketoprofen/tramadol 25 mg/75 mg: Randomised double-blind trial in moderate-to-severe acute pain after abdominal hysterectomy. BMC Anesthesiology. 2016;**16**:9

[59] McQuay HJ et al. Randomized clinical trial of dexketoprofen/tramadol 25mg/75mg in moderate-to-severe pain after total hip arthroplasty. British Journal of Anaesthesia. 2016;**116**:269-276

[60] Gay-Escoda C et al. Tramadol/dexketoprofen (TRAM/DKP) compared with tramadol/paracetamol in moderate to severe acute pain: Results of a randomised, double-blind, placebo and active-controlled, parallel group trial

in the impacted third molar extraction pain model (DAVID study). BMJ Open. 2019;**9**:e023715

[61] Hurley RW, Cohen SP, Williams KA, Rowlingson AJ, Wu CL. The analgesic effects of perioperative gabapentin on postoperative pain: A meta-analysis. Regional Anesthesia and Pain Medicine. 2006;**31**:237-247

[62] Dong J, Li W, Wang Y. The effect of pregabalin on acute postoperative pain in patients undergoing total knee arthroplasty: A meta-analysis. International Journal of Surgery. 2016;**34**:148-160

[63] Laskowski K, Stirling A, McKay WP, Lim HJ. A systematic review of intravenous ketamine for postoperative analgesia. Canadian Journal of Anaesthesia. 2011;**58**:911-923

[64] Loftus RW, Yeager MP, Clark JA, Brown JR, Abdu WA, Sengupta DK, et al. Intraoperative ketamine reduces perioperative opiate consumption in opiate-dependent patients with chronic back pain undergoing back surgery. Anesthesiology. 2010;**113**:639-646

[65] McNicol ED, Schumann R, Haroutounian S. A systematic review and meta-analysis of ketamine for the prevention of persistent postsurgical pain. Acta Anaesthesiologica Scandinavica. 2014;**58**:1199-1213

[66] Simpson JC, Bao X, Agarwala A. Pain management in enhanced recovery after surgery (ERAS) protocols. Clinics in Colon and Rectal Surgery. 2019;**32**(2):121-128. DOI: 10.1055/s-0038-1676477

[67] Dworkin RH, O'Connor AB, Audette J, et al. Recommendations for the pharmacological management of neuropathic pain: An overview and literature update. Mayo Clinic Proceedings. 2010;**85**(3 Suppl):S3-S14

[68] Gatti A, Sabato AF, Occhioni R, et al. Controlled-release oxycodone and pregabalin in the treatment of neuropathic pain: Results of a multicenter Italian study. European Neurology. 2009;**61**(3):129-137

[69] Gilron I, Bailey JM, Tu D, et al. Morphine, gabapentin, or their combination for neuropathic pain. The New England Journal of Medicine. 2005;**352**(13):1324-1334

[70] Hanna M, O'Brien C, Wilson MC. Prolonged-release oxycodone enhances the effects of existing gabapentin therapy in painful diabetic neuropathy patients. European Journal of Pain. 2008;**12**(6):804-813

[71] Varrassi G, Yeam CT, Rekatsina M, Pergolizzi JV, Zis P, Paladini A. The expanding role of COX inhibitor/opioid receptor agonist combination in the management of pain. Drugs. 04 August 2020. DOI: 10.1007/s40265-020-01369-x

Chapter 13

The Role of Cupping Therapy in Pain Management: A Literature Review

Asma Al-Shidhani and Abdulaziz Al-Mahrezi

Abstract

Cupping therapy is an ancient method which has been used for centuries for various painful conditions. It is performed by applying cups to selected skin points most commonly in the back aiming to create areas of sub-atmospheric pressure. It has been classified as either dry or wet type of therapy. Its mechanism of action is not well understood but several proposed mechanisms are described in the literature. It is relatively safe with a few reported side effects which include scar formation and skin infection. In this paper, a review of the literature will be presented to determine its potential benefits in pain management particularly in musculoskeletal conditions such as low back and neck pain.

Keywords: cupping therapy, chronic pain, complimentary therapies, low back pain, pain management

1. Introduction

Cupping therapy is one of the oldest methods of complimentary therapies which has been used in early human civilization. Evidence shows that it was first practiced by the Ancient Egyptians more than 5500 years ago and then it was introduced to the Greek, the Romans, and the rest of the world [1]. The main postulated aim of this therapy is the extraction of harmful substances or toxins from the body by creating negative pressure in a cup [2]. Cupping was described by Razi as a process in which blood from superficial small vessels located in muscles is released [3]. It has been traditionally used for the treatment of painful conditions but has also been used to treat chronic diseases such as cardiovascular disorders, skin diseases, inflammatory disorders, and metabolic diseases [4, 5]. Its exact mechanism of action is not well-understood but several theories have been proposed [6].

2. Description of cupping therapy

Cupping therapy is done by applying small round cups which are made of glass, bamboo, ceramic or plastic to the area of pain. The cup has a rolled rim to ensure tight contact with skin to preserve the negative pressure created [7]. The mouth of the cup is placed firmly over the preferred location against the skin. The negative pressure is generated by heat or by other vacuums like manual pumps. This negative pressure fixes the cup onto the skin and creates suction effect which pulls the skin upwards into the cup. Sometimes, the therapist uses lubricants to facilitate the movement of the cups to cover a wider area [8]. The common application sites are the back, chest, abdomen, buttock, and areas of abundant muscle. Traditionally, the cupping therapy is done in sets of four, six or ten [9]. The cups are usually kept in place for 5 to 20 minutes [6]. The common side-effects of cupping therapy are erythema, edema, and ecchymosis in the area where the cup rim was placed. These effects may take several days to weeks to disappear [4, 10]. The cupping therapy process usually consists of the following five main steps:

1. The therapist assigns and disinfects the designated area for cupping therapy.

2. A suitable sized cup is positioned on the selected area and the therapist uses a method of suction to suck the air inside the cup. The cup will be left on the skin for 3–5 minutes. If it is wet cupping, then superficial incisions are performed on the skin by a scalpel blade (No. 15 to 21) or by puncturing the skin with a needle, or an auto-lancing device or a plum-blossom needle [11].

3. The cup is placed again on the skin for 3–5 minutes.

4. The cup is removed.

5. The treated area is cleaned, disinfected, and a dressing is applied. The dressing is usually kept for 48 hours following the session of therapy [6].

3. Mechanism of action

While the exact mechanism of action of cupping therapy is not well-understood, multiple theories have been proposed. Six mechanisms of action have been suggested to describe the various effects of cupping therapy. Three of these theories are addressing the biological and mechanical basis of pain relief which results from cupping therapy. These theories are as follows: the pain-gate, the conditioned pain modulation, and the reflex zone. The remaining three proposed mechanisms of action are meant to explain the beneficial effects of cupping therapy which include an increase in blood circulation, immunomodulatory effects, and the removal of toxins and wastes [6]. The former three theories which are related to pain relief will only be discussed here.

3.1 Pain-gate theory

This theory proposes that cupping therapy could reduce pain intensity by influencing the communication routes of pain transmission from a stimulated area to the brain and backward [4]. Following a painful stimulus, pain signals are carried by both the small-diameter (A-delta and C) and the large-diameter (A-beta) nociceptive nerve fibers to synapse into a transmission cell in the dorsal horn of the spinal cord [12]. In this area pain modulation takes place through a network of interneurons and presynaptic pain gates [13]. The small fibers have an obstructive effect on the inhibitory cells thus allowing the flow of the transmission signals to the spino-thalamo-cortical pain pathway and then to the brain. While the large fibers stimulate the inhibitory cells and tend to inhibit transmission of pain signals. Thus, pain intensity is expected to be reduced when large nerve fibers are stimulated by touch or pressure or vibration. Based on this theory, both small and large nerve fibers are stimulated during cupping therapy [14]. During the initial stage of cupping therapy, the afferent large nerve fibers will partially close the presynaptic gate as a result of the application of pressure to the skin [13]. As the stimulus intensity is increased, the number of activated units of nerve fiber increases. The subsequent positive and negative effects of the small and large nerve fibers responses tend to counteract each other. However, prolonged stimulation will lead to adaptation of the large fibers which will eventually result in opening of the presynaptic pain gates [13]. This adaptation can be modulated by employing additional stimuli during cupping therapy such as vibration and scratching to stimulate the large fibers again [15]. This increased activity will lead to the closure of the pain gates and experiencing further pain relief [15]. More research is needed to validate the application of this theory in cupping therapy.

3.2 Conditioned pain modulation

This theory has been also known by the term "Diffuse Noxious Inhibitory Controls (DNICs)." It is based on the assumption that "pain inhibits pain," or one type of pain masks another [16]. DNIC comprises a spinal-medullary-spinal pathway that is activated when two concomitant painful stimuli are applied at the same time [16]. The activation of this pain pathway, which is triggered by a distant noxious stimulus, causes inhibition of the primary pain at the level of the nociceptive spinal neurons [16]. This pain inhibitory system has been successfully demonstrated in animal studies [17]. Furthermore, findings from clinical studies on the idiopathic pain syndromes such as irritable bowel syndrome, temporomandibular disorders, fibromyalgia, and tension-type headache had confirmed the relevance of this theory to chronic pain in humans [16]. According to this theory, local vibration or scratching done during cupping therapy causes a nociceptive stimulus that triggers the activation of DNICs which eventually lead to the relief of the primary pain [6].

3.3 Reflex zone theory

Reflex Zone Theory proposes that there is an existing link between one organ of the body and another one. This link is mediated by interaction between nerves, chemicals, and muscles [18]. Thus, a disturbance in one organ causes external manifestations which can be detected at a site distal to the disturbed organ. The external manifestations are dependent on the organ manifesting them. For example, skin can become cold and pale due to vasoconstriction or it can become warm and red due to vasodilatation. The organ functions are affected due to a reduction in the circulating blood and tissue fluids [19]. Animal studies showed that somatic stimulation of the skin or the peripheral joints could lead to significant effects on the cardiovascular, urinary, and gastrointestinal functions [20]. These reflexes can be either excitatory or inhibitory in terms of organ function. Their main action is attained through spinal pathways, supra-spinal and cortical centers [20]. Therefore, it is hypothesized that the application of the cupping therapy cups over the skin result in the stimulation of the skin receptors which will eventually lead to an improvement in the blood circulation through the neural connections to the affected organ [21].

4. Classification of cupping therapy

Cupping was broadly classified into dry and wet cupping, but in 2016 Al-Bedah *et al* introduced a new classification which consisted of six categories, namely, technical types, power of suction, method of suction, materials inside cups, area treated, and other cupping types [22]. Aboushanab *et al* made additional modifications of these categories to become as follows [23]:

4.1 Technical types

This category of cupping is classified according to the cupping technique which is used. It includes four types; dry cupping, flash cupping, wet cupping and massage cupping [22].

4.1.1 Dry cupping

Dry cupping is also known as static cupping or retained cupping [24]. In dry cupping, negative pressure is generated inside the cups by different ways of suction like fire, manual pump or electrical suction. The cups are usually kept on the skin for up to 15 minutes [22]. When a manual pump is used, the pressure inside the cup is controlled by the number of suctions. As the number increases, the negative pressure inside the cup will increase [2]. Similarly, when fire is used, prolongation of fire exposure will increase the negative pressure inside the cup. This negative pressure leads to protrusion of the skin [22].

4.1.2 Flash cupping

Flash cupping is also known as empty cupping [24]. It involves performing quick suctions of medium to light pressure over the targeted area. The cup is applied for a very short time of less than 30 seconds to stimulate the area. It can be done by using only one cup or four medium-sized cups. This method can be used in situations where dry cupping is not recommended. For example, in young people and females [22].

4.1.3 Wet cupping

Wet cupping is also known as full cupping, bloodletting cupping, and bleeding cupping. It is commonly used in traditional medicine [24]. It involves scraping of the skin by a surgical instrument before applying the cups to suck the blood. The main side-effects of this method include higher risk of infection, vasovagal attacks, and scars development [22].

4.1.4 Massage cupping

Massage cupping is also known as moving cupping, dynamic cupping, and gliding cupping [2]. It is performed by applying oil over the skin and moving the cups over the treated area by using weak suction. Different types of oils are used such as olive oil, peppermint oil, and lavender oil. This type of cupping can be used for both young and elderly people [22]. **Figure 1** contains images of the four technical types.

4.2 Power of suction

This category of cupping is classified according to the negative pressure level created inside the cups. The pressure levels used are light, medium, strong or pulsatile pressure [22].

4.2.1 Light cupping pressure

Light cupping pressure is defined as a pressure level between 100 and less than 300 millibar (mb). The therapist generates weak suctions in the cup using one to two full manual pump suctions [2, 25]. It is mainly used for children, elderly patients, and for sensitive body parts like the face. Light cupping pressure can be used in conjunction with massage, dry, and flash cupping techniques. Its main

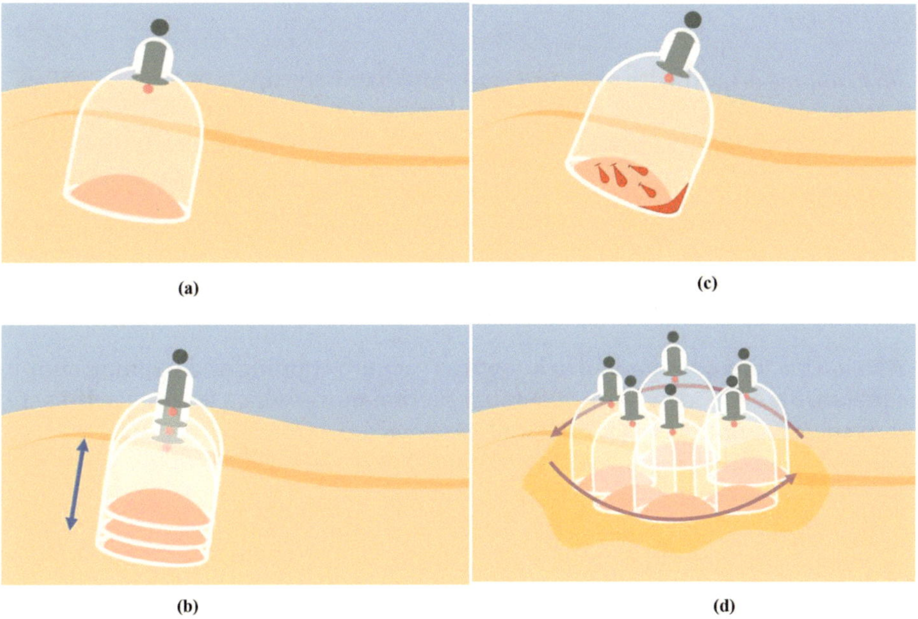

Figure 1.
Images representing the four technical types of cupping; (a) dry cupping, (b) flash cupping, (c) wet cupping, (d) massage cuppin.

advantage that it leaves most patients with no cupping marks. However, because of the light pressure, the cup tends to fall during the therapy session [22].

4.2.2 Medium cupping pressure

Medium cupping pressure is used for common purpose cupping [25]. The pressure level used is between 300 and less than 500 mb. It is created by 3–4 full manual pump suctions. Unlike light cupping, medium cupping can leave cupping marks over the body parts. It is not recommended for use over sensitive body areas such as the face [22].

4.2.3 Strong cupping pressure

Strong cupping pressure involves using a pressure level of above 500 mb [2]. It is usually generated by 5 or more full manual pump suctions. It is not recommended for children and elderly people. It can cause inflammation, dermatitis, skin burns, and pain [22].

4.2.4 Pulsatile cupping

Pulsatile cupping is when variable pulses of pressure are used. It is created by a mechanical device. One pulse is generated every 2 seconds. Therapists might use flexible silicone and plastic cups. The generated pressure level is usually between 100 and 200 mb. Its use has been limited to symptomatic pain relief in patients with knee osteoarthritis [26].

4.3 Methods of suction

The classification here is based on the method used to create the negative pressure inside the cups. These are as follows:

4.3.1 Fire cupping

Fire cupping is used with glass, ceramic, and bamboo cups that have no valves as the valve is used to control the air flow through the cup. Traditionally in China, a piece of paper or cotton is used either alighted and inserted into the cup directly, or soaked with 95% alcohol and attached to the end of a stick and then burned. The burning stick is used to make the cup hot and is removed later. This method is associated with a risk of burn [1, 22].

4.3.2 Manual vacuum cupping

Manual vacuum cupping is also known as vacuum cupping and opening cupping. The pressure is created by using a manual suction pump which is either self-suction cups or squeeze rubber top [1, 27]. Studies showed that manual vacuum cupping is superior to fire cupping in terms of causing greater blood flow to the treated area [1].

4.3.3 Electrical vacuum cupping

Electrical vacuum cupping is an electrical suction pump. It is used where the negative pressure can be easily adjusted and can be connected to several cups at the same time. Moreover, it is also used with pulsatile cupping because of its ability to generate pressure pulses [27].

4.4 Added therapy types:

This classification is done according to the additional material used in combination with the cups. It includes the following types [22, 23]:

4.4.1 Needle cupping

Needle cupping involves the combined use of acupuncture and cupping. Therapists usually apply acupuncture needles first followed by cupping therapy [27]. In this type, it is crucial to use small short needles and avoid specific body areas such as the abdomen and the chest to avoid any risk of organ penetration [22].

4.4.2 Hot cupping or Moxa cupping

Hot cupping or Moxa cupping is cupping combined with heat and a herb called Moxa [28]. Moxa is made up of dried Mugwort leaves. During the cupping process, the therapist will initially warm a needle with Moxa and applies a cup over it. A thin aluminum layer is used as a barrier before putting the hot Moxa to prevent skin burns [22].

4.4.3 Herbal cupping

Herbal cupping is also known as medicinal cupping. In this type, the therapist will boil a herbal solution for about 30 minutes and then bamboo cups will be soaked in the solution for five minutes before applying the cups to the skin [29]. To avoid skin burns, the cups will be left for one minute to cool down before applying them to the treated area [22].

Magnetic cupping is done by using magnetic cupping sets which have magnets inside. It is commonly used to treat joint-related diseases affecting big joints such as knees and elbows. It is presumed that the electromagnetic stimulation enhances the therapeutic effectiveness of cupping [30].

4.4.4 Laser cupping

Laser cupping is a new cupping device which is used in combination with cupping therapy. An acupuncture laser probe is inserted inside the cups in order to stimulate specific acupuncture points as an additive effect to the cupping. The advantage of this method is that it provides the 'double effect' of both cupping therapy and laser acupuncture [31].

4.4.5 Electric stimulation cupping

Electric stimulation cupping uses transcutaneous electrical nerve stimulation (TENS) with cupping. It has also a dual effect like laser cupping therapy as both electric and cupping stimulate the treated area. It is mainly used for the stimulation of specific points and in cases of muscular pain [30].

4.4.6 Water cupping

Water cupping is done with cups containing warm water. The therapist will fill a third of a cup with warm water and then a burning cotton wool will be inserted into the cup prior to placing the cup over the skin [11].

4.4.7 Aquatic cupping

Aquatic cupping is a combination of cupping therapy with aquatic therapy where the cupping is performed underwater since it is presumed that muscles can be stretched more underwater [32]. It is commonly used for rehabilitation, and musculoskeletal problems [32].

5. Common clinical indications for cupping therapy

5.1 Low back pain

Low back pain (LBP) is a common clinical problem which has an estimated one-year prevalence of 38% in the general population [33]. The current management options include bed rest during the acute phase, analgesia, physiotherapy, traction, alternative treatments, and health education on prevention of future episodes [34]. Cupping therapy has been used for a long time for both acute and chronic low back pain. Studies have shown significant reduction in pain intensity scores and improvement in functional outcome tools with cupping compared to other modalities of treatment like usual care or medications [34, 35]. Wang *et al* conducted a meta-analysis of six randomized controlled trials (RCTs). The total number of participants was 458 (230 received cupping *versus* 228 who received usual care). Five RCTs included patients with non-specific low back pain and a single RCT included post-partum women with low back pain. Different types of cupping were used in these trials (3 dry cupping, 2 wet cupping, 1 moving cupping). Pain was measured by different tools (1 visual analogue scale (VAS), 2 VAS + Oswestry pain disability index (ODI), 2 the McGill pain index (MPPI) + ODI, 1 VAS + MPPI). The meta-analysis concluded that cupping therapy was more effective compared to other modalities on reducing the VAS scores, and ODI scores. However, this positive effect was not captured on the MPPI.

Teut *et al* conducted a three-armed RCT in patients with chronic LBP to investigate the effectiveness of two different forms of cupping (dry pulsatile and minimal) compared to medication (paracetamol) on demand alone. A total of 110 subjects were enrolled in the study. Both forms of cupping were found to be effective compared to the control group after 4 weeks of therapy based on VAS scores. After 12 weeks, subjects who were in the pulsatile cupping group only reported beneficial effects as documented by the VAS scores and the physical component scale of the health quality of life short-form questionnaire (SF-36) [36]. Most of the studies which included patients with LBP investigated the short-term effects of cupping and were conducted for 2 to 12 weeks only [34, 37]. In addition, all of these studies suffered from major limitations which included high heterogeneity, small sample size, different inclusion criteria, different assessment tools, different types of cupping therapy, and different number of treatment sessions. Despite these limitations, the available literature supports the use of cupping therapy in patients with LBP but high-quality randomized clinical trials of longer duration and utilizing standardized assessment tools are needed to confirm these short-term beneficial effects.

5.2 Neck pain

The lifelong prevalence of neck pain varies from 14.2% to 71% and it is more dominant in the high activity age groups, mainly individuals aged 35 to 49 years [38]. It was found to be associated with increased medical costs and adverse effects on personal productivity [39]. The commonly used therapies for neck pain include the use of analgesics and physiotherapy. In addition, surgery might be of help in some specific situations. However, these options are not always effective, and sometimes are associated with serious side-effects. Therefore, people have been always looking for other alternative options which include traditional medicine [40]. Cupping is one of the methods used commonly by people to relieve neck pain especially for the non-specific types. Studies conducted in patients with this condition investigated the effectiveness of cupping by measuring the following outcomes: pain intensity, disability scores, and quality of life [41]. The current available evidence indicates that cupping is effective for patients with chronic non-specific neck pain in terms of reduction in pain scores, improvement in disability scores, and quality of life indices compared to no treatment or active controls (physical therapy, non-steroidal anti-inflammatory drugs (NSAIDs), heat pack therapy, and acupuncture) [41]. Kim *et al* conducted a systematic review and meta-analysis which included 18 studies, out of which 7 studies used wet cupping while 11 studies used dry cupping as an intervention [41]. The number of subjects in each study ranged between 40 to 240 [41]. The subjects in the cupping group were reported to have significant reduction in pain scores, and significant improvement in terms of function and quality of life compared with no intervention or active control groups [41]. Leem *et al* studied the effects of cupping in patients with chronic neck pain for up to 2 years and reported sustainable positive effects on physical function and quality of life for the whole period of time unlike the effects on pain intensity which were not maintained [42]. In conclusion, the current evidence supports the use of cupping therapy to treat neck pain but it is not conclusive because of the low quality of available studies. Future better designed studies are required to confirm the beneficial effects of cupping in this group of patients.

5.3 Arthritis

Arthritis is a commonly seen clinical problem in medical practice. It is a manifestation of many joint disorders like osteoarthritis, gout, rheumatoid arthritis and others. Cupping therapy has been used to reduce the joint pain associated with osteoarthritis (OA), gout and ankylosing spondylitis. OA is a common chronic degenerative joint disease. The commonly affected joints are knees, hips and shoulders. It may present with pain, stiffness, and decreased mobility due to the effects on joint function and stability [43]. Li J *et al* concluded that the use of a combination of cupping therapy and Western medicine (physical therapy and use of analgesics) is more effective compared to Western medicine alone in patients with knee OA in terms of pain and stiffness reduction and improvement in physical function domains of Western Ontario and McMaster Universities Osteoarthritis Index (WOMAC) [44]. Yet, the use of cupping therapy alone compared to Western medicine therapy was not superior in decreasing pain intensity [44].

Gout is an inflammatory arthritis which results from deposition of monosodium urate crystals in the joint space. It typically presents with painful joint inflammation, mainly in the first metatarsophalangeal joint [45]. A single study which was conducted in China investigated the combined effects of cupping and herbal medicine in comparison to the use of NSAIDs in acute gouty arthritis. The investigators reported that the therapeutic effects of both cupping and herbal medicine were comparable to NSAIDs but the differences were not statistically significant [46].

Ankylosing spondylitis (AS) is a chronic inflammatory disorder which causes chronic back pain. The common presenting symptoms are back pain and stiffness due to spinal fusion and ankylosis [47]. Ma *et al* conducted a systematic review and meta-analysis which included 5 RCTs, each with a sample size for each trial ranging from 42 to 280. Most of these trials were of low methodological quality [48]. It was concluded that the use of a combination therapy of cupping and Western medicine was more effective compared to Western medicine alone in terms of pain and stiffness reduction, improvement in physical function, disease activity, and serum levels of inflammatory markers (ESR and CRP) [48].

In conclusion, there is a weak evidence which supports the use of cupping therapy for pain management in different types of arthritis. Further research is required with better designed clinical trials to overcome the methodological problems, and the risk of bias with the present studies.

5.4 Post-herpetic neuralgia

Post-Herpetic Neuralgia (PHN) is a persistent neuropathic type of pain which develops as a complication of herpes zoster infection. It may occur in 20% of herpes zoster patients and it can persist for 90 days after the acute phase of the rash [49]. The aim of the treatment of PHN is to control the pain by using topical and systemic drugs like topical lidocaine or capsaicin and oral gabapentin, pregabalin, or tricyclic anti-depressants [50]. Cao *et al* conducted a systematic review of RCTs to evaluate the effects of wet cupping therapy in patients with PHN. Wet cupping therapy was found to be significantly better than medications, on rash healing (RR 2.49, 95%CI 1.91 to 3.24, $p < 0.00001$), pain reduction (RR 1.15, 95%CI 1.05 to 1.26, $p = 0.003$) and reduction in the incidence rate of post-herpetic neuralgia (RR 0.06, 95%CI 0.02 to 0.25, $p = 0.0001$) [51]. Tian *et al* reported that the use of wet cupping was significantly superior to pregabalin in terms of reduction in pain and reduction in peripheral and local serum substance P level [52]. A study by Wu *et al* found that the use of wet cupping was significantly more effective than herbal thermal compressing therapy and vitamin B12 intra-muscular injections in relieving the PHN pain [53]. Findings from these studies should be taken with caution because of the major limitations which included small sample size, methodological issues, and possibility of publication bias since all of the studies were conducted in a single country [51]. Further research with better designed studies and longer follow-up periods is warranted.

5.5 Carpel tunnel syndrome

Carpal tunnel syndrome (CTS) is a peripheral nerve entrapment due to the compression of the median nerve in the carpal tunnel of the wrist joint. It usually manifests as numbness and burning pain in the palm and the first three fingers (sensory involvement), and reduction in the grip strength (motor involvement) [54]. The beneficial effects of cupping therapy were observed when used in combination with physiotherapy or alone. Mohammadi *et al* studied the effects of cupping in combination with physiotherapy compared to physiotherapy alone on CTS patients. Modified cups were used in this study to accommodate the anatomical shape of the wrist joint. The pressure level used during the treatment sessions was 50 mmHg and the cups were applied for 4 minutes. A total of 10 sessions were done and the effects were assessed after completion of all the sessions. Four CTS-related parameters were measured: symptom severity, functional status, distal sensory latency, and distal motor latency. The study concluded that there was a significant improvement in the symptom severity scale and reduction in the distal sensory latency in the cupping group compared to the control group. In addition, subjects in the cupping group had an improvement in the functional status scale and reduction in the distal motor latency but the differences were not statistically significant. The limitations of the study included the lack of regular time intervals to assess the effects, and the uneven distribution of patients with severe disease between the two arms of the study [55]. Furthermore, two case reports had documented the beneficial effects of cupping in CTS patients [56, 57]. The first case report used wet cupping and reported profound reduction in pain, numbness and paresthesia. These clinical findings were confirmed by significant improvement in the electrophysiological measures as demonstrated by both nerve conduction velocity and electromyography [56]. The second case report used self-applied cupping at least once daily for 3 to 5 minutes for a period of 3 months in a patient with mild CTS symptoms. The patient reported an improvement in the symptoms after 1 week of treatment and complete resolution of all symptoms after 6–8 weeks. The nerve conduction study showed that median distal latency had returned back to the normal range after 3 months [57].

5.6 Fibromyalgia

Fibromyalgia is a disorder characterized by chronic generalized pain, fatigue, cognitive disturbances, sleep disorder, and pronounced somatic and psychological distress [58]. The main aim of treatment for fibromyalgia patients is to relieve pain and to improve the patients' quality of life [59]. Few studies were conducted to investigate the effects of cupping in fibromyalgia. Lauche *at al* reported that cupping therapy was more effective than usual care in patients diagnosed with the fibromyalgia syndrome after 18 days from treatment in terms of reduction in pain intensity and improvement in quality of life [60]. Moreover, the other studies were conducted to evaluate the effectiveness of a combination therapy of cupping and acupuncture together with conventional medications (anti-depressants) compared to medications alone [61, 62]. A total of 242 patients were included in both studies. Significant reduction in pain scores (MD −1.65, 95%CI −2.10 to −1.31, $P < 0.00001$) were reported in the combination group compared to the control group [29]. Further research with better quality studies is needed to determine the effectiveness of cupping in this group of patients.

6. Contraindications

Cupping therapy is a process where suction with or without scarification is done as a treatment for different types of pain and medical problems. Direct application of cupping on specific sites of the body is contraindicated as the negative pressure created during cupping therapy might be harmful [23]. These sites are veins, arteries, nerves, inflamed and injured skin, body orifices, eyes, lymph nodes, varicose veins, bone fractures, and sites of deep vein thrombosis [23]. Ahmedi et *al* classified the contraindications into absolute, relative and with cautions [5]. The contraindications are summarized in **Table 1**.

7. Infection control measures

Prevention of infection by following strict infection control measures is an essential aspect of clinical care. In cupping therapy, such measures are of paramount importance since the therapy necessitates direct contact with the skin and body fluids. Several infection control measures should be considered. These measures include hand hygiene and washing, and wearing personal protective equipment like gloves, masks, protective eyewear and gowns. Disinfection of the patient's skin with approved disinfectants is required before starting the procedure. Also, disinfection of the patient's bed or use of disposable bed covers is needed. It is recommended to use disposable cups, vacuum pumps, and surgical blades to avoid cross-transmission of infection. Lastly, adhering to proper medical waste segregation system is crucial [63, 64].

Absolute contraindication	Relative contraindication	Caution
Cancer	Acute infection	Active psoriasis
Organ failure (heart, renal, hepatic)	Severe chronic disease (e.g. heart disease)	Keloid scars
Patients using pacemaker	Pregnancy, puerperium	Children
Bleeding disorders like hemophilia	Anti-coagulant therapy	Anti-platelet therapy
Active cellulitis/erysipelas/abscess	Recent wet cupping session or recent blood donation	Peripheral vascular disease
Undiagnosed/suspicious lump	Menstruation	Anemia
Ulcer	Recent wet cupping session or recent blood donation	
Thrombophlebitis	Medical emergencies	
Deep vein thrombosis		
Cauda equina		
Stroke — unstable or evolving		
Fracture site		
Suspected osteomyelitis or septic arthritis		
Life threatening asthma		
Chemotherapy		

Table 1.
Contraindications to cupping therapy (adapted from Ahmedi et al *[5]).*

8. Complications of cupping

Cupping therapy is generally considered as a safe treatment with minor side-effects and complications [23, 65]. However, the safety of cupping therapy is under-reported. Most of the studies which were conducted primarily addressed its efficacy but only a few studies reported its complications. Generally, the complications can be divided into preventable and non-preventable [23]. The commonly recognized side-effects are erythema, edema, and ecchymosis which are directly caused by cupping. Skin burns have also been reported [65]. They may occur because of the following reasons: excessive use of alcohol, prolonged exposure to cupping therapy, sensitive skin especially in elderly people, and the use of fire [23, 65]. Separation of the epidermal layer from the dermal base of the skin may occur due to prolonged exposure of more than 20 minutes to high vacuum pressure during cupping therapy. This complication was specifically reported with pumping cupping therapy [23]. In one case report, application of cupping therapy for about 40 minutes over the lower back resulted in severe pain immediately after removal of the cups and the patient developed bullae and crusting over the application site later [66]. Change in atmospheric pressure has been reported as a risk factor for skin injury as seen in a patient who was traveling in an airplane. This resulted in multiple blisters and shades of redness, petechiae, and ecchymosis [67]. Exposure to blood-borne infections may occur if infection control measures are not followed strictly. For example, cases of factitial panniculitis and herpes simplex virus infection have been reported after cupping therapy [68, 69]. Possible complications of cupping therapy are summarized in **Figure 2**.

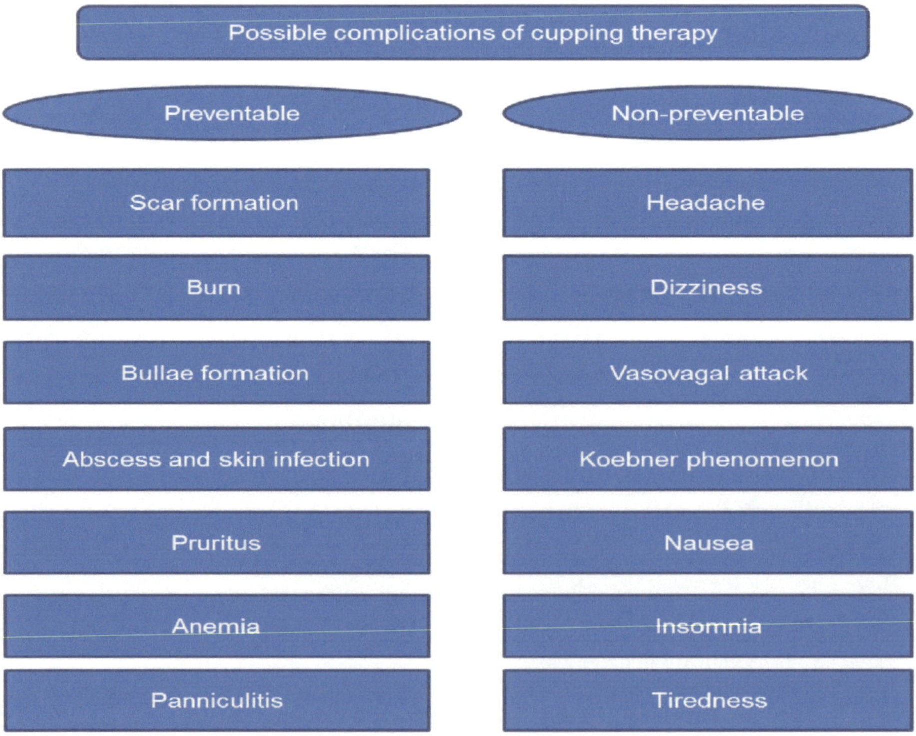

Figure 2.
Possible complications of cupping therapy (adapted from Aboushanab et al *[23]).*

9. Future directions

Cupping therapy is a complimentary type of therapy which is widely used all over the world for the treatment of chronic medical problems, especially for pain-related conditions. Although, there are several proposed theories which attempt to explain its mechanism of action in the management of chronic pain, the exact mechanism is still not clearly understood. Future research could focus on trying to find clear answers for the most likely mechanism of action and to validate the current theories in clinical trials. There is an emerging evidence of the promising benefits of cupping therapy in patients with common chronic painful conditions. However, despite the large number of clinical trials which were conducted, the evidence is still inconclusive due to major limitations. Future clinical trials of good quality are required. Such trials should ideally have a large sample size, better methodology and design, standardized treatment and reporting protocols, standardized assessment tools, and long follow-up periods.

10. Conclusions

Cupping therapy is an ancient complementary medicine practice which has been used for thousands of years for a variety of common medical problems. The current evidence is suggesting that cupping therapy may be effective in treating common chronic painful conditions for a short period. Yet, most of available studies have major limitations like small sample size, and different outcome assessment tools, duration of treatment, and treatment regimens. Publication bias is another important drawback, as most of the available studies were conducted in a single country. Future good quality, multicenter clinical trials utilizing standardized protocols are needed.

Author details

Asma Al-Shidhani and Abdulaziz Al-Mahrezi*
Department of Family Medicine and Public Health, College of Medicine and Health Sciences, Sultan Qaboos University, Muscat, Oman

*Address all correspondence to: abdulaziz@squ.edu.om

References

[1] Huang T, Zhang W, Huang X, Tian Y, Wang G, Zhang Y, et al. Comparing the efficacy of traditional firecupping and high-tech vacuum-cupping using laser doppler imaging at an acupuncture clinic in Beijing. Medical Acupuncture. 2011;23(1):13-18.). doi: 10.1089/acu.2010.0770.

[2] Tham LM, Lee HP, Lu C. Cupping: From a biomechanical perspective. Journal of Biomechanics. 2006;39(12):2183-2193. https://doi.org/10.1016/j.jbiomech.2005.06.027.

[3] Razi AMBZ. Kitab Al Mansoori. Translated by the Central Council for Research in Unani Medicine. New Delhi: Ministry of Health and Family Welfare, Govt. of India. 2002: 284, 391-394.

[4] Yoo SS., Tausk F. Cupping: east meets west. Int J Dermatol. 2004;43:664-665. 9. doi: 10.1111/j.1365-4632.2004.02224.x.

[5] Ahmedi M, Siddiqui MR. The value of wet cupping as a therapy in modern medicine e an Islamic perspective. Webmedcentral 2014;5(12). WMC004785.

[6] Al-Bedah AMN, Elsubai IS, Qureshi NA, Aboushanab T, Ali G, El-Olemy A, et al. The medical perspective of cupping therapy: Effects and mechanisms of action. Journal of Traditional and Complementary Medicine. 2019;9(2):90-97. DOI: 10.1016/j.jtcme.2018.03.003

[7] Kravetz RE. Cupping glass. Am J Gastroenterol. 2004;99(8):1418. doi:10.1111/j.1572-0241.2004.40696.x

[8] Turk JL, Allen E. Bleeding and cupping. Ann R Coll Surg Engl. 1983;65(2):128-131.

[9] Kouskoukis CE, Leider M. Cupping. The art and the value. Am J Dermatopathol. 1983;5(3):235-239.

[10] Manber H, Kanzler M. Consequences of Cupping. N Engl J Med 1996; 335:1281. DOI: 10.1056/NEJM199610243351705

[11] Al-Rubaye KQ. The clinical and histological skin changes after the cupping therapy (Al- Hijamah). J Turk Acad Dermatol. 2012;6(1):1261a. DOI:10.6003/JTAD.1261A1

[12] Staud R. Peripheral pain mechanisms in chronic widespread pain. Best Pract Res Clin Rheumatol. 2011;25(2):155-164. doi:10.1016/j.berh.2010.01.010

[13] Melzack R, Wall PD. On the nature of cutaneous sensory mechanisms. Brain. 1962;85:331-356. DOI: 10.1093/brain/85.2.331

[14] Michalsen A, Bock S, Lüdtke R, Rampp T, Baecker N, Bachmann J, et al. Effects of traditional cupping therapy in patients with carpal tunnel syndrome: a randomized controlled trial. J Pain. 2009;10(6):601-608. doi:10.1016/j.jpain.2008.12.013

[15] Tiran D, Chummun H. The physiological basis of reflexology and its use as a potential diagnostic tool. Complement Ther Clin Pract. 2005;11(1):58-64. doi:10.1016/j.ctnm.2004.07.007

[16] van Wijk G, Veldhuijzen DS. Perspective on diffuse noxious inhibitory controls as a model of endogenous pain modulation in clinical pain syndromes. J Pain. 2010;11(5):408-419. doi:10.1016/j.jpain.2009.10.009

[17] Le Bars D, Dickenson AH, Besson JM. Diffuse noxious inhibitory controls (DNIC). I. Effects on dorsal horn convergent neurones in the rat. Pain. 1979;6(3):283-304. doi:10.1016/0304-3959(79)90049-6

[18] Schouenborg J, Dickenson A. The effects of a distant noxious stimulation on A and C fibre-evoked flexion reflexes and neuronal activity in the dorsal horn of the rat. Brain Res. 1985;328:23-32. 1. 25. doi.org/10.1016/0006-8993(85)91318-6

[19] Ann Lett RM. Reflex Zone Therapy for Health Professionals. first ed. 2000. pp. 2-20.

[20] Sato A., Sato Y., Schmidt RF. The impact of somatosensory input on autonomic functions. Rev Physiol Biochem Pharmacol. 1997;130:257-262.

[21] Shaban T. Cupping therapy Encyclopedia. 1st Ed. California: On-Demand Publishing; 2013. P55

[22] Al-Bedah A, Aboushanab T, Alqaed M, Qureshi N, Suhaibani I, Ibrahim G et al. Classification of Cupping Therapy: A Tool for Modernization and Standardization. Journal of Complementary and Alternative Medical Research. 2016;1(1):1-10.DOI: 10.9734/jocamr/2016/27222.

[23] Aboushanab T, AlSanad S. Cupping Therapy: An Overview from a Modern Medicine Perspective. Journal of Acupuncture and Meridian Studies. 2018;11(3):83-87. DOI: 10.1016/j.jams.2018.02.001

[24] Cao H, Han M, Li X, Dong S, Shang Y, Wang Q, et al. Clinical research evidence of cupping therapy in China: A systematic literature review. BMC Complementary and Alternative Medicine. 2010;10(1):70. doi: 10.1186/1472-6882-10-70

[25] Al-Shamma YM, Abdil Razzaq A. Al- Hijamah cupping therapy. Kufa Med J. 2009;12(1)

[26] Teut M, Kaiser S, Ortiz M, Roll S, Binting S, Willich SN,et al. Pulsatile dry cupping in patients with osteoarthritis of the knee - a randomized controlled exploratory trial. BMC Complement Altern Med. 2012;12:184. Published 2012 Oct 12. doi:10.1186/1472-6882-12-184

[27] Duh FC, Chiu YH. Vacuum cupping under various negative pressures: An experimental investigation. Vacuum. Journal of Multidisciplinary Engineering Science and Technology (JMEST). 2015;(2)7

[28] Anees S, Arafath Y, Naaz A, Khan MQ. Hijamah (Cupping therapy) as a preventive medicine-a retro-prospective analytical study. International Journal of AYUSH. 2015;4(2):88-100.

[29] Cao, H., Li, X., Han, M. and Liu, J., 2013. Acupoint Stimulation for Fibromyalgia: A Systematic Review of Randomized Controlled Trials. Evidence-Based Complementary and Alternative Medicine, 2013, pp.1-15. DOI: 10.1155/2013/362831.

[30] Chirali, Ilkay Z. Traditional Chinese medicine cupping therapy. Elsevier Health Sciences. 2014;11,14,127,129

[31] Lin ML, Wu HC, Hsieh YH, Su CT, Shih YS, Lin CW, et al. Evaluation of the effect of laser acupuncture and cupping with ryodoraku and visual analog scale on low back pain. Evidence-Based Complementary and Alternative Medicine; 2012

[32] International Cupping Therapy Association (ICTA). Baguanfa treatments [Internet]. 2005. Available from: www.cuppingtherapy.org/pages/applications.html.

[33] Manchikanti L, Singh V, Falco FJ, Benyamin RM, Hirsch JA. Epidemiology of low back pain in adults. Neuromodulation. 2014; 17(Suppl 2): 3

[34] Wang YT, Qi Y, Tang FY, Li FM, Li QH, Xu CP, et al. The effect of cupping therapy for low back pain: A meta-analysis based on existing

randomized controlled trials. J Back Musculoskelet Rehabil. 2017;30(6):1187-1195. doi:10.3233/BMR-169736.

[35] Moura CC, Chaves ÉCL, Cardoso ACLR, Nogueira DA, Corrêa HP, Chianca TCM. Cupping therapy and chronic back pain: systematic review and meta-analysis. Rev Lat Am Enfermagem. 2018;26:e3094. doi: 10.1590/1518-8345.2888.3094.

[36] Teut M, Ullmann A, Ortiz M, Rotter G, Binting S, Cree M, et al. Pulsatile dry cupping in chronic low back pain -a randomized three-armed controlled clinical trial. BMC Complement Altern Med. 2018;18(1):115.

[37] Cramer H, Klose P, Teut, M, Rotter G, Ortiz M, Anheyer D, et al. Cupping for patients with chronic pain: A systematic review and meta-analysis. J Pain. 2020;S1526-5900(20)30003-1. doi:10.1016/j.jpain.2020.01.002

[38] Hoy DG, Protani M, De R, Buchbinder R. The epidemiology of neck pain. Best Pract Res Clin Rheumatol. 2010;24(6):783-792. doi:10.1016/j.berh.2011.01.019

[39] Fejer R, Kyvik KO, Hartvigsen J. The prevalence of neck pain in the world population: a systematic critical review of the literature. Eur Spine J 2006;15:834-848.

[40] Yuan QL, Guo TM, Liu L, Sun F, Zhang YG. Traditional Chinese medicine for neck pain and low back pain: a systematic review and meta-analysis. PLoS One. 2015;10(2):e0117146. DOI: 10.1371/journal.pone.0117146

[41] Kim S, Lee SH, Kim MR, Kim EJ, Hwang DS, Lee J, et al. Is cupping therapy effective in patients with neck pain? A systematic review and meta-analysis. BMJ Open. 2018;8(11):e021070. DOI: 10.1136/bmjopen-2017-021070

[42] Leem J. Long-term effect of cupping for chronic neck pain. Integr Med Res. 2014;3(4):217-219. doi:10.1016/j.imr.2014.10.001

[43] Ebell MH. Osteoarthritis: Rapid Evidence Review. Am Fam Physician. 2018;97(8):523-526.)

[44] Li JQ, Guo W, Sun ZG, Huang QS, Lee EY, Wang Y, et al. Cupping therapy for treating knee osteoarthritis: The evidence from systematic review and meta-analysis. Complement Ther Clin Pract. 2017;28:152-160. doi:10.1016/j.ctcp.2017.06.003

[45] Hainer BL, Matheson E, Wilkes RT. Diagnosis, treatment, and prevention of gout. Am Fam Physician. 2014;90(12):831-836.).

[46] Zhang S, Liu J, He K. Treatment of Acute Gouty Arthritis by Blood-letting Cupping plus Herbal Medicine. Journal of Traditional Chinese Medicine. 2010;30(1):18-20. DOI: 10.1016/s0254-6272(10)60005-2

[47] Jones G. What's new in osteoarthritis pathogenesis?. Intern Med J. 2016;46(2):229-236. doi:10.1111/imj.12763

[48] Ma SY, Wang Y, Xu JQ, Zheng L. Cupping therapy for treating ankylosing spondylitis: The evidence from systematic review and meta-analysis. Complement Ther Clin Pract. 2018;32:187-194. doi:10.1016/j.ctcp.2018.07.001

[49] Johnson RW, Rice AS. Clinical practice. Postherpetic neuralgia. N Engl J Med. 2014;371(16):1526-1533. doi:10.1056/NEJMcp1403062

[50] Saguil A, Kane S, Mercado M, Lauters R. Herpes Zoster and Postherpetic Neuralgia: Prevention and Management. Am Fam Physician. 2017;96(10):656-663.).

[51] Cao H, Zhu C, Liu J. Wet cupping therapy for treatment of herpes zoster: a systematic review of randomized controlled trials. Altern Ther Health Med. 2010;16(6):48-54.).

[52] Tian H, Tian YJ, Wang B, Yang L, Wang YY, Yang JS. [Impacts of bleeding and cupping therapy on serum P substance in patients of post herpetic neuralgia]. Zhongguo Zhen Jiu. 2013;33(8):678-681

[53] Wu X, Hu H, Guo L, Wang H. [Clinical observation of post-herpetic neuralgia treated with TCM herbal cupping therapy]. Zhongguo Zhen Jiu. 2013 ;33(2):141-144).

[54] Kostopoulos D. (2004). Treatment of carpal tunnel syndrome: A review of the nonsurgical approaches with emphasis in neural mobilization. Journal of Bodywork and Movement Therapies. 2004;8:2-8. https://doi.org/ 10.1016/ S1360-8592(03)00068-8)10.1016/ S1360-8592(03)00068-8).

[55] Mohammadi S, Roostayi MM, Naimi SS, Baghban AA. The effects of cupping therapy as a new approach in the physiotherapeutic management of carpal tunnel syndrome. Physiother Res Int. 2019;24:e1770. https://doi.org/10.1002/pri.1770)

[56] Aboonq M. Al-hijamah (wet cupping therapy of prophetic medicine) as a novel alternative to surgery for carpal tunnel syndrome. Neurosciences. 2019;24(2):137-141. DOI: 10.17712/nsj.2019.2.20180036

[57] Sucher B. Suction Decompression of the Carpal Tunnel. The Journal of the American Osteopathic Association. 2019;119(7):464. DOI: 10.7556/jaoa.2019.083

[58] Wolfe F, Clauw DJ, Fitzcharles MA, Goldenberg DL, Katz RS, Mease P, et al. The American College of Rheumatology preliminary diagnostic criteria for fibromyalgia and measurement of symptom severity. Arthritis Care Res (Hoboken). 2010;62(5):600-610. doi:10.1002/acr.20140

[59] Argoff CE. Pharmacologic management of chronic pain. J Am Osteopath Assoc. 2002;102(9 Suppl 3): S21-S27.

[60] Lauche R, Spitzer J, Schwahn B, Ostermann T, Bernardy K, Cramer H, et al. Efficacy of cupping therapy in patients with the fibromyalgia syndrome-a randomised placebo controlled trial. Sci Rep. 2016;6:37316. doi:10.1038/srep37316

[61] Cao JY. Li Y. Combination of acupuncture and antidepressant medications in treating of 56 cases of fibromyalgia. Chin Arch Trad Chi Med. 2003;21:813-817.

[62] Jiang ZY, Li CD, Qiu L, Guo JH, He LN, Yue Y,et al. Combination of acupuncture, cupping and medicine for treatment of fibromyalgia syndrome: a multi-central randomized controlled trial. Zhongguo Zhen Jiu. 2010;30(4):265-269.

[63] Kim TH, Kang JW. A good policy for guaranteed safe practice of complementary and alternative medicine, usage of disposable cupping cups. Evid Based Complement Alternat Med 2015;2015:970327.

[64] CCAOM Clean Needle Technique Manual. 7th Ed. Maryland: Council of Colleges of Acupuncture and Oriental Medicine; 2016. p. 36-37).

[65] Rozenfeld E, Kalichman L. New is the well-forgotten old: The use of dry cupping in musculoskeletal medicine. Journal of Bodywork and Movement Therapies. 2016;20(1):173-178. DOI:10.1016/j.jbmt.2015.11.009.

[66] Tuncez F, Bagci Y, Kurtipek GS, Erkek E. Suction bullae as a

complication of prolonged cupping. Clin Exp Dermatol. 2006;31(2):300-301. doi:10.1111/j.1365-2230.2005.02005.x

[67] Lin CW, Wang JT, Choy CS, Tung HH. Iatrogenic bullae following cupping therapy. J Altern Complement Med. 2009;15(11):1243-1245. doi:10.1089/acm.2009.0282

[68] Lee JS, Ahn SK, Lee SH. Factitial panniculitis induced by cupping and acupuncture. Cutis. 1995;55(4):217-218.

[69] Jung YJ, Kim JH, Lee HJ, Bak H, Hong SP, Jeon SY, et al. A herpes simplex virus infection secondary to acupuncture and cupping. Ann Dermatol. 2011;23(1):67-69. doi:10.5021/ad.2011.23.1.67

Chapter 14

Analgesics

Mihai Botea

Abstract

It is the responsibility of the professional care team to develop an effective person-centred Pain Management strategy which appropriately assesses patients, analyses the results of the assessment and devises a person centred plan to manage pain while allowing the person to remain as independent and functional as possible. The medications useful in treating acute pain are similar to those used in treating other types of pain. The World Health Organization (WHO) analgesic ladder developed for treating patients with cancer pain also provides a useful approach to treat acute pain. At the lowest level (mild pain) are recommended nonopioid analgesics such as paracetamol or/plus nonsteroidal anti-inflammatory drugs (NSAIDs) (e.g. ibuprophen). Such drugs have an analgesic ceiling; above a certain dose, no further analgesia is expected. For moderate pain, are recommended combining paracetamol and/or a NSAID with an opioid (a weak opoid). The inclusion of paracetamol limits the amount of opoids that should be used within 24 hour period, with many benefits which will be discussed later in the chapter. For severe level of pain, a strong opoid such as morphine is a better choice; such opoids have no analgesic ceiling. Most postoperative or trauma patients initially respond better to a morphine-equivalent opoid. At the moment when the patient is eating and drinking, a combination of oral analgesics including opoids and paracetamol plus/minus NSAID are most of the time an adequate choice.

Keywords: pharmacology, pharmacokinetics, doses, effects, interactions, side effects

1. Introduction

Pain is inevitable, suffering is optional.

(Dalai Lama)

Pain-related complaints represent as many as 70% of presenting concerns for patients in the A&E departments or GP setting [1–3]. A wide variety of options are available for the treatment of pain, from which the most known and used are the analgesics.

The approach to patients in pain should use a division of pain patients into four specific treatment groups: acute pain, chronic pain, recurrent pain and chronic pain of malignancy. In this chapter we will address mostly to the acute pain management.

Pain treatment should be initiated promptly, titrated to an acceptable level of relief, and continued during the cause's investigation. It is inappropriate to delay analgesics use until a diagnosis has been made. There is no evidence that the administration of adequate doses of opioid analgesia to establish patient comfort impairs the medical ability to rich a diagnose of an emergency condition. To the contrary, administration of analgesia may enhance the accuracy of physical examination and patient assessment [4, 5].

The medications useful in treating acute pain are similar to those used in treating other types of pain [1]. The World Health Organisation (WHO) analgesic ladder (**Figure 1**) developed for treating patients with cancer pain also provides a useful approach to treat acute pain. At the lowest level (mild pain) are recommended nonopioid analgesics such as paracetamol or/plus nonsteroidal anti-inflammatory drugs (NSAIDs) (e.g. ibuprofen). Such drugs have an analgesic ceiling; above a certain dose, no further analgesia effect is expected [1]. For moderate pain, are recommended combining paracetamol and/or a NSAID with an opioid (a weak opioid). The inclusion of paracetamol limits the amount of opioids that should be used within 24 hour period, with many benefits which will be discussed later in the chapter. For severe level of pain, a strong opioid such as morphine is a better choice; such opioids have no analgesic ceiling. Most postoperative or trauma patients initially respond better to a morphine-equivalent opioid. By the moment the patient is eating, drinking and ready for discharge, a combination of oral analgesics including opioids and paracetamol plus/minus NSAID are most of the time an adequate option.

Not all types of pain respond equally to the same medication. Usually NSAIDs and steroids are highly effective in controlling soft tissue and bone pain. Bone pain may be helped partially by opioids [1]. But overall, the combination of NSAIDs, paracetamol and opioids is synergistic in treating the most types of pain. Opioid analgesics are useful in controlling somatic and visceral pain. Neuropathic pain, often described as pain with a burning and hyperaesthesia characteristic, which responds well to a diverse group of drugs, called adjuvants, including low dose of antidepressants (amitriptyline), anticonvulsants (carbamazepine and clonazepam), antiarrhythmics (mexiletine), baclofen and alfa-adrenergic agonists (clonidine). Opioids may also be helpful [1]. Most of the time, analgesia is improved after 1–2 days of using adjuvant drugs. Adjuvants were not developed initially as analgesics but recent studies show they poses benefits in a better pain control. Drugs that control pain by different mechanisms of action may be synergistic, when used together. Also, by lower doses of two or more different agents, the patient may have better pain control with fewer side effects. This is the basic background for the multimodal analgesia concept.

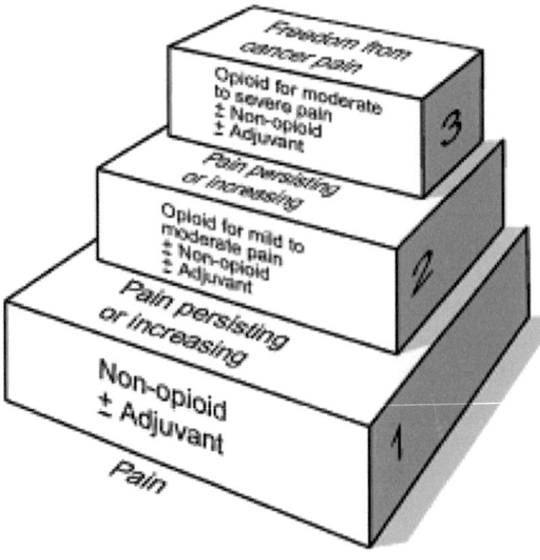

Figure 1.
WHO analgesic ladder.

2. Nonopioid analgesic agents

2.1 Paracetamol

Paracetamol is the first-line agent for the treatment of both acute and chronic pain. It is one of the pain killers with the highest profile of safety and is a first pharmacologic option for controlling pain in children and adults. It has a high toxic-to-therapeutic ratio and has very few significant drug interactions compared with other analgesics [2].

It can be given orally, rectally or parentally, has small anti-inflammatory activity, and is an effective analgesic and antipyretic.

Although paracetamol has been in use since 1880, its pharmacologic mechanism of action is not fully known. It has a rapid absorption from the small intestine after oral administration. Paracetamol has lower protein binding than NSAIDs (and hence fewer potential drug interactions) and higher volume of distribution [6].

Paracetamol is the active metabolite of the earlier (more toxic) drugs acetanilide and phenacetin. The recommended dose in adults is 0.5–1 g oral, iv or rectal every 4–6 hours when necessary, without exceeding a total daily dose of 4 g [6].

Paracetamol has a CNS action, where inhibits prostaglandin synthesis. In clinical doses it has insignificant peripheral anti-inflammatory action. Unlike morphine, paracetamol has no apparent biding sites, and unlike NSAIDs it does not inhibit peripheral cyclo-oxygenase activity. But however, his mechanisms of action include, beside central COX-2 inhibition [2, 7], inhibition of a central cyclo-oxygenase, COX-3, that is selectively susceptible to paracetamol, and modulation of descending serotonergic pathways that suppresses spinal cord nociceptive transmission. There is also evidence of agonism at the cannabinoid receptor CB_1 [2, 8]. There are, other evidences that paracetamol may inhibit prostaglandin endoperoxidase H_2 production at the cellular level, independent of cyclooxygenase activity [2, 6].

The most recent Cochrane review [9] of RCTs of single-dose oral analgesic for acute postoperative pain in adults reported a NNT of 3·6 with 1 g paracetamol, when morphine 10 mg IM has 2.9, ibuprofen 400 mg - 2.4 and codeine 60 mg - 16.7. Efficiency of paracetamol is improved in combinations with other analgesics, such as 400 mg ibuprofen, 60 mg codeine and 10 mg oxycodone (NNT 1·5, 2·2 and 1·8 respectively) [6, 9].

So, paracetamol is an effective analgesic, with potency somewhat less than standard dose of morphine. Paracetamol is an efficient adjunct to opioid analgesia, and regular administration after surgery produce an opioid sparing effect, because reduce opioid requirements by 20–30%. Paracetamol proved to be an integral component of multimodal analgesia in combination with NSAIDs and opioids. Paracetamol has less side effects than the NSAIDs and can be used when the latter are contraindicated.

A significant concern regarding paracetamol use relates to the development of hepatotoxicity; however, current data suggest this is unlikely to develop at therapeutic doses [10]. However, doses of more than 150 mg/kg of paracetamol taken within 24 hours may result in severe liver damage, hypoglycaemia and acute tubular necrosis, especially when associated with dehydration and chronic malnutrition [11]. Individuals taking enzyme-inducing agents are more susceptible. So, important caution should be taken in overdoses due to the risk of liver damage and less frequently renal damage. Nausea and vomiting, the only early features of poisoning, usually settle within 24 hours. Persistence beyond this time, often associated with the onset of a right-side subcostal pain and tenderness, usually indicates development of hepatic necrosis.

Side effects	Rare	Frequency not known
General	Acute generalised exanthematous pustulosis Malaise Skin reactions • Steven-Johnson syndrome • Toxic epidermal necrolysis	Blood disorders: leucopoenia neutropenia, thrombocytopenia as is bone marrow suppression
Specific	With iv use, flushing and tachycardia	With iv use, hypotension

Table 1.
Paracetamol side effects.

Paracetamol is metabolised in the liver primarily through conjugation to sulphate or glucuronides [2]. A minor pathway for the oxidative metabolism of paracetamol produces the toxic metabolite N-acetyl-P-benzoquinone (NAPQI) [2]. NAPQI requires glutathione for detoxification and elimination. Hepatic toxicity can occur when glutathione pathways are overwhelmed by an increase in NAPQI or decrease in glutathione.

Paracetamol is generally well tolerated with rare side effects when the right doses are prescribed (**Table 1**) [2, 4].

2.2 Interactions

It is associated with several important drug interactions. Many anticonvulsants, including phenytoin, barbiturates and carbamazepine induces hepatic microsomal enzymes. Increased conversion of paracetamol to its toxic metabolite may occur in patients who are taking anticonvulsants, but this rarely leads to concerning consequences in the context of the usual doses for pain management [2, 6].

Although uncommon, drug interaction resulting in an increased INR is reported for patients taking both paracetamol and warfarin, particularly among patients taking high doses of paracetamol (> 9 g/week) [2, 12, 13]. Long term use of paracetamol should be avoided in patients with hepatic or renal impairment. Patients with a history of salicylate hypersensitivity characterised by urticaria have a 11% cross-reactivity to paracetamol, and the agent should be used with caution in this group [2, 7].

3. Nonsteroidal anti-inflammatory drugs

The NSAIDs share several properties with aspirin and may be considered together.

NSAIDs are particularly used for the treatment of patients with chronic disease accompanied by pain and inflammation.

Some of them are also used for acute pain management and in the short-term treatment of mild to moderate pain including transient musculoskeletal pain. They are also suitable for the pain control in dysmenorrhoea and to release pain caused by secondary bone tumours, many of which produce lysis of bone and increase prostaglandins synthesis. Many of the NSAIDs are also used for postoperative analgesia as part of the multimodal analgesia strategy. Selective inhibitors of COX2 may be used in preference to non-selective NSAIDs for patients at high risk of developing serious gastro-intestinal side-effects.

There are some limited and low quality evidences against the use of NSAIDs in bone pathology, suggesting that prostaglandins promote bone formation and that NSAID might impair this process [14, 15], theory not proven through properly conducted studies. There is no evidence that NSAIDs administration on short term after fracture is detrimental to healing [2].

3.1 Mechanism of action

3.1.1 Prostaglandin synthesis inhibition

These agents inhibit cyclooxygenase (COX) and, as result, the synthesis of prostaglandin, a key mediator of inflammation, in the peripheral tissues, CNS and nerves – leading to an effective raise in the threshold of nociceptors stimulation. Aspirin acetylates and irreversibly inhibits cyclo-oxygenase, while NSAIDs work by competitive inhibition, being reversible. The prostaglandins are part of the eicosanoid's family, oxygenated metabolites of arachidonic acid and other polyunsaturated fatty acids that include leukotrienes [6].

The rate of prostaglandin synthesis is usually low, being regulated by trauma and tissue stimuli, which activates phospholipases to free arachidonic acid, from which prostaglandins are produced. Prostaglandins have several physiological roles, including gastric mucosal protection, bronchodilation and maintenance of renal tubular function, renal vasodilatation, regulation of tubular electrolytes and modulation the action of renal hormones [2, 6]. The side effects on the renal system of chronic NSAIDs is well known. In certain clinical settings when there are high plasma concentration of the vasoconstrictors rennin, noradrenaline, angiotensin and vasopressin, intrarenal vasodilators including prostacyclin are produced and renal function can be affected by NSAIDs administration [2]. The concomitant use of other potential nephrotoxic drugs, such as gentamicin, can worsen the renal effect of these drugs [2]. Nevertheless, with careful patient selection and closed monitoring the incidence of NSAID-renal damage is low.

Triggering bronchospasm is a recognised phenomenon in patients with asthma, rhinitis and nasal polyps [2]. Such "aspirin induce asthma" can be severe, and goes up to 10–15% as incidence with a feature cross sensitivity with NSAIDs. A known history of aspirin induce asthma should band the administration of NSAIDs perioperatively. The mechanism is unclear, but practice shown the reaction increases with the potency of the COX inhibition [2].

Endothelial released prostacyclin induces vasodilatation and prevents platelet adhesion, and platelet thromboxane produces aggregation and vasospasm. In addition to prostaglandins, cyclooxygenase induces prostacyclin synthesis, a vasodilator that also increases GI mucosal perfusion. Also, in the gastric tissue, COX-1 increases mucus and bicarbonate production, valuable feature for stomach mucosal protection [2]. Inhibition of COX-1 is affecting this protection, predisposing to ulcerations and bleeding, which can be exacerbated by concomitant NSAID-induced platelet dysfunction [2].

3.1.2 Cyclo-oxygenase isoenzymes

Two subtypes of cyclo-oxygenase enzyme have been identified. These are constitutional COX-1 and inducible COX-2, the last one triggered by inflammation and trauma. The COX-1 is present in all cells and regulates various roles in homeostatic function. NSAIDs, like aspirin, are non-selective cyclo-oxygenase inhibitors that act on both COX-1 and COX-2, which results in multiple beneficial effects (reduction in inflammation, pain and fever) but also some important side effects.

These two COX isoenzymes have 75% aminoacid homology, with almost identical enzymes kinetics.

COX-1 is a membrane bound haemoglycoprotein found in the endoplasmic reticulum of prostaglandin-inducing cells. The COX active site is a long hydrophobic channel. NSAIDs block COX-1 halfway down the channel by hydrogen bounding in a reversible fashion. Aspirin acetylates serine, irreversibly preventing access for arachidonic acid [6].

COX-2 has similar sites to COX-1 for the attachment of arachidonic acid, and a similar three-dimensional structure to COX-1.

Under physiological condition COX-1 activity predominates, to produce prostaglandins that regulate rapid physiological responses such as vascular homeostasis, gastric function, platelet activity and renal function. The concentration of the COX-1 isoenzyme is low, but it may increase 2 to 4-fold, triggered by grow hormones and various hormones stimulation. Low concentration of COX-2 can normally be detected in the brain, kidney and the pregnant uterus. COX-2 mRNA expression by synovial cells, fibroblasts, monocytes may be increased 10 to 80-fold when stimulated by cytokines, bacterial lipopolysaccharides or growth factors [6] These triggers increase COX-2 synthesis and tissue PGE2 concentration, resulting in inflammation and pain.

Inhibition of COX-1 induces antiplatelet activity that might be cardioprotective by inhibition of thromboxane synthesis more than prostacyclin. Inhibition of COX-2 inhibits prostacyclin synthesis more than thromboxane and may induce prothrombotic effects, leading to a higher risk of cardiovascular events [2]. In the case of nonselective COX inhibitors, both effects appear to be in balance each other out, resulting in minimal changes in cardiovascular risk [2]. But instead, the action of COX-2 inhibitors may result in result in an increased cardiovascular risk [16, 17].

Prostaglandins released by COX-1 is also a factor on keeping a good glomerular filtration rate (GFR) by renal vasodilatation that maintain renal blood flow. Inhibition of COX-1, especially in dehydrated patients can lead to affect GFR and even to an acute kidney injury [2]. Other condition that might worsen under NSAIDs treatment is congestive heart failure, due to sodium and water retention, hyperkalaemia, hypertension and acute renal failure.

The most common adverse effect of NSAIDs is GI mucosal erosion. In patients taking chronic NSAIDs (continuously for 1 year) 10 to 60% will experience abdominal pain, nausea, dyspepsia, and a 2 to 4% will end up with a symptomatic peptic ulcers [18]. Between the risk factors are known: age, concomitant use of corticosteroids and warfarin, coronary artery disease, congestive heart failure and diabetes mellitus. Several studies proved the efficiency of some protective agents as misoprostol and proton pump inhibitors [19]. The relative risk for causing GI effects under the NSAIDs treatment are shown in **Table 2** on below.

3.2 Side effects

This category of drugs is widely used, being very efficient medicines, but responsible for more serious drugs-related side effects than any other class of analgesic drugs [20]. The main side effect of NSAIDs as stated earlier is gastric erosion with the risk of GI bleeding, but also platelets dysfunction, renal failure and anaphylaxis or bronchospasm in individuals who have "aspirin – induced asthma" [2].

Single dose of NSAIDs such as diclofenac and ketorolac inhibit platelet function (prolong skin bleeding time and inhibit platelet function in vitro), but do not tend to increase bleeding in normal patients. However, when concomitant anticoagulation treatment or presence of subclinical bleeding diathesis occurs, then there is an increased risk of surgical bleeding [2].

Conversely, NSAIDs and COX-2 inhibitors have a small prothrombotic tendency. The risk is increasing by prolonged administration and by the dose taken, and for the more selective agents (COX-2) but also for diclofenac [2]. Studies shows that diclofenac 150 mg has similar risk to etoricoxib. Ibuprofen in a daily dose of 2400 mg also

NSAID	*Relative risk of serious GI toxicity*
COX-2 inhibitor	0.6
Ibuprofen	1.0
Diclofenac	1.8
Naproxen	2.2
Indomethacin	2.4
Piroxicam	3.8
Ketoprofen	4.2
Ketorolac	24.7
Risk reduction when added to ibuprofen	Proton pump inhibitor
0.09	Misoprostol
0.57	

Table 2.
Risk of serious gastrointestinal effects of NSAIDs [18, 19].

represents a high risk for thrombosis. But reduced doses to 1200 mg a day Ibuprofen and Naproxen 1 g daily are not associated with an increase risk [21, 22].

3.3 Contraindications of NSAIDs

There are many contraindications of this drug class presented on below (**Table 3**) [23].

3.4 Efficiency of the NSAIDs

The number needed to treat (NNT, basically the number of patients in a study to whom the drug must be given to show a benefit) for diclofenac 50 mg 2.3, ketorolac 10 mg is 2.6 and ibuprofen 400 mg 2.4. For comparison, the NNT of morphine 10 mg

Relative contraindications	**Absolute contraindication**
Impaired hepatic function, diabetes, bleeding or coagulation disorder, vascular disease	History of GI bleeding or ulceration
Surgery with a high risk of intraoperative haemorrhage (cardiac, vascular, etc.)	Known allergy to NSAIDs
Surgery where an absence of bleeding is important (eye surgery or neurosurgery)	Sever liver dysfunction
	Cardiac failure (risk of sodium, potassium and water retention)
Concurrent use of ACE inhibitors, potassium sparing diuretics, anticoagulants, methotrexate, cyclosporin, gentamicin	Dehydration, hypovolemia, hypotension
Pregnant and lactating women	Hyperkalaemia
Age >65 years (risk of kidney impairment)	Pre-existing renal impairment
Uncontrolled hypertension	
Aspirin-induced asthma	

Table 3.
NSAIDs contraindications.

IM is 2.9 and codeine 60 mg PO is 16.7. When given in combination with opioids, NSAIDs optimise the pain control and decrease opioid consumption by 25–50% [2]. NSAIDs are insufficient as a single pain killer use for relief of very severe pain.

COX-2 inhibitors produce less clinically significant peptic ulceration than other NSAIDs. So, COX-2 inhibitors are not far from any incidence of this adverse event, and there still debates on COX-2 inhibitors use in patients who have various risk factors for gastric erosion.

Platelets do not produce COX-2 (only COX-1) and so, COX-2 selective inhibitors do not affect platelet function. Studies have proved the lack of and antiplatelet effect of COX-2 inhibitors, and a reduction in surgical bleeding in comparison to other NSAIDs.

COX-2 is resident (constitutive) in some tissues including the renal, and COX-2 inhibitors have similar adverse effects on renal function to the non-selective NSAIDs (**Table 4**) [2].

3.5 Drug interactions

Aspirin. NSAIDs may impair the cardioprotective feature of aspirin, but this subject is still debatable lacking of strong evidences against use of NSAIDs for acute pain or inflammation in a patient on chronic daily aspirin use [24, 25].

Oral Anticoagulants. NSAIDs have an antiplatelet effect, added to the anticoagulant properties of warfarin, is exponential increasing the risk of significant bleeding complications, especially from the GI ulcers. Furthermore, NSAIDs displace protein-bound warfarin and is leading to increase the prothrombin times during a constant warfarin dose [18]. NSAIDs should be avoided in patients who are taking warfarin.

ACE Inhibitors. Concomitant use of NSAIDs with ACE inhibitors may impair kidney function and may prejudice the antihypertensive effect of ACE inhibitors.

Diuretics. Patients on diuretics have a higher risk of developing renal failure because of NSAIDs-mediated decreased kidney blood perfusion. Also, the natriuretic response to diuretics is in relation with prostaglandin-mediated vasodilatation.

Glucocorticoids. Patients on corticosteroids possess a higher risk of peptic ulcer. NSAIDs should be avoided in patients concomitantly taking corticosteroids unless closely supervised.

	NSAIDs	**COX-2**
Efficacy for moderate to severe acute pain (numbers to treat – NNT)	Diclofenac 50 mg (2.3) Ibuprofen 400 mg (2.4) Ketorolac 10 mg (2.6)	Celecoxib 200 mg (4.5) Parecoxib 20 mg (3.0) Etoricoxib 120 mg (1.8)
Renal function	Can impair renal function postoperatively	Similar adverse effects
Gastrointestinal	Acute gastrointestinal damage and bleeding can occur. Risk increased with higher doses, history of GI ulceration, long term use, and elderly	Less clinically significant peptic ulceration
Platelet function	Inhibit platelet function but do not significantly increase surgical blood loss in normal patients. Associated with higher incidence of post-tonsillectomy bleeding	Do not impair platelet function
Aspirin-exacerbated respiratory disease	10–15% of asthmatics affected when given aspirin. Cross-sensitivity with NSAIDs	Do not produces bronchospasm
Bone healing	Impaired in animal studies. No strong evidences that clinically important	Similar to NSAIDs

Table 4.
Comparison of non-selective NSAIDs and COX-2 inhibitors.

Lithium. NSAIDs increase lithium reabsorption and may reduce lithium excretion, and cause subsequently increases lithium levels. CNS manifestations (confusion, drowsiness, vertigo, tremors, seizures), QRS complex widening and cardiac arrhythmias are warning signs of lithium toxicity. The lithium doses should be reduced in patient concurrently taking NSAIDs.

Methotrexate. Chronic use of NSAIDs and methotrexate have resulted in prolonged, increased levels of methotrexate, leading to severe toxicity. A possible mechanism is accountable due to decreased renal blood supply, slowing down the elimination of methotrexate.

4. Opioid analgesic agents

In 1680, Sydenham wrote "Among the remedies it has pleased Almighty God to give to man to relive his suffering, none is so universal and so efficacious as opium" [2, 26]. Hundreds of years later, this statement is still valid, and opioids are the cornerstone of pain management. The beneficial effects have been well studied for centuries, as their toxicity and also the potential for abuse.

Opioid analgesics are usually used to relieve moderate to severe pain particularly of visceral origin. Repeated administration may cause dependence and tolerance, but this is not deterrent in the pain control of terminal illness. Regular use of a potent opioid may be appropriate for certain cases of chronic non-malignant pain; treatment should be supervised by medical staff and the patient should be assessed regularly. However, due to concerns about inducing opioid toxicity or addiction and sometimes due to poor understanding of the pharmacology features of these drugs, opioids are often inadequate used in clinical practice [27, 28].

4.1 Mechanism of action and toxic effects

Opioids bind to specific endorphin system receptors located throughout the nervous system but not only. Opioid receptors are G-protein-coupled transmembrane receptors. These exist throughout the CNS, with particularly high concentration in thalamus and spinal cord. They are also present outside the CNS, and these are responsible for other opioids effects (gastrointestinal tract) and their postulated value in some peripheral anaesthetic techniques, such as intra-articular infiltrations [6]. The actions of various opioids are induced by the specific binding properties of the agent to the various receptors (**Table 5**).

Opioid receptor class	Effects	Associated endogenous endorphin
Miu 1	Euphoria, supraspinal analgesia, confusion, dizziness, nausea, low addiction potential	Beta-endorphin
Miu 2	Respiratory depression, CV and GI effects, miosis, urinary retention	Beta-endorphin
Delta	Spinal analgesia, CV depressions, decreased brain and myocardial activity, physical dependence	Enkephalin
Kappa	Spinal analgesia, dysphoria, psychotomimetic effects, feedback inhibition of the endorphin system	Dynorphin, Beta-endorphin
Epsilon	Hormone	Beta-endorphin
Gamma	Dysphoria, psychotomimetic effects	Beta-endorphin

Table 5.
Opioids receptors end their effects.

Opioids decrease the medullary sensitivity to CO_2, which may cause respiratory depression and also, suppress the medullary cough centre, for this reason some studies advocate for its use as an antitussive. Opioids can activate the chemoreceptor trigger zone, causing nausea or vomiting, but this is relatively infrequent. This drug class decrease bowel motility and smooth muscle function, responsible for constipation, and rarely, urinary retention. To a varying degree, some opioids destabilise mast cells in a dose dependent fashion, causing histamine release, manifested with pruritus, urticaria and sometimes, orthostatic hypotension.

4.2 Clinical effect

Opioid agonist agents cause a range of mainly depressant and some stimulant actions of the CNS through specific receptors (**Table 6**). These drugs have little capacity to produce amnesia, do not alter seizure threshold and have no anticonvulsant activity [6].

Opioids given systemically produce analgesia through actions at two anatomically distinct regions: supraspinal and spinal sites. They efficiently reduce the intensity of pain and the associated fear. This is achieved by raising the pain threshold, modifying the reaction to pain, and inducing sleep. They are efficient for controlling dull pain rather than sharp intermittent pain. Opioids are less effective for the treatment of neuropathic pain.

Opioids actions are also towards reduction in the level of consciousness and eventually produce sleep, with the loss of responsiveness to verbal stimulation. In anaesthesia combinations, they produce a dose related decrease in the MAC for volatile anaesthetics, with a ceiling of 60–70% decrease in MAC [6]. Another important feature in the combination with the volatile agents is increase in cerebral vasoconstriction [6]. Opioids do not cause a loss of cerebral autoregulation or reactivity to CO_2. During EEC recording, there is a ceiling effect, with a slowing EEG frequency and the production of high-voltage (delta) waves [6].

4.3 Cardiovascular effects

In normovolemic patients, opioids barely influence haemodynamic parameters, with minimal cardiac depression, no baroreceptors inhibitions and modest reduction in preload and afterload. Haemodynamic compromise may be detected in subjects whose cardiovascular integrity is dependable on a high level of sympathetic tone, because opioids decrease central sympathetic outflow when even small doses can cause hypotension and circulatory collapse [6]. Morphine has the greatest effect on the vascular system. Morphine has the greatest effect on histamine release and subsequent indirect effect on catecholamine release. This may lead to tachycardia with a reduction in systemic vascular resistance (SVR) and mean arterial pressure (MAP). This risk can be prevented by pre-treatment with an antihistaminic drug and volume loading [6].

Opioids induce a negative chronotropic effect through a central vagal stimulation. Pethidine, however, has a homology with atropine and can trigger tachycardia, and it is the only opioid to induce significant direct myocardial depression when used at high doses. Myocardial depression is observed also after extraordinary high doses of morphine and fentanyl, as during cardiovascular anaesthesia. Morphine has indirect positive inotropic effects at doses of 1–2 mg/kg, and blocks neurally and hormonally mediated venoconstriction to reduce preload, rendering it useful in the management of left ventricular failure [6].

Opioids preserve circulatory stability to a greater extent than most other anaesthetic agents [6].

System		Effect
Musculoskeletal	Gait	Decrease physical performance Ataxia Decrease spinal cord reflexes
	Rigidity	Muscular rigidity occurs 60–90 seconds post-injection and abolish after 10–20 minutes Mainly thoracoabdominal and arms muscles, higher risk with advanced age, high speed of injection, increased dose, use of N_2O Mediated via nucleus raphe magnus
	Multifocal myoclonus	Non-convulsive related, higher risk with pethidine
Neural	Central	Spectrum from abnormal eye movement, to contraction of extremities, to tonic-clonic movements Euphoria: especially for opioids which cross the blood-brain barrier quickly Dysphoria in some individuals Subjective feelings of body warmth and heavy extremities Apathy Decreased level of consciousness Decreased concentration and orientation
	EEG	Effects vary between different opioids: slowing of frequency, production of high voltage & waves No capacity to induce EEG silence
Vision	Edinger-Westphal nucleus	Miosis (via a decrease in inhibition to the nucleus) except pethidine Reversed by hypoxia and atropine
Cerebrovascular	SSEPs	No effect
	ICP	No effect
	CBF	No effect, but increased vasoconstriction with vasodilators No loss of autoregulation or CO_2 reactivity $CMRO_2$ reduced by up to 10–25%
Thermoregulation	Response	Decrease thermoregulation response (as for volatile agents)
	Peripheral effects	Promote hypothermia via decreased BMR (10–20%), venodilation, muscle relaxation

SSEPs – somatosensory evoked potential, ICP – intracranial pressure, $CMRO_2$ – cerebral metabolic rate of oxygen consumption.

Table 6.
Opioids effects on the CNS [6].

4.4 Effects on other organ systems

Opioids are the most efficient of all pain analgesics drugs for attenuating the stress response associated with pain, laryngoscopy and airway manipulation. The plasma concentration of stress hormones (cortisol, catecholamines, vasopressin, aldosterone and growth factor) increases during trauma, anaesthesia or surgery. This produce increased myocardial work, tissue catabolism and hyperglycaemia – effects associated with increased morbidity and mortality. Opioids reduce nociception inhibiting the pituitary-adrenal axis, decreasing central sympathetic outflow and influencing centrally mediated neuroendocrine response. Fentanyl and its congeners are the most efficacious in this action (**Table 7**).

System		Effect
Cardiovascular	Heart rate	Sinus bradycardia via central vagal stimulation Occasionally sinus arrest exacerbated by concomitant vagal excitation (e.g. laryngoscopy) and Beta-blockers
	Mean arterial pressure	Usually no effect or a slight decrease (unless significant bradycardia) Greater decrease if associated with histamine release
	Vascular system	No effect on SVR (unless histamine release) Mild venodilation with a decrease in preload (due to decrease of central sympathetic outflow)
	Myocardium	No effect on contractility (except for pethidine which is a depressant) No effect on metabolic rate Possible ischemic preconditioning
	Excitability	Decreased myocardial contractility Increased refractory period Increased VF threshold
Respiratory	Mechanics	Decrease in rate, tidal volume and minute ventilation at equianalgesic doses Increase pauses, irregular breathing and apnoea
	Control	Increased apnoeic threshold Decrease CO_2 sensitivity Decrease carotid body chemoreception and hypoxic drive Voluntary control of respiration remains intact No effect on hypoxic pulmonary vasoconstriction
	Airway reflexes	Decrease airway reflexes with improve tolerance to ETT Antitussive through central and peripheral actions Decrease mucociliary action Brief cough in up to 50% with pethidine bolus
Gastrointestinal	Stomach and bowel	Decrease peristalsis and secretions and increase tone causing dry stool and constipation Decrease gastric acid Decrease gastric emptying with increase antral tone and decrease lower oesophageal sphincter tone promoting high aspiration risk Increase tone of pyloric, ileocecal and anal sphincters
	Biliary tree	Increase bile duct pressure Sphincter Oddi contraction (little clinical significance)
	Chemoreceptor trigger zone	Nausea and vomiting
Genitourinary	Kidney	Antidiuresis as a result of decrease in renal blood flow and decrease in GFR (predominates) Decrease vasopressin release in response to osmotic triggers
	Bladder	Increased bladder and urethral tone Vesicular sphincter contraction
Immunity	Immune system	Decrease immunoglobulin production (uncertain significance) Reactivation of herpes simplex virus 2–5 days after neuraxial opioid

Table 7.
Opioid effects on major organ system [6].

4.5 Side effects

Side effects can be observed from minors to the most concerning ones and are individual and age depending beyond of disease extension, presence of organ dysfunction, concurrent administration of certain drugs, route of administration and prior of opioid exposure. Some side effects induced by the opioids are induced by the activation of the opioid receptors either peripherally or centrally, or even in both areas. Serious allergic reactions to opioids are extremely rare, although anaphylaxis has been reported.

At equianalgesic doses, all opioids produce equivalent degrees of respiratory depression through reducing the sensitivity to CO_2 of the breathing drive. The extreme ages, elderly and neonates are at the highest risk. Tolerance arises rapidly to this effect, and with chronic opioid exposure the risk of major respiratory depression is reduced. Apnoea may occur in conscious patients, but this is rare, and is usually associated with other signs of CNS depression. In such a condition, apnoeic patients can be instructed to breath as voluntary control of ventilation remains intact. Sleep or the concomitant use of other CNS depressants (except clonidine) potentiates this risk.

Opioid-induce depression of airway reflexes is usually regarded as an advantage side effect for the practitioner in some condition like airway manipulation. Although at the same time the mucociliary function depression can be detrimental. All opioids have an antitussive activity at less than analgesic doses, working via central and peripheral mechanisms.

The incidence of nausea after opioids use is reported to be between 10 and 60%, and this is markedly increased in pain-free and ambulatory patients (via opioid sensitisation of the vestibular nucleus). This reactivity is based on individual variability, but tolerance develops rapidly [6]. Switch to oral administration and substituting one opioid to another may reduce the incidence of nausea.

Constipation remains the most common side effect of chronic opioid treatment, and toxic megacolon may occur in patients with ulcerative colitis [6]. Tolerance, in this situation develops very slowly, as well as other smooth muscle effects. Loperamide is a synthetic agent, does not cross the blood brain barrier, used as an antimotility drug. All opioids are reported to increase bile duct pressure, with a spasmogenic action cause contraction of the sphincter of Oddi with effects on doses dependent activity [6]. Pethidine also, produces smooth muscle contraction via a direct action. Opioids effects on the biliary tract can be reversed by naloxone, nitroglycerine and glucagon.

Other effects on the smooth muscle target the genitourinary system, often leading to urinary retention and urgency. This effect is predominant in elderly and when administered neuraxially. This later feature explains a centrally mediated mechanism of action via receptors located at the sacral spinal cord.

There are some others centrally mediated opioids effects. Some of these are of no clinical benefit and usually unpleasant. Often, opioids may trigger pruritus with various ranges of severity, with mechanism of action not fully discovered. The pruritus predominantly affects nose, face and chest being independent of histamine release. Substituting opioids agents will decrease the incidence. Studies has shown that low dose of naloxone will alleviate this effect. Muscle rigidity is triggered at or just after the loss of consciousness and may manifest from hoarseness in mild cases to impossibility of ventilate in severe situations. It can be minimised by co-administration of induction agents and benzodiazepines. In anaesthetic practice may be prevented by pre-treatment priming with small doses of muscle relaxants. This side effect was reported to be with a higher incidence on concomitant use of nitrous oxide [6]. It is seen more commonly with Fentanyl and its congeners than with morphine and the risk is dose depended. In emergency situation of impossibility of ventilation can be reversed by administration of naloxone.

Opioids agents decrease thermoregulation thresholds, except pethidine, which is a unique in its ability to reduce shivering. Tramadol also has proved to be efficacious in this regard [6].

Histamine release and associated hypotension are variable in incidence and severity, and are with decreased incidence where is a slow IV administration and ameliorated by intravascular fluid loading. This effect is less with fentanyl and its subclass agents, except pethidine. The histamine release may be localised or generalised, often causing facial flushing and variable itch [6].

4.5.1 Opioid-specific effects

Pethidine has been described as a unique agent because of its non-opioid effects. It has a local anaesthetic effect of equivalent potency to cocaine and it has a quinidine-like effect on cardiac muscle to reduce cardiac irritability and arrhythmias [6]. Pethidine overdose produce a complex syndrome characterised by a cardiovascular collapse, seizures, hyperreflexia, mydriasis in addition to a respiratory depression [6].

The use of phenylpiperidines family (except remifentanil) in anaesthesia has been associated with postoperative respiratory depression after high doses, due secondary peaks in plasma levels, possible from the opioids release from the body stores. This action is responsible for the increase in peripheral perfusion and postoperative shivering.

4.6 Pharmacokinetics

4.6.1 Administrations

The choice of route of administration depends on the opioid being utilised, pain severity, the need for agent titration, potential side effects and contraindications to a particular route. The way of administration may activate the onset of peak analgesia and the side effects. For example, respiratory depression may be triggered 7 minutes after an IV dose of morphine, but not until 30 minutes after IM or 6–10 hours after a spinal administration.

There are various degree and length of pain relief effect conferred by certain routes. Spinal administration may produce a greater quality and potentially a longer duration of analgesia, with a lower incident of supraspinal effects. However, an increased incidence of specific side effects (nausea, itching, urinary retention) occurs.

No opioid agonist demonstrates dose-dependent pharmacokinetics. First pass metabolism of orally administrated opioids is made in the liver and the digestive tract wall (up to 50%). Opioids given IM or SC have 100% bioavailability, but peak plasma concentration may be variable up to fivefold influenced by body temperature, site of injection and hemodynamic status. IV administration results in a much restricted rage of plasma concentration [6].

The lung exerts an important first-pass effect on highly lipid-soluble opioids. Prior administration of other lipophilic amines, such propranolol decreases pulmonary uptake, by saturating biding sites [6].

4.6.2 Elimination

Opioids mainly sustain a liver metabolism with a renal excretion of the more hydrophilic metabolites. A few metabolites also take the biliary excretion route. Some amounts of the more hydrophilic agents may be excreted unchanged in the urine. Liver blood flow is the main factor influencing the plasma clearance for most opioids, because of their high hepatic extraction ratio [6].

Morphine. The biotransformation of morphine is unique among opioids agents. Glucuronidation is responsible for 60–80% of its metabolism, and is primarily undergone in the liver with production of high quantity morphine-3-glucoronide (M3G) and only 10% of morphine-6-glucoronide (M6G). The remainder undergoes sulphation (important feature in neonates where glucuronidation metabolism is immature), 5% is demethylated to normorphine, a small amount is converted to codeine, and 10% is excreted in the urine [6, 29]. In healthy subjects up to 10% of glucuronidation occurs in extrahepatic sites, such kidney and intestine. The excretion of the morphine metabolites is directly influenced by the creatinine clearance. 90% of conjugated morphine is excreted in the urine and 10% is excreted in bile, sweat and breast milk. M6G is 2–4 time more potent than morphine and has a longer elimination half-life [29]. Despite being more hydrophilic than morphine, M6G cross the blood-brain barrier, with a longer action due to slower elimination from this site. There is also an entero-hepatic recirculation of morphine and its metabolites, particularly under the chronic oral administration [29].

Diamorphine. Diamorphine is inactive and needs deacetylation in the CSF, liver, and plasma to its final metabolites 6-monoacetylmorphine and morphine. These active metabolites are more hydrophilic, and their ensuing metabolism is as for morphine [6].

Codeine. Codeine is suffering a hepatic metabolization to mainly codeine conjugates and norcodeine, with some urinary excretion of free codeine. Up to 10% of a dose is also metabolised to morphine. This biotransformation is responsible for analgesia produced by codeine. Due to genetic polymorphism, up to 8% of western Europeans are deficient of the enzyme implicated in the liver metabolism. These patients require higher doses, and they may still not experience effective pain relief. Furthermore, the variability may produce dangerous high morphine levels in breast milk [30].

Pethidine. Pethidine metabolism mainly involves hydrolysis to pethidinic acid, with small amount being freely excreted through urine (5%) of the prodrug – although this may be increased up to 25% with urinary acidification ($pH < 5$) [6]. One third of the metabolism takes the route to N-demethylation to norpethidine, which is finally hydrolysed to norpethidinic acid. Enzyme induction triggered by chronic pethidine use (sometimes also by carbamazepine therapy) induces high levels of transformed norpethidine [6].

Fentanyl and sufentanyl. The high lipid solubility of these agents is responsible for their large volume of distribution, which causes rapid and continued peripheral tissue uptake, limiting initial liver metabolism. This is leading to a greater variability in plasma concentration (13-fold range in fentanyl) during the elimination phase, particularly with fluctuations in muscles blood flow that may be responsible of the secondary peaks in plasma concentration after large doses. Fentanyl, sufentanyl and alfentanyl have a small unchanged renal excretion, being mainly metabolised in the liver. These inactive metabolites are taking the urinary route for excretion.

4.6.3 Patient factors influencing opioid pharmacokinetics and pharmacodynamics

The pharmacokinetics and dynamics of opioids may be altered in a number of physiological states as stated in **Table 8**.

4.7 Opioid drug interaction

This class of pain killers have limited but important interactions with other drugs. Their action is synergistically with other CNS depressant on the level of consciousness. Barbiturates, benzodiazepines and propofol produce effects on the loss of

Physiological states	Effect	Mechanism
Obesity	Overdosage	Central volume of distribution is not reflected by actual body weight Increased volume of distribution prolongs elimination half-life
Infant	Prolonged effect	Decreased conjugation capacity Immature renal function
Elderly	Increased sensitivity to opioid	Decreased neuronal cell mass Decreased central volume of distribution
	Prolonged effect of infusion	Decreased lean body mass with increase adipose tissue is responsible for an increase in total volume of distribution Decreased hepatic blood flow (by 40–50% by age of 75)
Hepatic failure	Increased sensitivity to opioids (in severe liver failure only)	Synergism if encephalopathic Altered integrity of blood-brain barrier Increased elimination half-life for pethidine and tramadol
Renal failure	Morphine toxicity	Accumulation of M6G Possible hydrolysis of glucuronides back to parent compound Uraemia potentiates CNS depression and increases blood-brain barrier permeability

Table 8.
Factors influencing opioid pharmacokinetics and pharmacodynamics.

consciousness with a synergic action from the opioids side and also increase the risk of cardiovascular depression. With anaesthetic use, opioids may decrease the concentration of volatile agents by up to 50% while ensuring amnesia and immobility, with the preservation of hemodynamic stability at low inhaled concentrations (≤1 MAC) [6].

The use of opioids (particularly pethidine and tramadol) with monoamine oxidase inhibitors (MAOI) may lead to serious and potentially fatal consequences as excitatory syndrome (type I) [2, 6]. This is complex syndrome characterised by excitatory phenomena including agitation, fever, rigidity, seizures and coma. This is triggered by the excessive CNS serotonin activity, since both MAOI and pethidine block serotonin reuptake. Rarely also can arise an inhibitory syndrome (type II) characterised by respiratory depression, coma and hypotension, which is the result of MAOI inhibition of hepatic microsomal enzymes leading to a pethidine accumulation.

A similar excitatory syndrome (serotoninergic) is found during the combination of tramadol and serotonin-noradrenaline reuptake inhibitors (SNRIs) [6].

Morphine has been recommended as the opioid of choice for use in these patients.

4.8 Opioid antagonists

The main opioid antagonist currently used in practice is naloxone.

Naloxone is an N-allyl derivate of oxymorphone. It is pure opioid antagonist, without an intrinsic pharmacological activity. It has a high affinity for miu opioid receptors but also blocks other receptors. Naloxone reverses the respiratory depression and analgesia of opioids but also precipitates the withdrawal syndrome in opioids addicts. Naloxone could also block the action of endogenous opioids. IV administration of 200–400 mcg of naloxone will reverse the respiratory depression, but incremental titration (1.5–3 mcg/kg) is referable in order to minimise the reversal of the analgesic effects of the opioids. Naloxone's action time is roughly 30 minutes, so further doses may be considered to avoid the return of respiratory depression effects of any agonist agent that outlasts the effect of naloxone. Naloxone is also efficient in releasing the pruritus and urinary retention of the intrathecal and epidural opioids. Naloxone has very small oral availability, only 2%, because and major first pass metabolism [6].

4.9 Tramadol

Tramadol is included in the opioids class of drugs, with unique and complex mode of action, only part of which is mediated through opioid receptors. Tramadol is an analogue of codeine and acts as a weak agonist at all types of opioid receptors, with some preference for the miu receptors. It has 10% of the potency of morphine. Tramadol blocks the reuptake of noradrenaline and 5-HT (serotonin) and facilitate the release of the later. By its effects, influences nociceptive transmission activating the descending inhibitory pathways in the CNS. Therefore, Naloxone only partially reverses the analgesic effects of tramadol. Effects on alfa2-adrenergic, NMDA and benzodiazepine receptors may be due to indirect effects secondary noradrenergic system effects [31].

Tramadol is recommended in the treatment of moderate to severe pain. It is well absorbed when given orally, with a bioavailability of 68% and only 20% protein bound. Tramadol is predominantly metabolised in the liver by demethylation and conjugation, with 90% being excreted in the urine. The elimination half-life is 4–6 hours. His metabolites have longer half-life (up to 9 hours) and 2–4 times greater analgesic potency than tramadol and precautions should be taken in hepatic and renal failure.

Tramadol exhibits small risk for respiratory depression when compared with equianalgesic doses of morphine. Also, cardiovascular effects are minimal. There is a low potency for abuse and physical dependence, but still reported. Tramadol's known side effects include: dizziness, nausea, sedation, dry mouth, sweating and skin rashes.

Concomitant use of MAOIs is contraindicated and co-administration with carbamazepine may decrease the concentration and effect of tramadol.

5. General pain management principles

- A - ask about pain regularly
- B - believe the patient's/resident's and family's reports of pain and what relieves it
- C - choose appropriate pain control options
- D - deliver interventions in a timely, logical and coordinated fashion
- E - empower patients

6. Pharmacological intervention

As a result of a nationwide effort to reduce unnecessary opioid use and reduce incidents of patient abuse, clinicians are encouraged to carefully assess their patient's pain, limit the number of prescribed opioids analgesics and limit further prescribing by evaluating the patient's pain relief and increased functional ability.

The trend to lower usage has had a tremendous impact on opiod use worldwide over the last years. By 2016, paracetamol/hydrocodone, which had been the leading medication prescribed for pain, had dropped from first most prescribed pain medication to the fourth most prescribed drug in the nation, with the volume of prescriptions down to 7.2% in 2015, from 34% in 2012.

In order to facilitate this continuing trend, it is recommended that the following WHO decision ladder and in-depth patient assessment be utilised before requesting or prescribing opioid compounds.

7. Multimodal analgesia

Multimodal analgesia is defined as the use of more than one pharmacological class of analgesic medication targeting different receptors along the pain pathway with the goal of improving analgesia while reducing individual class-related side effects. Evidence today supports the routine use of multimodal analgesia in the perioperative period to eliminate the over-reliance on opioids for pain control and to reduce opioid-related adverse events. A multimodal analgesic protocol should be surgery-specific, functioning more like a checklist than a recipe, with options to tailor to the individual patient.

Elements of this protocol may include opioids, non-opioid systemic analgesics like paracetamol, non-steroidal anti-inflammatory drugs, gabapentins, ketamine, and local anaesthetics administered by infiltration, regional block, or the intravenous route [32–37]. While implementation of multimodal analgesic protocols perioperatively is recommended as an intervention to decrease the prevalence of long-term opioid use following surgery, the concurrent crisis of drug shortages presents an additional challenge. Anaesthesiologists and acute pain medicine specialists will need to advocate locally and nationally to ensure a steady supply of analgesic medications and in-class alternatives for their patients' perioperative pain management.

8. Conclusion

The recommendations are on the basis of the underlying premise that optimal management begins with the patient assessment and development of a plan of care tailored to the individual and the medical status or the surgical procedure involved, with follow-up assessments and adjustments as needed. The evidences support the use of multimodal regimens in many situations, although the exact components of effective multimodal care will vary depending on the patient, setting, and surgical procedure or the medical condition. Therefore, it is important that clinicians consider their patients' pain in the context of: biological, social and psychological factors.

Author details

Mihai Botea[1,2]

1 University of Oradea, Pelican Clinic Hospital, Romania

2 Senior Clinical Fellow at St Bartolomew's Hospital, London, UK

*Address all correspondence to: drmob78@yahoo.com

References

[1] James C. Duke, Brian M Keech. Duke's Anaesthesia secrets. 5th Edition. Elsevier Saunders. 2016

[2] John A. Marx, Robert S. Hockberger, Ron M. Walls and all. *Rosen's Emergency Medicine Concepts and Clinical Practice*. 8th Edition. Elsevier Saunders. 2014

[3] Todd KH, et al: Pain in the emergency department: Results of the pain and emergency medicine initiative (PEMI) multicenter study. J Pain 2007; 8:460-466

[4] Bijur PE, Kenny MK, Gallagher EJ: Intravenous morphine at 0.1 mg/kg is not effective for controlling severe acute pain in the majority of patients. Ann Emerg Med 2005; 46:362-367.

[5] Birnbaum A, Esses D, Bijur PE, Holden L, Gallagher EJ: Randomized double-blind placebo-controlled trial of two intravenous morphine dosages (0.10 mg/kg and 0.15 mg/kg) in emergency department patients with moderate to severe acute pain. Ann Emerg Med 2007; 49:445-453, e441-e442.

[6] Ted Lin, Tim Smith and Collin Pinnock and all. *Fundamentals of Anaesthesia*. 4th Edition. Cambridge University Press. 2017

[7] Asero R: Risk factors for acetaminophen and nimesulide intolerance in patients with NSAID-induced skin disorders. Ann Allergy Asthma Immunol 1999; 82:554-558.

[8] Schwab JM, Schluesener HJ, Laufer S: COX-3: Just another COX or the solitary elusive target of paracetamol? Lancet 2003; 361:981-982.

[9] Moore RA, Derry S, Aldington D, Wiffen PJ. Single dose oral analgesics for acute postoperative pain in adults – an overview of Cochrane reviews. Cochrane Database Syst Rev 2015; (9) CD008659.

[10] Dart RC, Bailey E. Does therapeutic use of acetaminophen cause acute liver failure? Pharmacotherapy 2007; 27: 1219-1230.

[11] British National Formulary. Online www.bnf.org

[12] Hylek EM: Paracetamol (acetaminophen) and warfarin interaction: Unraveling the pivotal role of the vitamin K cycle. Thromb Haemost 2004; 92:672-673.

[13] Hylek EM, Heiman H, Skates SJ, S heehan MA, Singer DE: Acetaminophen and other risk factors for excessive warfarin anticoagulation. JAMA 1998; 279:657-662.

[14] Hernandez-Diaz S, Garcia-Rodriguez LA: Epidemiologic assessment of the safety of conventional nonsteroidal anti-inflammatory drugs. Am J Med 2001; 110(Suppl 3A):20S–27S.

[15] Reuben SS, Ablett D, Kaye R: High dose nonsteroidal antiinflammatory drugs compromise spinal fusion. Can J Anaesth 2005; 52:506-512

[16] Bhattacharyya T, Smith RM: Cardiovascular risks of coxibs: The orthopaedic perspective. J Bone Joint Surg Am 2005; 87:245-246.

[17] Fischer LM, Schlienger RG, Matter CM, Jick H, Meier CR: Current use of nonsteroidal antiinflammatory drugs and the risk of acute myocardial infarction. Pharmacotherapy 2005; 25:503-510.

[18] Battistella M, Mamdami MM, Juurlink DN, Rabeneck L, Laupacis A: Risk of upper gastrointestinal hemorrhage in warfarin users treated with nonselective NSAIDs or COX-2 inhibitors. Arch Intern Med 2005; 165:189-192

[19] Raskin JB, et al: Misoprostol and ranitidine in the prevention of NSAID-induced ulcers: A prospective, double-blind, multicenter study. Am J Gastroenterol 1996; 91:223-227.

[20] Hersh EV, Pinto A, Moore PA: Adverse drug interactions involving common prescription and over-the-counter analgesic agents. Clin Ther 2007; 29(Suppl):2477-2497.

[21] US Food and Drug Administration (2004). FDA public health advisory: safety of Vioxx. M http://www.fda.gov/drugs/drugsafety/post market drug safety information for patients and providers/ucm106274.htm.

[22] Medicines and Healthcare Products Regulatory Agency. MHRA public assessment report. Non-steroidal anti-inflammatory drugs and cardiovascular risks in the general population, January 2010. M http://www.mhra.gov.uk/safety-public-assessment-reports/CON105663

[23] Keith G. Allman, Iain H. Wilson, Aidan M O'Donnell. *Anaesthesia Oxford Handbook*, 4th Edition. Oxford University Press. 2016

[24] Corman SL, Fedutes BA, Ansani NT: Impact of nonsteroidal antiinflammatory drugs on the cardioprotective effects of aspirin. Ann Pharmacother 2005; 39:1073-1079.

[25] MacDonald TM, Wei L: Effect of ibuprofen on cardioprotective effect of aspirin. Lancet 2003; 361:573-574

[26] Gutstein HB, Akil H: Opioid analgesics. In: Hardman JG, Limbird LE, Gilman AG, eds. Goodman & Gilman's The Pharmacological Basis of Therapeutics, ed 10. New York: McGraw-Hill; 2001:569-619.

[27] Todd KH, Samaroo N, Hoffman JR: Ethnicity as a risk factor for inadequate emergency department analgesia. JAMA 1993; 269:1537-1539.

[28] Brown JC, Klein EJ, Lewis CW, Johnston BD, Cummings P: Emergency department analgesia for fracture pain. Ann Emerg Med 2003; 42:197-205.

[29] O'Connor AB, Lang VJ, Quill TE: Underdosing of morphine in comparison with other parenteral opioids in an acute hospital: A quality of care challenge. Pain Med 2006; 7:299-307.

[30] Turturro MA, Paris PM, Yealy DM, Menegazzi JJ: Hydrocodone versus codeine in acute musculoskeletal pain. Ann Emerg Med 1991; 20:1100-1103.

[31] Hewitt DJ, Todd KH, Xiang J, Jordan DM, Rosenthal NR: Tramadol/acetaminophen or hydrocodone/acetaminophen for the treatment of ankle sprain: A randomized, placebo-controlled trial. Ann Emerg Med 2007; 49:468-480, e461-e462.

[32] Gustafsson UO, Scott MJ, Hubner M, Nygren J, Demartines N, Francis N et al. Guidelines for perioperative care in elective colorectal surgery: Enhanced Recovery After Surgery (ERAS®) Society recommendations: 2018. World J Surg 2019; 43: 659-695.

[33] Nelson G, Bakkum-Gamez J, Kalogera E, Glaser G, Altman A, Meyer LA et al. Guidelines for perioperative care in gynecologic/oncology: Enhanced Recovery After Surgery (ERAS) Society recommendations – 2019 update. Int J Gynecol Cancer 2019; 29: 651-668.

[34] Low DE, Allum W, De Manzoni G, Ferri L, Immanuel A, Kuppusamy M et al. Guidelines for perioperative care in esophagectomy: Enhanced Recovery After Surgery (ERAS®) Society recommendations. World J Surg 2019; 43: 299-330.

[35] Thorell A, MacCormick AD, Awad S, Reynolds N, Roulin D, Demartines N et al. Guidelines for perioperative care in bariatric surgery: Enhanced Recovery After Surgery

(ERAS) Society recommendations. World J Surg 2016; 40: 2065-2083.

[36] Temple-Oberle C, Shea-Budgell MA, Tan M, Semple JL, Schrag C, Barreto M et al. Consensus review of optimal perioperative care in breast reconstruction: Enhanced Recovery After Surgery (ERAS) Society recommendations. Plast Reconstr Surg 2017; 139: 1056e–1071e

[37] Shen H, et al: Analgesic action of acetaminophen in symptomatic osteoarthritis of the knee. Rheumatology (Oxford) 2006; 45:765-770.

Chapter 15

NSAIDs, Opioids, and Beyond

Coti Phillips, Edwin Contreras and Jessica Oswald

Abstract

Medications are prescribed throughout the world for a variety of reasons including pain. NSAIDs, opioids, and other non-opioid modalities have been used to treat both acute and chronic pain. In this chapter we will discuss the pharmacokinetics, indications, function and associated complications for commonly used pain medications to include NSAIDs, opioids, antidepressants, cannabinoids, and ketamine.

Keywords: acute pain, chronic pain, NSAIDs, opioids, antidepressants, cannabinoids, ketamine

1. Introduction

Acute and chronic pain is a complex disease process that can be difficult to treat. Despite new developments in medications and technology, nonsteroidal anti-inflammatory drugs (NSAIDs) and opioids are among the most widely prescribed medications in the world [1, 2]. In addition to NSAIDs and opioids, adjunctive pharmacologic agents to include antidepressants, cannabinoids and ketamine have increased in popularity. This chapter aims to review commonly prescribed pain medications with a focus on their classification categories, mechanisms of action, and major side effect profiles.

2. NSAIDs

Nonsteroidal anti-inflammatory drugs (NSAIDs) were first introduced in the 1960s and are the most prescribed medication class in the world. The United States issues more than 100 million prescriptions annually [3] with approximately 20% of its citizens using NSAIDs on a frequent monthly basis at some point during their lifetime [4].

NSAIDs are a diverse group of compounds with varying chemical structures that possess anti-inflammatory, antipyretic, and analgesic properties [5]. They represent a class of drugs with a primary mechanism of action that involves inhibition of the pro-inflammatory cyclooxygenase (COX) enzymes. This includes both non-selective COX inhibitors (COX-1 and COX-2) including aspirin, indomethacin, and ibuprofen as well as the newer selective COX-2 inhibitors such as celecoxib. NSAIDs have an established short-term efficacy in the treatment of osteoarthritis (OA) and associated chronic low back pain as well as an opioid sparing effect when combined with most chronic pain management regimens [6, 7]. Despite the well-documented efficacy of NSAIDs, there are serious side effects associated with routine use that include gastrointestinal irritation (gastritis and ulceration of the stomach and small

IntechOpen

intestine), cardiovascular events (myocardial infarction, hypertension exacerbation) and renal toxicity (acute renal failure, electrolyte and fluid abnormalities).

2.1 Mechanism of action

Prostaglandins are lipid compounds that are physiologically active and have a diverse range of homeostatic and inflammatory effects in the human body that modulate fever and pain. They are the primary mediators of inflammatory cascades resulting in peripheral sensitization, hyperalgesia and chronic pain. Prostaglandin H_2 (PGH_2) is a common precursor for prostaglandins (PGE_2, PGI_2, and PGF_2) and thromboxane. It is synthesized from arachidonic acid via the rate limiting enzyme cyclooxygenase (COX) (**Figure 1**). By inhibiting the cyclooxygenase (COX) enzymes and thus inhibiting prostaglandin synthesis, NSAIDs are able to produce their analgesic and anti-inflammatory effects. COX exists in two isoforms, COX-1 and COX-2. COX-1 is expressed throughout the body and is a normal component of most cells. It is a necessary in the production of protective gastric mucosal secretions and regulation of gastric acid, promotion of platelet aggregation and the maintenance of renal blood flow [9]. COX-2, however, is minimally expressed and tightly regulated under normal conditions but is induced with the pro-inflammatory stimuli seen with cellular injury (IL-1, TNF-alpha tumor necrosis factor–alpha, and cytokines) [10]. Given some of the beneficial aspects of COX-1 and the specific pro-inflammatory aspect of COX-2, newer NSAIDs are directly targeted at selective

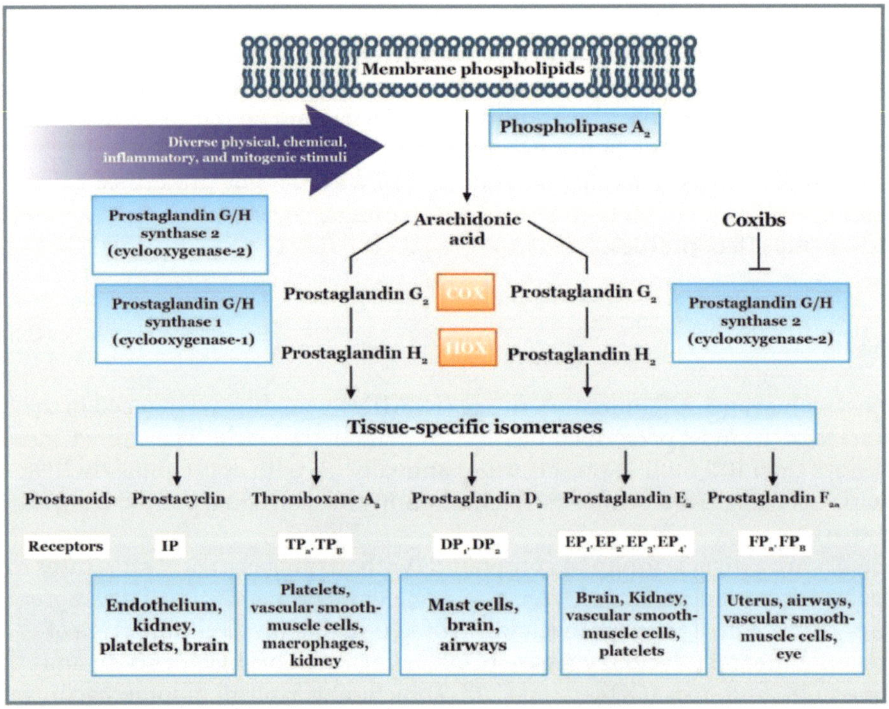

Arachidonic acid, a 20-carbon fatty acid containing four double bonds, is liberated from the *sn*2 position in membrane phospholipids by phospholipase A_2, which is activated by diverse stimuli. Arachidonic acid is converted by cytosolic prostaglandin G/H synthases, which have both cyclooxygenase (COX) and hydroperoxidase (HOX) activity, to the unstable intermediate prostaglandin H_2. The synthases are colloquially termed cyclooxygenases and exist in two forms, cyclooxygenase-1 and cyclooxygenase-2. Coxibs selectively inhibit cyclooxygenase-2. Prostaglandin H_2 is converted by tissue-specific isomerases to multiple prostanoids. These bioactive lipids activate specific cell-membrane receptors of the superfamily of G-protein–coupled receptors. Some of the tissues in which individual prostanoids exert prominent effects are indicated. IP denotes prostacyclin receptor, TP thromboxane receptor, DP prostaglandin D_2 receptor, EP prostaglandin E_2 receptor, and FP prostaglandin $F_{2\alpha}$ receptor.

Figure 1.
Production and actions of prostaglandins and thromboxane (adapted from [8]).

inhibition of COX-2 and are collectively referred to as coxibs. NSAIDs are otherwise non-selective in their inhibition of COX-1 and COX-2 although with varying affinity (**Table 1**).

2.2 Side effects

The same mechanism of action that provides the therapeutic effect of NSAIDs is also most commonly responsible for the side effects associated with chronic use. By inhibiting prostaglandin synthesis, NSAIDs increase the risk of gastrointestinal bleeding [12–16], thrombosis [17], and myocardial infarction [18]. COX-1 mediated synthesis of PGE_2 is responsible for gastric mucosa integrity. Inhibiting PGE_2

NSAID	COX-2 selectivity•	Gastrointestinal risk	Cardiovascular risk	Clinical use
Aspirin	Low	Moderate	Low	Prevention of cardiovascular events, mild pain, and inflammation
Ibuprofen	Moderate	Low	Moderate to high	Osteoarthritis, rheumatoid arthritis, fever, dysmenorrhea, mild to moderate pain, headache, migraine, myalgia
Diclofenac	High	Moderate	High	Osteoarthritis, rheumatoid arthritis, fever, dysmenorrhea, mild to moderate pain, migraine
Indomethacin	Low	Moderate to high	Moderate to high	Osteoarthritis, rheumatoid arthritis, bursitis, tendinitis, mild to moderate pain, or severe pain
Naproxen	Low	Moderate to high	Low	Gouty arthritis, mild to moderate pain, tendonitis, fever, rheumatoid disorders, osteoarthritis, dysmenorrhea, migraine prevention
Meloxicam	High	Low	Moderate to high	Osteoarthritis, rheumatoid arthritis
Celecoxib	High	Low	Moderate to high	Osteoarthritis, ankylosing spondylitis, rheumatoid arthritis, acute pain, dysmenorrhea

Adapted from [11].
**Only generic names provided. List not all inclusive. Keep in mind NSAIDs carry varying risks of rare liver toxicity and renal failure.*
•Selectivity is based on in vitro assay studies and should be interpreted with caution as different assay methods give different results. No assay method can predict what will happen when the drug is given to patients. Clinical studies are the best way to determine the effects of NSAIDs in patients.

Table 1.
*Safety comparison of some of the most commonly used NSAIDs.**

production with traditional non-selective NSAIDs results in gastric mucosal impairment and injury. Gastroduodenal ulcers are commonly identified with endoscopy after chronic non-selective NSAID use with double-blind trials showing incidence as high as 46% after 24 weeks of ibuprofen use [19]. Extra care must be taken with NSAID use in special populations including the elderly and those with underlying gastric irritation, stress related gastric mucosal injury (SRMD), and portal hypertensive gastropathy.

Given the side effects associated with inhibition of COX-1, especially the GI toxicity noted above, selective COX-2 inhibiting NSAIDs were created with the intention of avoiding harmful GI events while continuing to retain the anti-inflammatory and analgesic benefits of COX-2 antagonism. The selective COX-2 inhibition that occurs with coxibs (celecoxib, rofecoxib) was, however, believed to be associated with increased cardiovascular (CV) events including hypertension and thrombosis. The CV side effects are attributed to the imbalance in vascular tone and clotting hemostasis that is in part regulated by arachidonic metabolites; with COX-1 mediated TXA_2 being an inducer of platelet aggregation and COX-2 mediated PGI_2 being an inhibitor of platelet aggregation [20]. This is highlighted with PGI_2 receptor deficient mice being more prone to thrombosis then wild type mice [21]. Ultimately, large randomized controlled trials showed that celecoxib in moderate doses was non-inferior to naproxen or ibuprofen (non-selective NSAIDs) in regards to a primary outcome of cardiovascular causes of death [22].

3. Opioids

Opioids have been used for the management of pain since the earliest records of human history. The Sumerians of Mesopotamia were the first to cultivate the poppy plant [23]. Further refinement paralleled the advancement of human growth with the first extraction of morphine from opium occurring in 1803 [24]. New formulations, concentrations, and routes of delivery were developed and there was a simultaneous increase in medicinal as well as recreational use. Opiate use peaked between 1999 and 2017 and was responsible for approximately 400,000 overdose related deaths [25]. This has culminated into the current state of affairs where narcotic prescription abuse has become a national crisis with strict regulations on prescribing now in place. The fine balance between proper medical uses for the treatment of acute and chronic pain versus inappropriate overprescribing is being heavily scrutinized requiring careful consideration of the appropriateness of initiating opioids and the risks and benefits of chronic use. The importance of this is demonstrated with meta-analysis showing roughly 5% of patients prescribed an opioid for pain developing iatrogenic opioid dependence or abuse [26]. One must have an intimate understanding of the various opioid medications available and take a careful and strategized approach to prescribing a chronic regimen to suitably navigate this dilemma. Nonetheless, opioids remain a mainstay in the treatment of acute and chronic cancer related pain. This is in contrast to the benefit of opioids used in chronic non-malignant pain with studies continuing to show little to no benefit in quality of life or functional capacity [27, 28].

3.1 Mechanism of action

The classification of *opioid* commonly refers to all compounds that bind to the opiate receptors. This includes the naturally occurring alkaloids derived from the opium poppy (morphine, codeine), semi-synthetic opioids which are synthesized from naturally occurring opiates (oxycodone, heroin) and fully synthetic opioids (methadone, fentanyl). Opioids as a class are similar in that they all cause analgesia and have a common side effect profile. Opioid drugs impart their effects primarily through three receptors: Mu (μ), Delta (δ), and Kappa (κ) (**Table 2**). These receptors are found both peripherally and centrally and can be activated all along the neuroaxis including the cortex, brainstem, interneurons of the spinal cord and the nociceptors at the level of the primary sensory neurons. Activation of these receptors is responsible for both the analgesic properties of opioids as well as the major side effects. All opioid receptors are G-protein coupled receptors that inhibit adenylyl cyclase, decreasing conductance of voltage-gated Ca++ channels and/or opening rectifying K+ channels (**Figure 2**). This ultimately prevents calcium influx and the release of pronociceptive neurotransmitters (glutamate, substance P, and calcitonin gene-related peptide from the nociceptive fibers) [31]. By preventing the release of these pain-promoting neurotransmitters, opioids are able to impart their analgesic properties.

3.2 Opioid receptors

Mu receptors are largely thought of as the primary receptor responsible for analgesia with opioids; thus, the term "mu agonist" is often used to describe opioids used for the management of pain. Mu opioid receptors (MOR) are found in high density at the periaqueductal gray (PAG) of the midbrain. Agonism of MOR in this region is thought to eliminate a tonic gamma aminobutyric acid (GABA) tone thus

	Mu (μ)	**Delta (δ)**	**Kappa (κ)**
	Mu 1: Analgesia Mu 2: Sedation, vomiting, respiratory depression, pruritus, euphoria, anorexia, urinary retention, physical dependence	Analgesia, spinal analgesia	Analgesia, sedation, dyspnea, psychomimetic effects, miosis, respiratory depression, euphoria, dysphoria, dyspnea
Endogenous peptides			
Enkephalins	Agonist	Agonist	
Beta-endorphin	Agonist	Agonist	
Dynorphin A	Agonist		Agonist
Agonists			
Morphine	Agonist		Weak agonist
Codeine	Weak agonist	Weak agonist	
Fentanyl	Agonist		
Meperidine	Agonist	Agonist	
Methadone	Agonist		
Antagonists			
Naloxone	Antagonist	Weak antagonist	Antagonist
Naltrexone	Antagonist	Weak antagonist	Antagonist
Adapted from [29, 30].			

Table 2.
Analgesic effects at opioid receptors.

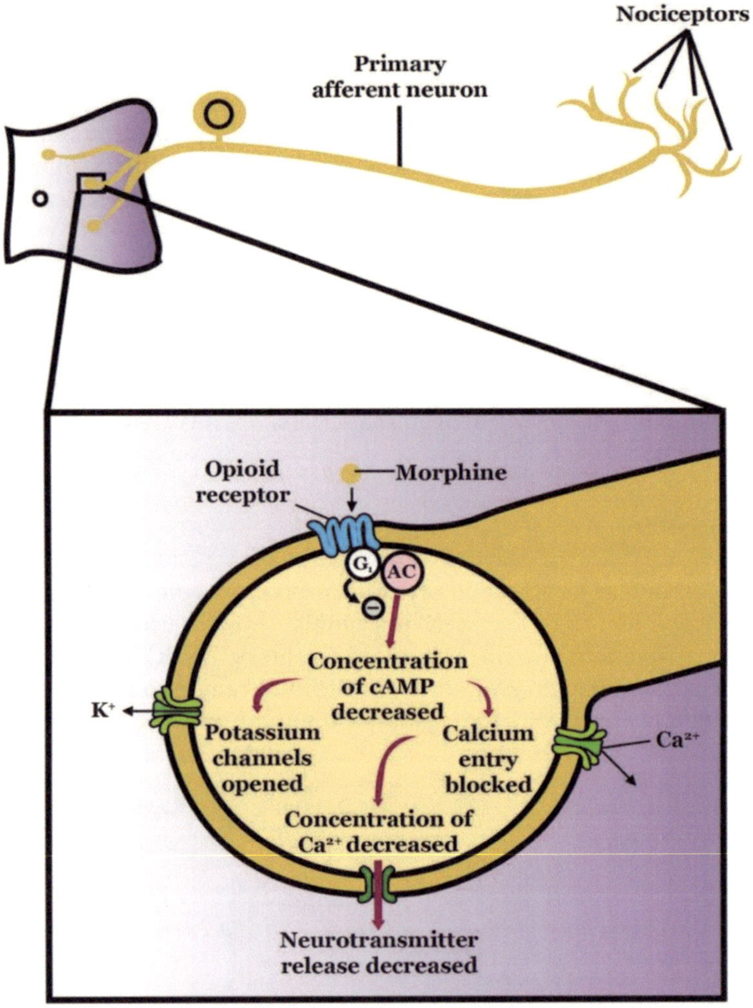

Figure 2.
Mechanisms of opioid action in the spinal cord.

indirectly stimulating descending inhibitory pathways at the level of the spinal cord [32]. MOR receptors are also in high density on dorsal horn neurons and elicit their analgesic effect through inhibition of glutamine release decreasing the transmission of nociceptive information from A-delta and C nerve fibers.

The drugs that are able to fully activate these mu receptors in a dose dependent fashion are referred to as full agonists. This is in contrast to the drugs that are either weak agonists at the mu receptor (while preventing other full agonists from binding) or are antagonists at the mu receptor while being an agonist at another receptor. These are referred to as agonist-antagonist drugs and include buprenorphine+naloxone (suboxone), nalbuphine, and pentazocine. Reversal of the effects caused by mu agonists is accomplished with competing antagonists (naloxone), which are crucial in the medical management of opioid overdoses and the associated respiratory depression. Kappa and delta receptors also contribute to analgesia and the other clinical effects seen with acute and chronic use including respiratory depression and sedation. Kappa receptors, in particular, are localized in the brain stem and spinal cord and are chiefly responsible for providing spinal analgesia [29]. Opioid receptors also bind to endogenous opioid peptides (endorphins, enkephalins, and dynorphins), which are important in overall pain modulation.

The clinical use of opioids is dependent upon more than just the receptor specificity and relies on deep understanding of the pharmacokinetics of these drugs for optimal use. In a basic sense, opioids can be classified into either short or long acting agents although this terminology inappropriately simplifies complex pharmacodynamic and pharmacokinetic properties of these drugs.

3.3 Side effects

The interaction between exogenous opioids and opioid receptor activation has a diverse side effect profile with variable differences seen with acute and chronic use. These side effects include constipation, nausea and vomiting, hyperalgesia, opioid induced hormonal changes, and respiratory depression. Opioid induced constipation (OIC) is one of the most commonly seen side effects with roughly one half of patients experiencing OIC with long-term use [33]. OIC can cause significant morbidity with associated adverse effects including fecal impaction with obstruction, reflux, dyspepsia, cramping/pain, and lengthened hospitalization [34]. For this reason, all chronic opioid regimens should include prophylactic laxatives. Mu opioid receptors are abundant in the respiratory rhythm generating regions of the brainstem and pons. Agonism of these receptors causes opioid induced breathing alterations including significant reduction in respiratory rate and minute ventilation with associated hypercapnia. This can ultimately lead to fatal apnea, especially with lipophilic opioids and intravenous administration that allows for quick equilibration at the effect compartment (central respiratory centers) [35]. Given the euphoria that occurs with opioids, addiction is another potential iatrogenic side effect seen with acute and chronic use. This can be associated with tolerance to opioids, which is defined as a decreased objective and subjective effect with a stable dose over time as well as requiring increasing amount of an opioid to achieve the same effect. Increasing tolerance also develops to the other effects of opioids including respiratory depression [24]. This is problematic in patients abusing opioids given the tendency for relapse back to a previous dose that will now cause profound respiratory depression due to the loss of tolerance during abstinence.

4. Antidepressants

Antidepressants have a long established efficacy in the treatment of neuropathic predominant chronic pain disorders [36]. Neuropathic pain disorders develop from a multitude of disease processes that directly arise from lesions or other damage to the central or peripheral somatosensory nervous system [37]. Associated diseases and processes include diabetes mellitus (diabetic peripheral neuropathy), HIV (HIV polyneuropathy), herpes zoster (post-herpetic neuralgia), and medical interventions (e.g., post-mastectomy pain, chemotherapy). Tricyclic antidepressants (TCAs) including amitriptyline, imipramine, and nortriptyline are routinely used as first line options in the management of neuropathic pain [36, 38]. TCAs can be started and maintained at doses lower than the doses used in depression thus reducing some of the side effects commonly seen at depression doses such as dry mouth, sedation, urinary retention and orthostatic hypotension. TCAs must be used cautiously in patients taking other serotonergic drugs or in patients with a history of cardiovascular disorders, glaucoma, or urinary retention given the anticholinergic side effects TCAs can produce. Of note, TCAs are beneficial to both depressed and non-depressed patients as well as having the added value of helping with depression in the depressed subpopulation [36]. Serotonin-norepinephrine reuptake inhibitors (SNRIs) are also commonly used in the management of chronic pain with duloxetine having FDA approval for the management of fibromyalgia and venlafaxine showing superiority to placebo in the treatment of diabetic neuropathy [39, 40].

The primary mechanism of action of TCAs in the treatment of neuropathic pain involves the reuptake inhibition of norepinephrine (NE) and serotonin (5-hydroxytryptamine [5-HT]), which causes a blockade of the neuronal membrane ion channels and increases the activation of descending inhibitory pathways in the midbrain and spinal cord [41, 42]. SNRIs also elicit their effect through inhibition of NE and 5-HT blocking their role in descending pain pathways.

5. Cannabinoids

The term cannabinoid is used to collectively describe all naturally occurring and synthetic compounds that are structurally similar to and elicit similar effects as the cannabinoid plants, most notably *cannabis*. In addition to the cannabinoids derived from plants (phytocannabinoids), there are also endogenously produced cannabinoids (endocannabinoids) and synthetic cannabinoids now being produced for medical use. Endocannabinoids are fundamental in human homeostasis with established behavioral, metabolic, immunologic, and physiologic functions [43]. Cannabinoids bind to two isotypes of G protein coupled receptors, CB_1 and CB_2 [44]. The CB_1 receptor is found predominantly in the CNS including the brain, spinal cord, and the sensory nerve terminals and along primary pain pathways. Activation of CB_1 receptors at these sites results in membrane hyperpolarization and the modulation of nociceptive neurotransmitters contributing to both the pain relief and psychotomimetic properties of cannabinoids [45]. This reduced pain with cannabinoid receptor agonists can occur at multiple levels of the CNS both peripherally and centrally. CB_2 receptors are concentrated in the hematopoietic cells of the immune system and are involved in a diverse range of immunomodulatory effects including the inhibition of cytokine release [46, 47].

Cannabis contains over 500 chemical compounds including over 150 phytocannabinoids with the most studied being Δ^9-tetrahydrocannabinol (THC) and cannabidiol (CBD). THC is the chief psychotropic compound of *cannabis* and is found in varying concentrations in different strains of the plant. THC has a strong affinity for CB_1, which is regarded as the primary receptor responsible for the psychoactive effects seen with cannabis. In contrast, CBD does not activate CB_1 so it does not produce psychoactive effects and is associated more with the anti-inflammatory effects of cannabinoids [48]. There are currently three cannabinoid drugs available for use in the United States. Epidolex® is a CBD based drug used to treat epileptic disorders and is derived from cannabis. Dronabinol and Nabilone are synthetic THC compounds approved for use in chemotherapy associated nausea and as an appetite stimulant in HIV/AIDS [49]. Molecular and preclinical evidence continues to support the anti-nociceptive properties of cannabinoids although experimental human studies are more heterogeneous with varying results although ongoing research is being conducted [50]. With major legislative changes in the USA, thirty-three states and the District of Columbia have passed laws broadly legalizing cannabis in some form at the time of this writing.

6. Ketamine

Ketamine is a dissociative analgesic and amnestic medication that acts as a non-competitive antagonist of the N-Methyl-D-Aspartate (NMDA) receptor in the central nervous system [51]. It has been used since the 1960s as an anesthetic agent and continues to be studied and adapted for novel psychiatric and anesthetic purposes. Ketamine has multiple sites of drug action but its principal nociceptive effects occur at the NMDA receptors. NMDA receptors have dense expression in the temporal cortex, hippocampus, basal ganglia, cerebellum and brain stem and are known to contribute to the neuronal process that mediate nociception via activation by glutamate, an excitatory amino acid [52]. By targeting this receptor, ketamine has profound attenuating effects on ascending nociceptive transmission and amplification of descending inhibitory pathways [52, 53]. Ketamine is currently utilized in the management of many diseases and other applications including the management of chronic pain disorders (e.g., complex regional pain syndrome, phantom limb pain, fibromyalgia), acute pain, conscious sedation, and intraoperatively for antihyperalgesia and induction of anesthesia [54].

7. Conclusions

NSAIDs have been used historically to treat both acute and chronic pain. They possess analgesic, antipyretic, and anti-inflammatory properties through the inhibition of the pro-inflammatory cyclooxygenase (COX) enzymes. Their mechanism of action allows them to establish efficacy in treating a variety of pain diseases but also allows their routine use to produce serious side effects. COX-1 receptors are expressed throughout our body and its inhibition can lead to gastric mucosal injury including gastroduodenal ulcers. Selective COX-2 inhibitors were created with hopes of avoiding the side effects connected with non-selective COX-inhibitors; however, they are associated with their own complications which include an increased risk for cardiovascular events (thrombosis and hypertension).

Opioids remain a popular option in treating pain due to their effect on the Mu (μ), Delta (δ), and Kappa (κ) receptors. By activating these receptors, opioids can prevent the release of pain-promoting neurotransmitters providing their analgesic effects. However, the activation of the same receptors is also responsible for the associated side effects. These side effects vary depending on either acute or chronic use but can be life-threatening in some cases. This includes respiratory depression which can lead to fatal apnea. Chronic opioid use is associated with opioid induced constipation that can cause significant morbidity. It is therefore recommended to include prophylactic laxatives with chronic regimens. It is important to remember that addiction and tolerance is associated with opioid use due to its euphoric effect. Therefore, the clinical use of these medications should not only depend on their mechanism of action but also on understanding the potential severe complications that arise with their use.

Neuropathic chronic pain disorders have been effectively treated with antidepressants. These disorders include, but are not limited to, diabetic peripheral neuropathy, HIV polyneuropathy, and post-herpetic neuralgia. One of the first line options are the tricyclic antidepressants (TCAs) which are usually started and maintained at lower doses versus the depression doses. This helps reduce some of their side effects including urinary retention, sedation, and dry mouth. Other antidepressants include serotonin-norepinephrine reuptake inhibitors that are also used in the management of neuropathic disorders.

Cannabinoids exhibit their effects by binding to CB_1 and CB_2 receptors, two isotypes of G-protein coupled receptors. The agonism of these receptors is responsible for cannabinoids' anti-inflammatory and analgesic effects. CB_1 receptor agonism is also predominately responsible for the psychoactive effect. Preclinical evidence supports anti-nociceptive effects and with recent legalization of cannabis, the use of cannabinoids to treat pain disorders will expand with ongoing research.

Ketamine has many uses in treating both acute and chronic pain including fibromyalgia. It is also used for conscious sedation due to both its dissociative and amnestic properties. Ketamine has multiple sites of interactions but it exhibits its principle nociceptive effect by acting as a non-competitive antagonist of the N-Methyl-D-Aspartate (NDMA) receptor.

Author details

Coti Phillips[1*], Edwin Contreras[2] and Jessica Oswald[1,3,4]

1 Department of Anesthesiology, University of California San Diego, La Jolla, United States

2 Department of Emergency Medicine, Kaiser Permanente Southern California, San Diego, United States

3 Center for Pain Management, University of California San Diego, La Jolla, United States

4 Department of Emergency Medicine, University of California San Diego, La Jolla, United States

*Address all correspondence to: cotiphillips@gmail.com

References

[1] Alam, A. and D.N. Juurlink, *The prescription opioid epidemic: an overview for anesthesiologists.* Canadian Journal of Anesthesia/Journal canadien d'anesthésie, 2016. 63(1): p. 61-68.

[2] Laine, L., *Approaches to nonsteroidal anti-inflammatory drug use in the high-risk patient.* Gastroenterology, 2001. 120(3): p. 594-606.

[3] and, A.A.C., t.D.S.a.R.M. Advisory, and Committee, *FDA Briefing Document: Joint Meeting of the Arthritis Advisory Committee and the Drug Safety and Risk Management Advisory Committee* A. Division of Anesthesia, and Addiction Products (DAAAP) Editor. 2018.

[4] Paulose-Ram, R., et al., *Frequent monthly use of selected non-prescription and prescription non-narcotic analgesics among U.S. adults.* Pharmacoepidemiology and Drug Safety, 2005. 14(4): p. 257-266.

[5] Vane, J.R., *The fight against rheumatism: from willow bark to COX-1 sparing drugs.* J Physiol Pharmacol, 2000. 51(4 Pt 1): p. 573-86.

[6] Bjordal, J.M., *Non-steroidal anti-inflammatory drugs, including cyclo-oxygenase-2 inhibitors, in osteoarthritic knee pain: meta-analysis of randomised placebo controlled trials.* 2004. 329(7478): p. 1317-0.

[7] Romsing, J., et al., *Reduction of opioid-related adverse events using opioid-sparing analgesia with COX-2 inhibitors lacks documentation: A systematic review.* Acta Anaesthesiologica Scandinavica, 2005. 49(2): p. 133-142.

[8] Fitzgerald, G.A. and C. Patrono, *The Coxibs, Selective Inhibitors of Cyclooxygenase-2.* New England Journal of Medicine, 2001. 345(6): p. 433-442.

[9] Matsui, H., et al., *The pathophysiology of non-steroidal anti-inflammatory drug (NSAID)-induced mucosal injuries in stomach and small intestine.* 2011. 48(2): p. 107-111.

[10] Crofford, L.J., *COX-1 and COX-2 tissue expression: implications and predictions.* J Rheumatol Suppl, 1997. 49: p. 15-9.

[11] *Managing NSAID risks.* Pharmacist's Letter, 2015. September.

[12] *Vascular and upper gastrointestinal effects of non-steroidal anti-inflammatory drugs: meta-analyses of individual participant data from randomised trials.* The Lancet, 2013. 382(9894): p. 769-779.

[13] García Rodríguez, L. and H. Jick, *Risk of upper gastrointestinal bleeding and perforation associated with Individual non-steroidal anti-inflammatory drugs.* 1994. 343(8900): p. 769-772.

[14] Harirforoosh, S., W. Asghar, and F. Jamali, *Adverse Effects of Nonsteroidal Antiinflammatory Drugs: An Update of Gastrointestinal, Cardiovascular and Renal Complications.* Journal of Pharmacy & Pharmaceutical Sciences, 2014. 16(5): p. 821.

[15] Hernández-Díaz, S. and L.A.G. Rodríguez, *Association Between Nonsteroidal Anti-inflammatory Drugs and Upper Gastrointestinal Tract Bleeding/Perforation.* Archives of Internal Medicine, 2000. 160(14): p. 2093.

[16] Laine, L., K. Takeuchi, and A. Tarnawski, *Gastric Mucosal Defense and Cytoprotection: Bench to Bedside.* 2008. 135(1): p. 41-60.

[17] Kearney, P.M., et al., *Do selective cyclo-oxygenase-2 inhibitors and*

traditional non-steroidal anti-inflammatory drugs increase the risk of atherothrombosis? Meta-analysis of randomised trials. BMJ, 2006. 332(7553): p. 1302-1308.

[18] Davis, A. and J. Robson, *The dangers of NSAIDs: look both ways.* 2016. 66(645): p. 172-173.

[19] Hawkey, C., et al., *Comparison of the effect of rofecoxib (a cyclooxygenase 2 inhibitor), ibuprofen, and placebo on the gastroduodenal mucosa of patients with osteoarthritis: A randomized, double-blind, placebo-controlled trial.* Arthritis & Rheumatism, 2000. 43(2): p. 370.

[20] Zarraga, I.G.E. and E.R. Schwarz, *Coxibs and Heart Disease.* Journal of the American College of Cardiology, 2007. 49(1): p. 1-14.

[21] Cheng, Y., *Role of Prostacyclin in the Cardiovascular Response to Thromboxane A2.* Science, 2002. 296(5567): p. 539-541.

[22] Nissen, S.E., et al., *Cardiovascular Safety of Celecoxib, Naproxen, or Ibuprofen for Arthritis.* New England Journal of Medicine, 2016. 375(26): p. 2519-2529.

[23] Schiff, P.L., *Opium and its alkaloids.* Vol. 66. 2002. 186-194.

[24] Rosenblum, A., et al., *Opioids and the treatment of chronic pain: controversies, current status, and future directions.* Experimental and clinical psychopharmacology, 2008. 16(5): p. 405-416.

[25] Scholl, L., et al., *Drug and Opioid-Involved Overdose Deaths - United States, 2013-2017.* MMWR. Morbidity and mortality weekly report, 2018. 67(5152): p. 1419-1427.

[26] Higgins, C., B.H. Smith, and K. Matthews, *Incidence of iatrogenic opioid dependence or abuse in patients with pain who were exposed to opioid analgesic therapy: a systematic review and meta-analysis.* British Journal of Anaesthesia, 2018. 120(6): p. 1335-1344.

[27] Eriksen, J., et al., *Critical issues on opioids in chronic non-cancer pain: an epidemiological study.* Pain, 2006. 125 (1-2): p. 172-9.

[28] Stein, C., H. Reinecke, and H. Sorgatz, *Opioid use in chronic noncancer pain: guidelines revisited.* Curr Opin Anaesthesiol, 2010. 23(5): p. 598-601.

[29] Trescot, A.M., et al., *Opioid pharmacology.* Pain Physician, 2008. 11(2 Suppl): p. S133-53.

[30] *Miller, Ronald D. Miller's Anesthesia. 7th ed. Philadelphia, PA: Churchill Livingstone/Elsevier, 2010.*

[31] Stein, C. and C. Zollner, *Opioids and sensory nerves.* Handb Exp Pharmacol, 2009(194): p. 495-518.

[32] Williams, J., *Basic Opioid Pharmacology.* Reviews in Pain, 2008. 1(2): p. 2-5.

[33] Neefjes, E.C., et al., *Clinical evaluation of the efficacy of methylnaltrexone in resolving constipation induced by different opioid subtypes combined with laboratory analysis of immunomodulatory and antiangiogenic effects of methylnaltrexone.* BMC Palliative Care, 2014. 13(1): p. 42.

[34] Webster, L.R., *Opioid-Induced Constipation.* Pain Medicine, 2015. 16(suppl 1): p. S16-S21.

[35] Boom, M., et al., *Non-analgesic effects of opioids: opioid-induced respiratory depression.* Curr Pharm Des, 2012. 18(37): p. 5994-6004.

[36] O'Connor, A.B. and R.H. Dworkin, *Treatment of Neuropathic Pain: An Overview of Recent Guidelines.* 2009. 122(10): p. S22-S32.

[37] Pain, I.A.f.t.S.o. *Taxonomy.* Taxonomy#Neuropathicpain 2016 December 14, 2017 [cited 2019 June 26th].

[38] Wright, M.E. and D. Rizzolo, *An update on the pharmacologic management and treatment of neuropathic pain.* Jaapa, 2017. 30(3): p. 13-17.

[39] Arnold, L.M., et al., *A double-blind, multicenter trial comparing duloxetine with placebo in the treatment of fibromyalgia patients with or without major depressive disorder.* Arthritis & Rheumatism, 2004. 50(9): p. 2974-2984.

[40] Rowbotham, M.C., et al., *Venlafaxine extended release in the treatment of painful diabetic neuropathy: a double-blind, placebo-controlled study.* Pain, 2004. 110(3): p. 697-706.

[41] Beal, B.R. and M.S. Wallace, *An Overview of Pharmacologic Management of Chronic Pain.* Medical Clinics of North America, 2016. 100(1): p. 65-79.

[42] Jan, H.V., *Mechanisms and Treatment of Neuropathic Pain.* Central Nervous System Agents in Medicinal Chemistry, 2009. 9(1): p. 71-78.

[43] Amin, M.R. and D.W. Ali, *Pharmacology of Medical Cannabis.* Adv Exp Med Biol, 2019. 1162: p. 151-165.

[44] Pertwee, R.G., *Pharmacological Actions of Cannabinoids*. Springer-Verlag. p. 1-51.

[45] Sharon, H. and S. Brill, *Cannabis-based medicines for chronic pain management: current and future prospects.* Curr Opin Anaesthesiol, 2019.

[46] Schatz, A.R., et al., *Cannabinoid Receptors CB1 and CB2: A Characterization of Expression and Adenylate Cyclase Modulation within the Immune System.* 1997. 142(2): p. 278-287.

[47] Pertwee, R.G., *The pharmacology of cannabinoid receptors and their ligands: an overview.* International Journal of Obesity, 2006. 30(S1): p. S13-S18.

[48] Klauke, A.L., et al., *The cannabinoid CB2 receptor-selective phytocannabinoid beta-caryophyllene exerts analgesic effects in mouse models of inflammatory and neuropathic pain.* European Neuropsychopharmacology, 2014. 24(4): p. 608-620.

[49] Urits, I., et al., *An Update of Current Cannabis-Based Pharmaceuticals in Pain Medicine.* Pain and Therapy, 2019. 8(1): p. 41-51.

[50] Lötsch, J., I. Weyer-Menkhoff, and I. Tegeder, *Current evidence of cannabinoid-based analgesia obtained in preclinical and human experimental settings.* European Journal of Pain, 2018. 22(3): p. 471-484.

[51] Moyse, D.W., et al., *Perioperative Ketamine Administration for Thoracotomy Pain.* Pain Physician, 2017. 20(3): p. 173-184.

[52] Niesters, M., et al., *Effect of Subanesthetic Ketamine on Intrinsic Functional Brain Connectivity.* 2012. 117(4): p. 868-877.

[53] Schwartzman, R.J., et al., *Neuropathic Central Pain.* Archives of Neurology, 2001. 58(10): p. 1547.

[54] Maher, D.P., L. Chen, and J. Mao, *Intravenous Ketamine Infusions for Neuropathic Pain Management.* Anesthesia & Analgesia, 2017. 124(2): p. 661-674.

Chapter 16

Analgesic Potential of Monoterpenes from Citrus Essential Oils

Ines Banjari, Jelena Balkić and Viduranga Yashasvi Waisundara

Abstract

Chronic pain is a noteworthy health issue with immense impact on global healthcare systems. Although this issue has not come into the limelight as other noncommunicable diseases, it should be highlighted that modern medicine still has no efficient treatment to curb chronic pain. In this aspect, essential oils have been used for the prevention of several disease conditions including pain management. These odorous products, obtained from botanically defined raw material, have a variable and complex composition. Their composition largely depends on the extraction technique used, from simple hydro-distillation, to supercritical or microwave-assisted extraction. Monoterpenoids are some of the most biologically active and highly researched compounds when it comes to antinociceptive effects. They are volatile oils, primarily composed of two isoprene units with highly distinctive aromas and flavors. More than 90% of the essential oils of medicinal plants consist of monoterpenoids like limonene, myrcene, α-terpineol, linalool, pinene, *p*-cymene, and nerol. Besides strong anti-inflammatory effect, all essential oils with high D-limonene content pose a significant free radical scavenging effect, predominantly disabling the production of reactive oxygen species. Further studies in humans are encouraged to determine the real long-term potential in treating chronic pain.

Keywords: chronic pain, essential oils, citruses, monoterpenes, limonene

1. Introduction

Chronic pain is defined as a long-term pain lasting 3–6 months after the normal healing period, and is described as continuous or recurrent [1]. The European Pain Federation (EFIC) in its Declaration on Pain identifies chronic pain as a distinct health issue, which has an immense financial impact on healthcare systems around the world [2]. In Europe, 20% of adults or one in five suffer from chronic pain, and about 34% of them describe their chronic pain as severe [3]. In the U.S., estimated prevalence among adults ranges from 11 to 40% [4]. Estimated total cost of the consequences of chronic pain across Europe is €300 billion [3], while the annual healthcare cost for back pain only was estimated to be £13.44 billion in Germany and £1 billion in UK [5].

Chronic pain alters all aspects of a patient's life inducing severe physical, psychological, and social impairments, while increasing consumption of opiates and analgesics. It eventually deteriorates an individual's quality of life [1, 3, 5].

The most common sites affected, according to a UK population study, are the lower back [30%], hip [25%], neck and shoulder (25%), and knee (24%) [6]. The underlying pathophysiology of chronic pain is usually complex, and can be explained by the presence of typical inflammation and neuropathy [7].

Modern medicine still has no efficient treatment to deal with chronic pain. Essential oils have been used to prevent and treat diseases for many centuries [8] and have been proven to pose antibacterial, antifungal, antiproliferative, anti-inflammatory, antioxidant, and anesthetic properties, although the exact mechanisms of action are still elusive [8, 9]. Recent meta-analysis by Lakhan et al. [10] found a significant positive effect of aromatherapy [compared with placebo or treatments as usual controls] in reducing pain intensity, with the strongest evidence for nociceptive and acute pain, unlike inflammatory and chronic pain. The aim of this chapter is to summarize the existing evidence on the effectiveness of Citrus essential oils, that is, their monoterpenes and especially limonene, for the treatment of chronic pain.

2. Essential oils

One of the modalities where plants have been put to use is aromatherapy, where they can be diffused aromatically, consumed internally, or applied topically to the skin [8, 11]. In general, the respiratory tract offers the most rapid way of entry of oils followed by the dermal pathway [12]. The main beneficial constituents present in essential oils are the monoterpenes, sesquiterpenes, and phenylpropanoids [9]. Citrus essential oils have been used for millennia to treat anxiety, agitation, stress, challenging behaviors, fatigue, and insomnia [11]. Composition of selected essential Citrus oils is given in **Table 1**, along with their beneficial health effects. The composition of a specific essential oil will vary significantly depending on the extraction technique used.

3. Extraction techniques of essential oils

There are several extraction techniques that are commonly used for the isolation and purification of bioactives from herbs used as pain medications. A summary of these techniques is shown in **Figure 1**. Most of these bioactives are extracted together with the essential oils of the herbs. It is important that the selected extraction technique is compatible with the bioactives as well as the herb, and is efficient in obtaining as much quantity as possible while preserving the functionality.

Techniques commonly employed for extracting essential oils include hydro-distillation, steam distillation, solvent extraction, head space analysis, and liquid CO_2 extraction [37]. Head space analysis is a potentially rapid method, which is used to extract essential oils and requires very little plant material, but a complete recovery may occur only for highly volatile materials. Conventional methods such as steam distillation and solvent extraction may result in severe losses of volatile materials because the liquid in which the oil is collected should be subsequently removed by evaporation. Application of heat in this instance is a disadvantage.

Ultrasound has been recently applied to improve the extraction of polysaccharides and essential oils from plant material that is used for pain medication, mainly through the phenomenon of cavitation [38–41]. Chemat et al. [41] prepared hexane extracts of two caraway seeds focusing on the carvone and limonene contents which were isolated in the process. The study demonstrated that the carvone yield and plant extract quality were better in ultrasound extraction compared with those obtained by conventional methodologies.

Essential oil		Main constituents	Health effects	Reference	Chemical structures of some key monoterpenes [13]
Common name	Latin name				
Sweet orange	*Citrus sinensis* L.	Limonene (66.8–80.9%), β-myrcene (3.76–6.28%), α-pinene (1.65–2.48%)	• High antioxidant activity in linoleic acid system	[14–17]	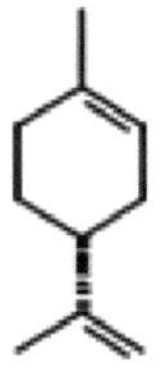 *d*-Limonene
Bitter orange	*Citrus aurantium* L.	Limonene (51.3–98.173%), α-pinene (0.476%), and β-pinene (0.176%)	• Mild sedative and hypnotic (calming) effect, motor relaxant effects, decreases the symptoms of anxiety • Gastroprotective properties • High free radical scavanging properties	[13, 18–21]	
Neroli	*Citrus aurantium* L.	Linalool (29%), linalyl acetate (20%), β-pinene (3%), limonene (5%), nerolidol (9%), E-farnesol (5.14%)	• Decreases the symptoms of anxiety, improves mood, and creates a sense of well-being by regulating serotonine receptors • Anti-inflammatory activity against acute and chronic inflammation • Central and peripheral antinociceptive effects (due to high linalool content) • Decreases the abdominal constriction via inhibition of prostaglandin production	[13, 21–23]	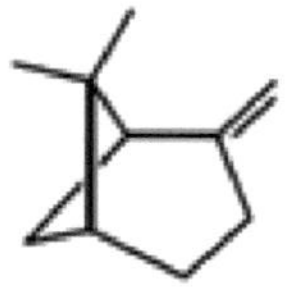 β-Pinene
Orange Petitgrain	*Citrus aurantium* L.	Linalyl acetate (28.94–50.0%), linalool (36.10%), α-terpineol (6.80%)	• Free radical scavanging ability	[13, 22, 24]	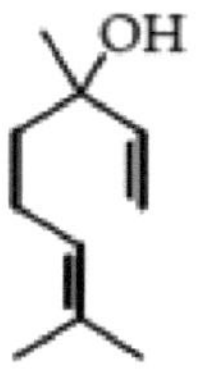 Linalool

Essential oil		Main constituents	Health effects	Reference	Chemical structures of some key monoterpenes [13]
Common name	Latin name				
Mandarin	*Citrus reticulata* Blanco	Limonene (64–71%), β-myrcene (3.27–4.05%), decanal (2.33–7.71%), linalool (1.10–2.56%)	• Moderate radical scavenging activity	[13–15]	
Bergamot	*Citrus aurantium subsp. bergamia* (Risso & Poit.)	Limonene (25–53%), linalool (2–20%), linalyl acetate (15–40%), bergamottin (furanocoumarins)	• Good radical scavenging activity	[25–28]	
Lemon	*Citrus limon* (L.) Osbeck	D-Limonene and L-limonene (52.77%), β-pinene (10.80%), myrcene (10.16%)	• Significant antioxidant effect (preventing lipoperoxidation especially at a high dose)	[9, 11, 16, 29]	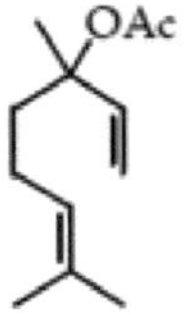 Linalyl acetate
Key Lime	*Citrus aurantifolia*	Limonene (52.2%), γ-terpinene (17.0%), α-pinene (3.2%), and β-pinene (13.0%)	• Relieve common cold, flu, asthma, arthritis • High radical scavenging activity • Anti-inflammatory effects via reduced cell migration, cytokine production, and protein extravasation	[13, 30–32]	

Essential oil		Main constituents	Health effects	Reference	Chemical structures of some key monoterpenes [13]
Common name	**Latin name**				
Sweet lime	*Citrus limetta*	Limonene (85–95%), camphene (1.78%), ρ-cymene (0.38%), geraniol (0.36%), α-terpinene (0.33%), α-terpineol (0.31%), neral (0.29%), β-bisabolene (0.12%)	• Strong antioxidant, antibacterial, and antifungal activity	[33]	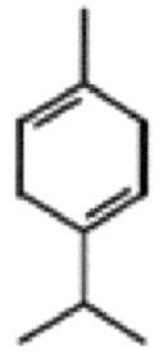 γ-Terpinene
Grapefruit	*Citrus paradisii* Macfady	Limonene (50.8–86.27%), β-myrcene (3.51–6.20%), α-terpinene (2.11%), linalool oxide (2.29–6.52%), nootkatone (8.47–25.4%)	• Moderate antioxidant activity in linoleic acid system	[14–16, 34]	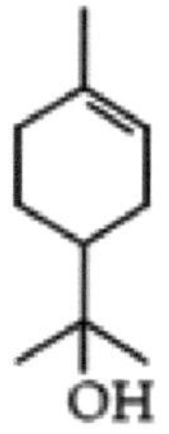 α-Terpineol
Yuzu or Yuja	*Citrus junos* Sieb. ex Tanaka	Limonene (63.1–68.1%), γ-terpinene (11.4–12.5%), β-phellandrene (4.6–5.4%), myrcence (3.0–3.2%), and α-pinene (2.3–2.7%)	• Anti-inflammatory properties (ability to inhibit the production of cytokines and ROS and reduces eosinophil migration) • Decreases total mood disturbance and tension-anxiety	[13, 35]	

Essential oil		Main constituents	Health effects	Reference	Chemical structures of some key monoterpenes [13]
Common name	Latin name				
Palestinian or Indian sweet lime	*Citrus limettioides* Tanaka	D-Limonene (89.089%), β-myrcene (2.933%), (±)-linalool (2.927%), α-pinene (0.865%), (E)-citral (0.749%)	• Antibacterial and antifungal activity • For acne control, for the treatment of various infectious diseases (e.g., typhoid fever), food poisoning, inflammation, sepsis, endocarditis, bladder, prostate, and epididymal infections	[36]	

Table 1.
Composition of selected essential Citrus oils and observed health effects.

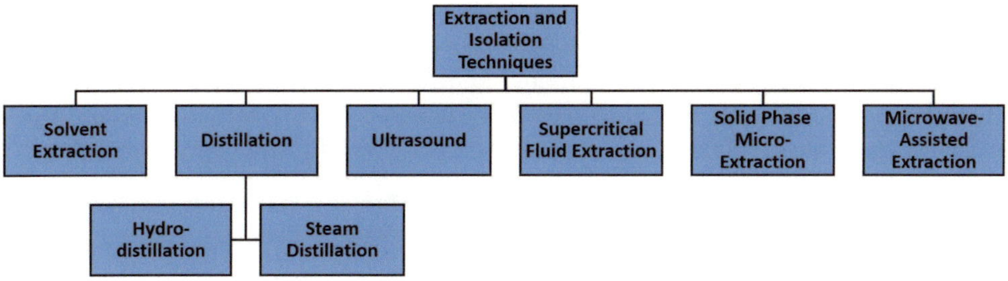

Figure 1.
Common extraction techniques used for the preparation of essential oils and their bioactives.

Supercritical extraction (SFE) of the compounds responsible for the mitigating pain contained in herbs is another favorable technique that can be used for industrial-scale yielding of the responsible bioactives [42, 43]. Microwave-assisted extraction (MAE) is another method that is typically used for the extraction of bioactives for pain medication [44]. This technique offers a rapid delivery of energy to a total volume of solvent and solid herb matrix with subsequent heating of the solvent and solid matrix, efficiently and homogeneously [40]. Accelerated solvent extraction (ASE) is a solid-liquid extraction process performed to isolate bioactives for pain medication at elevated temperatures, usually between 50 and 200°C and at pressures between 10 and 15 MPa [40]. Solvent-free microwave extraction (SFME) is considered as a green method for the extraction of essential oils from herbs for pain medication. The methodology is a combination of microwave heating and dry distillation performed at atmospheric pressure without any added solvent or water [45].

4. Bioactive components in essential oils

One of the most biologically active and best studied herbal compounds are monoterpenoids, which consist of two isoprene units, but contain a wide variety of structures. They are volatile oils with highly distinctive aromas and flavors. More than 90% of the essential oils of medicinal plants consist of monoterpenoids [46]. Most studies analyzing analgesic potential of essential oils were tested on animal models [47].

Out of all terpenoid compounds, limonene and carvone have shown to be effective in several tumors (stomach, pulmonary, and mammary) [48]. D-limonene and/or its metabolites have been found in serum, liver, lung, kidney, and other tissues such as adipose tissue and mammary glands, which may explain its positive effect on mammary gland carcinoma [49]. D-limonene is also an excellent solvent of cholesterol; so, it is used clinically to dissolve cholesterol-containing gallstones [49]. Because of its gastric acid neutralizing effect and its support of normal gastrointestinal motility, it has also been used for relief of heartburn [49].

5. Essential oils monoterpenes

5.1 Limonene

Limonene is a colorless liquid hydrocarbon classified as a monocyclic terpene [30], one of the main constituents found in essential oils extracted from citrus peels [50]. Out of the two isomers, D- and L-limonene, D-isomer is more common and possesses a strong orange odor [30, 50, 51], which is the reason for its wide application as a flavor and fragrance additive [49]. Health benefits of limonene include antioxidant, anti-inflammatory, vasorelaxant, anticarcinogenic, chemopreventive, and chemotherapeutic potentials [13, 52–54].

The analgesic effect is helpful in relieving headaches and stomach ache, relaxing the muscles, and preventing muscle stiffness. It also helps to overcome fatigue and it plays a vital role in relaxing and stabilizing the nervous system and, therefore, is used as a sedative [50, 52].

Yoon et al. [55] carried out a study to verify the pharmacological and biological effects of limonene on the production of pro-inflammatory cytokines and inflammatory mediators in RAW 264.7 macrophages and concluded that limonene effectively inhibited lipopolysaccharide-induced nitric oxide (NO) and prostaglandin E2 production that included dose-dependent decreases in the expression of inducible nitric synthase (iNOS) and cyclooxygenase-2 (COX-2) proteins. The same study also showed inhibition of macrophage-cytokine production [55]. A beneficial antioxidant effect via increased iNOS and COX-2 protein expression was found in ulcerative colitis rat models [53]. Moreover, systemic application of limonene reduced nociceptive behaviors via H_2O_2-induced TRPA1 activation, and this effect is related to the inflammatory pain [51]. Myrcene and limonene inhibit IL-1β-induced responses found in osteoarthritis [56].

In conclusion, D-Limonene presented significant antinociception in different models of nociception without opioid receptor stimulation [57]. Instead, it is more likely related to the appreciable anti-inflammatory activity of this compound [58].

5.2 Myrcene

Myrcene or β-myrcene is a monoterpene polyunsaturated acyclic found in nature, originally isolated from lemon grass oil (*Cymbopogon citratus*) [58]. Besides its effect on both central and peripheral sites through endogenous opioids and α2-adrenoreceptors, it was also shown to inhibit lipopolysaccharide [LPS]-induced inflammation including cell migration and production of NO, along with significant inhibition of c-interferon and IL-4 production [58, 59].

5.3 α-Terpineol

α-Terpineol is a volatile monoterpene alcohol, relatively nontoxic, and one of the major components of the essential oils of various plant species, being a nonirritant at 1–15%, and non-phototoxic [13]. There are three isomers, α-, β-, and γ-terpene, with the latter two differing only by the location of the double bond [51]. It is the third most representative monoterpene in citrus species [60]. It has insecticidal, antimicrobial, antispasmodic, anticonvulsant [47], antinociceptive, and immunostimulant properties, and it increases the skin's permeability to soluble compounds [60].

Studies have found that α-terpineol possesses peripheral and central analgesic properties [7]. A research conducted on mice, using carrageenan and TNF-α induced hypernociception, showed increase of the mechanical threshold of hypernociceptive behavior by α-terpineol, probably by the inhibition of inflammatory mediators (inhibiting the release of substance P and other inflammatory molecules such as serotonin, histamine, bradykinin, and prostaglandins) [60]. α-Terpineol showed an antioxidant activity as it was able to suppress the superoxide production by agonist-stimulated monocytes [7]. Moreover, α-terpineol showed higher COX-2 activity inhibition than aspirin, the most popular NSAID, and most potently inhibited the expression of pro-inflammatory cytokines and NF-κB activation [7, 61]. α-Terpineol also showed antinociceptive effect in the capsaicin (neurogenic origin), glutamate, and formalin-induced orofacial nociception tests [51, 62, 63].

Anti-inflammatory effects that α-terpineol from orange juice demonstrated *in vitro* (suppressed IL-6 and increased IL-10) were further analyzed by *ex vivo* experiments, and results have shown anti-inflammatory action in macrophages after incubation of human blood with α-terpineol [61]. Described effects were attributed to α-terpineol, while linalool and limonene had no significant action [61]. On the other hand, a research conducted on morphine-tolerant mice showed inhibitory effect of α-terpineol in low dosages on the induction of dependence on morphine and attenuated the signs of withdrawal syndrome without antinociceptive effect [46].

5.4 Linalool

Linalool is an acyclic oxygenated monoterpene reported to be the major volatile component of the essential oils of several aromatic species, including the Rutaceae family, with sedative, antidepressant, anticancer, antifungal, and pesticidal properties [13]. It is the most studied monoterpene in various painful conditions [58]. A research on adult female Swiss mice treated with a single intraperitoneal injection of (−)-linalool (50 or 200 mg/kg) or multiple treatments given chronically (twice daily for 10 days; 50 mg/kg, i.p.) showed that (−)-linalool significantly reduced CFA-induced mechanical hypersensitivity (complete Freund's adjuvant) and produced effective reduction in CFA-induced paw edema following the acute treatment [61, 64]. Following intraperitoneal administration in mice, linalool was found to produce antinociceptive and antihyperalgesic effects in different animal models in addition to its anti-inflammatory properties [65]. (−)-Linalool acts as analgesic on several receptors, including opioids, adenosine A1 and A2, cholinergic M2, and produces changes in K+ channels, thus exerting analgesic-like activity [58, 66].

Some recent studies demonstrate that (−)-linalool inhibits transient receptor potential A1 (TRPA1) and N-Methyl-D-aspartate (NMDA) channels and decreases the nociception induced by cinnamaldehyde or capsaicin [58, 67].

It is neither toxic nor irritable to skin and presents an extremely low risk of skin sensitization [13]. However, due to poor oral availability, despite the biological properties of (−)-linalool, its use in the treatment of painful and inflammatory disorders is still limited [51]. Nascimento et al. [68] used pure 95% linalool, complexed and noncomplexed in β-cyclodextrin (used to increase aqueous solubility and bioavailability of monoterpenes), in an animal model of fibromyalgia. They found that both formulations had an anti-hyperalgesic effect, with the complexed form being more effective and producing a longer lasting effect (for 24 h after administration) [68]. Analgesic effect of linalool on acute central nociception (hot plate), visceral (acetic acid), and chronic pain models of neuropathic origin, and the opioid and glutamatergic systems are probably involved in this action [51, 62, 67, 69]. One preclinical trial showed that linalool from rosewood was able to reduce the action potential amplitude assessed using an isolated nerve in the single sucrose gap technique, showing it blocked neuronal excitability [70].

5.5 Pinene

α-Pinene is an organic compound of the terpene class, one of two isomers of pinene, the other being β [30]. The effects of *Ugni myricoides* (Kunth) O. Berg essential oil and its major constituent, α-pinene [52.1%], were analyzed in inflammatory and neuropathic models of hypernociception in mice, and the results showed that the oil significantly prevented mechanical hypernociception induced by carrageenan or complete Freund's adjuvant (CFA), and those effects were attributed to α-pinene, which clearly has a potential role for the management of inflammatory and neuropathic pain [61]. Furthermore, the effect on inflammatory processes were observed in studies performed *in vivo*, in which repeated treatments with α-pinene [5–50 mg/kg, p. o.] were able to abolish the mechanical sensitization induced by CFA or by the partial ligation of the sciatic nerve [58]. In addition, it has been shown that α-pinene has anti-inflammatory and anti-catabolic activities in human chondrocytes [56].

β-Pinene is present in high amounts [5.1–13.1%] in lime citrus oil [32]. In animal models, β-pinene showed to be effective only on acute central nociception, yet, it was able to reverse the antinociceptive effect of morphine in tests equivalent to the effect of naloxone [58].

5.6 p-cymene

Biological precursor of carvacrol, p-cymene occurs in oranges and tangerines [51, 71]. Different behavioral tests of nociception in animal models showed that it exerted both peripheral and central antinociceptive action [51]. A study investigated the antinociceptive potential of p-cymene in mice models of orofacial nociception induced by formalin, capsaicin, and glutamate, and results showed that the treatment with p-cymene at all doses reduced the nociceptive behavior in all nociception tests, suggesting an action in both neurogenic and inflammatory pain [71]. Moreover, tests conducted on Swiss mice showed decreased mechanical hypernociception, reduced leukocyte and neutrophils migration, and reduced TNF-α level [51]. Like other previously mentioned terpenic compounds, p-cymene has a relatively short pharmacological half-life and bioavailability; so, complexation with β-cyclodextrin has shown to improve its analgesic and anti-inflammatory effects through improved bioavailability [72].

5.7 Nerol

This acyclic monoterpene alcohol is found in many essential oils, *Citrus aurantium* among them [51]. In the oxazolone-induced colitis model, González-Ramírez et al. [73], observed antinociceptive effect of nerol [30 mg/kg], which led to a significant reduction on expression of some pro-inflammatory cytokines, like IL-13 and TNF-α, which are highly characteristic for gastrointestinal tract disorders [51].

6. Analgesic potential of some essential oils

All essential oils with high D-limonene content pose significant free radical scavenging effect, predominantly disabling production of reactive oxygen species (ROS) [13]. Essential oils of sweet orange, lemon, and bergamot are most widely used to test analgesic effects in animal models. More recently, some essential oil blends were tested in various human cell models and showed significant positive effects on inflammation, immune modulation, cell cycle regulation, and other cellular functions [8].

7. Safety

Bioactive compounds found in essential oils are quickly absorbed after dermal, oral, or pulmonary administration, and are excreted by the kidneys in the form of phase-II conjugates [66]. Only a small fraction is eliminated unchanged by the lungs [66]. Generally speaking, Citrus essential oils are nontoxic, non-mutagenic, and noncarcinogenic, meaning that sweet orange, bitter orange, neroli, petitgrain, lemon, lime (both distilled and expressed), bergamot, and grapefruit oils have GRAS status [74].

However, a mixture of two optic isomers of limonene present in the essential oils of citrus fruits was shown to be hepatotoxic, have a sedative muscular relaxing effect in mice and be nephrotoxic only in male rats, cause small-scale irritation in rabbits, and be carcinogenic and teratogenic [75].

The fast metabolism and short half-life of active compounds have led to the belief that there is a minimum risk of accumulation in body tissues [12]. In humans, ingestion of D-limonene resulted in an excretion of 52–83% of the dose in the urine within 48 hours [49]. However, limonene at 20 g caused diarrhea and transient proteinuria in healthy volunteers [75]. Vapor inhalation caused respiratory disorders coupled with a decrease in vital capacity [75]. No neurological disorders occurred, but chronic exposure can induce irritation and allergy; therefore, it must be mentioned in the list of "ingredients" of cosmetics [75]. It is not acutely toxic, nephrotoxic, or carcinogenic for humans, but the oxidized D-limonene may carry some toxicity, hence, citrus oils should be stored in dark at 4°C [13]. Nevertheless, unoxidized D-limonene is listed as an allergen by the EU, and moderately allergenic in Germany [13].

8. Conclusions

All phytochemicals present in essential oils presented here may simultaneously target multiple mechanisms involved in chronic pain. Despite long history of therapeutic applications of essential oils for the treatment of pain, only recently more attention was given to their components and elucidating mechanisms behind their antioxidant, anti-inflammatory, and antinociceptive potential. Monoterpenes are key holders of analgesic potential in Citrus essential oils, especially D-limonene and linalool. Essential oils are generally considered as safe; however, due to low bioavailability and stability, monoterpenes are complexed with β-cyclodextrin to improve their analgesic activity [62, 69]. Further studies are encouraged to determine the analgesic potential of Citrus essential oils in managing daily activities of people with a long-term history of chronic pain.

Conflict of interest

The authors declare that the research was conducted in the absence of any commercial or financial relationships that could be construed as a potential conflict of interest.

Author details

Ines Banjari[1], Jelena Balkić[2] and Viduranga Yashasvi Waisundara[3]*

1 Department of Food and Nutrition Research, Faculty of Food Technology Osijek, Josip Juraj Strossmayer University of Osijek, Osijek, Croatia

2 Department for Dietetics and Nutrition, University Hospital Osijek, Osijek, Croatia

3 Australian College of Business and Technology – Kandy Campus, Peradeniya Road, Kandy, Sri Lanka

*Address all correspondence to: viduranga@gmail.com

References

[1] Treede RD, Rief W, Barke A, Aziz Q, Bennett MI, Benoliel R, et al. A classification of chronic pain for ICD-11. Pain. 2015;**156**:1003-1007. DOI: 10.1097/j.pain.0000000000000160

[2] European Pain Federation [EFIC]. Declaration on Pain. Available from: https: //www.europeanpainfederation.eu/ [Accessed: 08 June 2018]

[3] PAE. Survey on chronic pain. 2017. Available from: http: //www.pae-eu.eu/wp-content/uploads/2017/12/PAE-Survey-on-Chronic-Pain-June-2017.pdf

[4] Dahlhamer J, Lucas J, Carla Zelaya C, Nahin R, Mackey S, De Bar L, et al. Prevalence of chronic pain and high-impact chronic pain among adults — United States, 2016. CDC. 2018;**67**(36):1001-1006. DOI: 10.15585/mmwr.mm6736a2

[5] Phillips CJ. The cost and burden of chronic pain. Pain Reviews. 2009;**3**(1):2-5. DOI: 10.1177/204946370900300102

[6] Macfarlane GJ, Beasley M, Smith BH, Jones GT, Macfarlane TV. Can large surveys conducted on highly selected populations provide valid information on the epidemiology of common health conditions? An analysis of UK biobank data on musculoskeletal pain. British Journal of Pain. 2015;**9**:203-212. DOI: 10.1177/2049463715569806

[7] Khaleel C, Tabanca N, Buchbauer G. α-Terpineol, a natural monoterpene: A review of its biological properties. Open Chemistry. 2018;**16**:349-361. DOI: 10.1515/chem-2018-0040

[8] Han X, Parker TL, Dorsett J. An essential oil blend significantly modulates immune responses and the cell cycle in human cell cultures. Cogent Biology. 2017;**3**:1340112. DOI: 10.1080/23312025.2017.1340112

[9] Sarmento-Neto JF, Nascimento LG, Bezerra Felipe CF, de Sousa DP. Analgesic potential of essential oils. Molecules. 2016;**21**(1):E20. DOI: 10.3390/molecules21010020

[10] Lakhan SE, Sheafer H, Tepper D. The effectiveness of aromatherapy in reducing pain: A systematic review and meta-analysis. Pain Research and Treatment. 2016;**2016**:8158693. DOI: 10.1155/2016/8158693

[11] Ali B, Al-Wabel NA, Shams S, Ahamad A, Khan SA, Anwar F. Essential oils used in aromatherapy: A systemic review. Asian Pacific Journal of Tropical Biomedicine. 2015;**5**(8):601-611. DOI: 10.1016/j.apjtb.2015.05.007

[12] Djilani A, Dicko A. The therapeutic benefits of essential oils. Nutrition, well-being and health. In: Bouayed J, editor. Nutrition, Well-Being and Health. Rijeka, Croatia: IntechOpen; 2012. pp. 155-178. DOI: 10.5772/25344

[13] Dosoky NS, Setzer WN. Biological activities and safety of citrus spp. essential oils. International Journal of Molecular Sciences. 2018;**19**:1966. DOI: 10.3390/ijms19071966

[14] Kamal GM, Anwar F, Hussain AI, Sarri N, Ashraf MY. Yield and chemical composition of citrus essential oils as affected by drying pretreatment of peels. International Food Research Journal. 2011;**18**(4):1275-1282

[15] Kamal GM, Ashraf MY, Hussain AI, Shahzadi A, Chughtai MI. Antioxidant potential of peel essential oils of three Pakistani citrus species: Citrus reticulata, Citrus sinensis and Citrus paradisii. Pakistan Journal of Botany. 2013;**45**(4):1449-1454

[16] Ahmad MM, Rehman SU, Iqbal Z, Anjum FM, Sultan JI. Genetic variability to essential oil composition in four citrus fruit species. Pakistan Journal of Botany. 2006;**38**(2):319-324

[17] Egharevba HO, Oladosun P, Izebe KS. Chemical composition and anti-tubercular activity of the essential oil of orange [Citrus sinensis L.] peel from North Central Nigeria. International Journal of Pharmacognosy and Phytochemical Research. 2016;**8**(1):91-94

[18] Radan M, Parčina A, Burčul F. Chemical composition and antioxidant activity of essential oil obtained from bitter orange peel [Citrus aurantium L.] using two methods. Croatica Chemica Acta. 2018;**91**(1):125-128. DOI: 10.5562/cca3294

[19] Siddique S, Shafique M, Parveen Z, Jabeen Khan S, Khanum R. Volatile components, antioxidant and antimicrobial activity of citrus aurantium var. bitter orange peel oil. Pharmacologyonline. 2011;**2**:499-507

[20] Bakhsha F, Yousefi Z, Aryaee M, Jafari SY, Derakhshanpoor F. Comparison effect of lavender and Citrus aurantium aroma on anxiety in female students at Golestan University of Medical Sciences. Journal of Basic Research in Medical Sciences. 2016;**3**(4):4-11. DOI: 10.18869/acadpub.jbrms.3.4.4

[21] Carvalho-Freitas MIR, Costa M. Anxiolytic and sedative effects of extracts and essential oil from Citrus aurantium L. Biological & Pharmaceutical Bulletin. 2002;**25**:1629-1633

[22] Sarrou E, Chatzopoulou P, Dimassi-Theriou K, Therios I. Volatile constituents and antioxidant activity of peel, flowers and leaf oils of Citrus aurantium L. growing in Greece. Molecules. 2013;**18**:10639-10647. DOI: 10.3390/molecules180910639

[23] Khodabakhsh P, Shafaroodi H, Asgarpanah J. Analgesic and anti-inflammatory activities of Citrus aurantium L. blossoms essential oil [neroli]: Involvement of the nitric oxide/cyclic guanosine monophosphate pathway. Journal of Natural Medicines. 2015;**69**:324-333. DOI: 10.1007/s11418-015-0896-6

[24] Mondello L, Dugo G, Dugo P, Bartle KD. Italian citrus Petitgrain oils. Part I. composition of bitter orange Petitgrain oil. Journal of Essential Oil Research. 1996;**8**(6):597-609. DOI: 10.1080/10412905.1996.9701026

[25] Ferlazzo N, Cirmi S, Calapai G, Ventura-Spagnolo E, Gangemi S, Navarra M. Anti-inflammatory activity of Citrus bergamia derivatives: Where do we stand? Molecules. 2016;**21**:1273. DOI: 10.3390/molecules21101273

[26] Mannucci C, Navarra M, Calapai F, Squeri R, Gangemi S, Calapai G. Clinical pharmacology of Citrus bergamia: A systematic review. Phytotherapy Research. 2017;**31**:27-39. DOI: 10.1002/ptr.5734

[27] Lauro F, Ilari S, Giancotti LA, Morabito C, Malafoglia V, Gliozzi M, et al. The protective role of bergamot polyphenolic fraction on several animal models of pain. PharmaNutrition. 2016;**4S**:35-40

[28] Navarra M, Mannucci C, Delbò M, Calapai G. Citrus bergamia essential oil: From basic research to clinical application. Frontiers in Pharmacology. 2015;**6**:36. DOI: 10.3389/fphar.2015.00036

[29] Campêlo LML, Almeida AAC, Freitas RLM, Cerqueira GS, Sousa GF, Saldanha GB, et al. Antioxidant and antinociceptive effects of citrus

Limon essential oil in mice. Journal of Biomedicine & Biotechnology. 2011:678673. DOI: 10.1155/2011/678673

[30] Gobato R, Gobato A, Fedrigo DFG. Molecular electrostatic potential of the main monoterpenoids compounds found in oil lemon Tahiti – [citrus Latifolia Var Tahiti]. Parana Journal of Science and Education. 2015;**1**:1-10

[31] Md Othman S, Hassan M, Nahar L, Basar N, Jamil S, Sarker S. Essential oils from the Malaysian citrus [Rutaceae] medicinal plants. Medicine. 2016;**3**:13. DOI: 10.3390/medicines3020013

[32] Amorim JL, Simas DL, Pinheiro MM, Moreno DS, Alviano CS, da Silva AJ, et al. Anti-inflammatory properties and chemical characterization of the essential oils of four citrus species. PLoS One. 2016;**11**(4):e0153643. DOI: 10.1371/journal.pone.0153643

[33] Javed S, Ahmad R, Shahzad K, Nawaz S, Saeed S, Saleem Y. Chemical constituents, antimicrobial and antioxidant activity of essential oil of Citrus limetta var. Mitha [sweet lime] peel in Pakistan. African Journal of Microbiology Research. 2013;**7**(24):3071-3077. DOI: 10.5897/AJMR12.1254

[34] El Kamali HH, Burham BO, El-Egami AA. Essential oil composition of internal fruit Peel of Citrus paradisi from Sudan. AM Research. 2015;**1**(9):2079-2085. DOI: 10.6084/m9.figshare.1480470

[35] Lan-Phi NT, Shimamura T, Ukeda H, Sawamura M. Chemical and aroma profiles of yuzu [citrus junos] peel oils of different cultivars. Food Chemistry. 2009;**115**(3):1042-1047

[36] Vasudeva N, Sharma T. Chemical composition and antimicrobial activity of essential oil of citrus limettioides Tanaka. Journal of Pharmaceutical Technology and Drug Research. 2012:1-7. DOI: 10.7243/2050-120X-1-2

[37] Charles DJ, Simon JE. Comparison of extraction methods for the rapid determination of essential oil content and composition of basil. Journal of the American Society for Horticultural Science. 1990;**115**(3):458-462

[38] Mason TJ. Ultrasound in synthetic organic chemistry. Chemical Society Reviews. 1997;**26**:443-451. DOI: 10.1039/CS9972600443

[39] Vinatoru M, Toma M, Mason TJ. Ultrasound-assisted extraction of bioactive principles from plants and their constituents. Advances in Sonochemistry. 1999;**5**:209-247

[40] Wang L, Weller CL. Recent advances in extraction of nutraceuticals from plants. Trends in Food Science and Technology. 2006;**17**:300-312. DOI: 10.1016/j.tifs.2005.12.004

[41] Chemat S, Lagha A, AitAmar H, Bartels PV, Chemat F. Comparison of conventional and ultrasound-assisted extraction of carvone and limonene from caraway seeds. Flavour and Fragrance Journal. 2004;**19**:188-195. DOI: 10.1002/ffj.1339

[42] Reverchon E. Supercritical fluid extraction and fractionation of essential oils and related products. Journal of Supercritical Fluids. 1997;**10**(1997):1-37. DOI: 10.1016/S0896-8446[97]00014-4

[43] Fornari F, Vincente G, Vazquez E, Garcia-Risco MR, Reglero G. Isolation of essential oil from different plants and herbs by supercritical fluid extraction. Journal of Chromatography. A. 2012;**1250**:34-48. DOI: 10.1016/j.chroma.2012.04.051

[44] Kaufmann B, Christen P. Recent extraction techniques for natural products: Microwave-assisted extraction and pressurized solvent extraction.

Phytochemical Analysis. 2002;**13**: 105-113. DOI: 10.1002/pca.631

[45] Filly A, Fernandez X, Minuti M, Visinoni F, Cravotto G, Chemat F. Solvent-free microwave extraction of essential oil from aromatic herbs: From laboratory to pilot and industrial scale. Food Chemistry. 2014;**150**:193-198. DOI: 10.1016/j.foodchem.2013.10.139

[46] Parvardeh S, Moghimi M, Eslami P, Masoudi AR. α-Terpineol attenuates morphine-induced physical dependence and tolerance in mice: Role of nitric oxide. Iranian Journal of Basic Medical Sciences. 2016;**19**:201-208

[47] De Sousa DP, Quintans L, de Almeida RN. Evolution of the anticonvulsant activity of α-terpineol. Pharmaceutical Biology. 2007;**45**(1):69-70. DOI: 10.1080/13880200601028388

[48] Raphael TJ, Kuttan G. Immunomodulatory activity of naturally occurring monoterpenes carvone, limonene, and perillic acid. Immunopharmacology and Immunotoxicology. 2003;**25**(2):285-294. DOI: 10.1081/IPH-120020476

[49] Sun J. D-limonene: Safety and clinical applications. Alternative Medicine Review. 2007;**12**(3):259-264

[50] Chhikara N, Kour R, Jaglan S, Gupta P, Gata Y, Panghal A. Citrus medica: Nutritional, phytochemical composition and health benefits – A review. Food & Function. 2018;**9**:1978. DOI: 10.1039/c7fo02035j

[51] De Cássia da Silveira e Sá R, Cardoso Lima T, da Nóbrega FR, Medeiros de Brito AE, de Sousa DP. Analgesic-like activity of essential oil constituents: An update. International Journal of Molecular Sciences. 2017;**18**:2392. DOI: 10.3390/ijms18122392

[52] Nogueira de Melo GA, Grespan R, Fonseca JP, Farinha TO, Silva EL, Romero AL, et al. Rosmarinus officinalis L. essential oil inhibits in vivo and in vitro leukocyte migration. Journal of Medicinal Food. 2011;**14**:944-946. DOI: 10.1089/jmf.2010.0159

[53] Yu L, Yan J, Sun Z. D-limonene exhibits anti-inflammatory and antioxidant properties in an ulcerative colitis rat model via regulation of iNOS, COX-2, PGE2 and ERK signaling pathways. Molecular Medicine Reports. 2017;**15**:2339-2346. DOI: 10.3892/mmr.2017.6241

[54] Lima TC, Mota MM, Barbosa-Filho JM, Dos Santos MRV, De Sousa DP. Structural relationships and vasorelaxant activity of monoterpenes. Daru. 2012;**20**:23. DOI: 10.1186/2008-2231-20-23

[55] Yoon WJ, Lee NH, Hyun CG. Limonene Supresses lipopolysaccharide-induced production of nitric oxide, prostaglandin E2, and pro-inflammatory cytokines in RAW 246.7 macrophages. Journal of Oleo Science. 2010;**59**(8):415-421

[56] Rufino AT, Ribeiro M, Sousa C, Judas F, Salgueiro L, Cavaleiro C, et al. Evaluation of the anti-inflammatory, anti-catabolic and pro anabolic effects of E caryophyllene, myrcene and limonene in a cell model of osteoarthritis. European Journal of Pharmacology. 2015;**750**:141-150. DOI: 10.1016/j.ejphar.2015.01.018

[57] Do Amaral JF, Silva MIG, Neto MRA, Neto PFT, Moura BA, de Melo CTV, et al. Antinociceptive effect of the monoterpene R-[+]-limonene in mice. Biological & Pharmaceutical Bulletin. 2007;**30**:1217-1220

[58] Guimarães AG, Quintans JSS, Quintans-Júnior LJ. Monoterpenes with analgesic activity—A systematic review. Phytotherapy Research. 2013;**27**:1-15. DOI: 10.1002/ptr.4686

[59] Souza MC, Siani AC, Ramos MF, Menezes-de-Lima OJ, Henriques MG. Evaluation of anti-inflammatory activity of essential oils from two Asteraceae species. Pharmazie. 2003;**58**:582-586

[60] De Oliveira MG, Marques RB, de Santana MF, Santos AB, Brito FA, Barreto EO, et al. α-Terpineol reduces mechanical hypernociception and inflammatory response. Basic & Clinical Pharmacology & Toxicology. 2012;**111**:120-125. DOI: 10.1111/j.1742-7843.2012.00875.x

[61] De Cássia da Silveira e Sá R, Nalone Andrade L, Pergentino de Sousa D. A review on anti-inflammatory activity of monoterpenes. Molecules. 2013;**18**:1227-1254. DOI: 10.3390/molecules18011227

[62] Brito RG, Santos PL, Oliveira MA, Pina LTS, Antoniolli AR, da Silva Almeida JRG, et al. Natural Products as Promising Pharmacological Tools for the Management of Fibromyalgia Symptoms – A Review in Discussions of Unusual Topics in Fibromyalgia, Chapter 4. 2018:57-78. DOI: 10.5772/intechopen.70016

[63] Quintans-Júnior LJ, Oliveira MGB, Santana MF, Santana MT, Guimarães AG, Siqueira JS, et al. α-Terpineol reduces nociceptive behavior in mice. Pharmaceutical Biology. 2011;**49**(6):583-586. DOI: 10.3109/13880209.2010.529616

[64] Katsuyama SK, Towa AO, Amio SK, Ato KS, Agi TY, Ishikawa YK, et al. Effect of plantar subcutaneous administration of bergamot essential oil and linalool on formalin-induced nociceptive behavior in mice. Biomedical Research. 2015;**36**(1):47-54. DOI: 10.2220/biomedres.36.47

[65] Sakurada T, Kuwahata H, Katsuyama S, Komatsu T, Morrone LA, Corasaniti MT, et al. Intraplantar injection of bergamot essential oil into the mouse Hindpaw: Effects on capsaicin-induced nociceptive behaviors. International Review of Neurobiology. 2009;**85**:237-248. DOI: 10.1016/S0074-7742[09]85018-6

[66] De Sousa DP. Analgesic-like activity of essential oils constituents. Molecules. 2011;**16**:2233-2252. DOI: 10.3390/molecules16032233

[67] Batista PA, de Paula Werner MF, Oliveira EC, Burgos L, Pereira P, da Silva Brum LF. The antinociceptive effect of [-]-linalool in models of chronic inflammatory and neuropathic hypersensitivity in mice. The Journal of Pain. 2010;**11**(11):1222-1229. DOI: 10.1016/j.jpain.2010.02.022

[68] Nascimento SS, Camargo EA, DeSantana JM, Araújo AAS, Menezes PP, Lucca-Júnior W, et al. Linalool and linalool complexed in β-cyclodextrin produce anti-hyperalgesic activity and increase Fos protein expression in animal model for fibromyalgia. Naunyn-Schmiedeberg's Archives of Pharmacology. 2014;**387**(10):935-942. DOI: 10.1007/s00210-014-1007-z

[69] Quintans-Júnior LJ, Barreto RSS, Menezes PP, Almeida JRGS, Viana AFSC, Oliveira RCM, et al. β-Cyclodextrin-complexed [-]-linalool produces antinociceptive effect superior to that of [-]-linalool in experimental pain protocols. Basic & Clinical Pharmacology & Toxicology. 2013;**113**:167-172. DOI: 10.1111/bcpt.12087

[70] De Almeida RN, Araújo DAM, Gonçalves JCR, Montenegro FC, de Sousa DP, Leite JR, et al. Rosewood oil induces sedation and inhibits compound action potential in rodents. Journal of Ethnopharmacology. 2009;**124**(3):440-443. DOI: 10.1016/j.jep.2009.05.044

[71] Santana MF, Quintans-Júnior LJ, Cavalcanti SCH, Oliveira MGB, Guimarães AG, Cunha ES, et al.

p-cymene reduces orofacial nociceptive response in mice. Revista Brasileira de Farmacognosia. 2011;**21**(6):1138-1143. DOI: 10.1590/S0102-695X2011005000156

[72] Quintans-Júnior SS, Menezesa PP, Santosa MRV, Bonjardima LR, Almeidab JRGS, Gelainc DP, et al. Improvement of p-cymene antinociceptive and anti-inflammatory effects by inclusion in β-cyclodextrin. Phytomedicine. 2013;**20**:436-440. DOI: 10.1016/j.phymed.2012.12.009

[73] González-Ramírez AE, González-Trujano ME, Orozco-Suárez SA, Alvarado-Vásquez N, López-Muñoz FJ. Nerol alleviates pathologic markers in the oxazolone-induced colitis model. European Journal of Pharmacology. 2016;**776**:81-89. DOI: 10.1016/j.ejphar.2016.02.036

[74] Food and Drug Administration, Table of substances generally recognized as safe. 1998. Available from: //www.libertynatural.com/info/eoinfo/FDA_EO_GRAS.htm [Accessed: 28 November 2018]

[75] Vigan M. Essential oils: Renewal of interest and toxicity. European Journal of Dermatology. 2010;**20**(6):685-692. DOI: 10.1684/ejd.2010.1066